Bleeding During Pregnancy

Eyal Sheiner

Editor

Bleeding During Pregnancy

A Comprehensive Guide

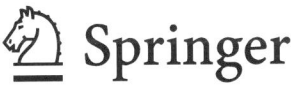 Springer

Editor
Eyal Sheiner, MD, PhD
Department of Obstetrics and Gynecology
Faculty of Health Sciences
Soroka University Medical Center
Ben-Gurion University of the Negev
Beer-Sheva, Israel
sheiner@bgu.ac.il

ISBN 978-1-4419-9809-5   e-ISBN 978-1-4419-9810-1
DOI 10.1007/978-1-4419-9810-1
Springer New York Dordrecht Heidelberg London

Library of Congress Control Number: 2011929988

Printed on acid-free paper

Springer is part of Springer Science+Business Media (www.springer.com)

Acknowledgments

Pregnancy-related bleeding is a clinical challenge. Obstetrical morbidity associated with bleeding is significant. Accordingly, I was pleased to have the opportunity to participate in the creation of this book and invite some of the world's experts on this topic to share their experience and knowledge. I thank all of the authors for their excellent chapters. I am most appreciative of their work. As always, the support of my beloved family was crucial and unwavering.

The book is dedicated to my mother, Zehava Sheiner (1945–2010), who passed away unexpectedly during the process of editing the book.

Beer-Sheva, Israel   Eyal Sheiner

Contents

Contributors

Frédéric Amant, MD, PhD Division of Gynecological Oncology,
Department of Obstetrics and Gynecology, University Hospitals of Leuven,
Leuven, Belgium

Cande V. Ananth, PhD, MPH Department of Obstetrics and Gynecology,
College of Physicians and Surgeons, Columbia University, New York, NY, USA

Nardin Aslih, MD Department of Obstetrics and Gynecology,
Hillel Yaffe Medical Center, Hadera, Israel; Faculty of Health Sciences,
The Technion University Medical School, Haifa, Israel

Lisa M. Barroilhet, MD Department of Obstetrics and Gynecology,
Brigham and Women's Hospital, Boston, MA, USA

Ruth Beer-Weisel, MD Department of Obstetrics and Gynecology,
Soroka University Medical Center, School of Medicine, Faculty of
Health Sciences, Ben-Gurion University of the Negev, Beer-Sheva, Israel

Ross S. Berkowitz, MD Brigham and Women's Hospital,
New England Trophoblastic Disease Center, Boston, MA, USA

Eran Bornstein, MD Department of Obstetrics and Gynecology,
Lenox Hill Hospital, New York, NY, USA

Joseph C. Canterino, MD, FACOG Division of Maternal Fetal Medicine,
Department of Obstetrics and Gynecology, Jersey Shore University
Medical Center, Neptune, NJ, USA; UMDNJ-Robert Wood Johnson
Medical School, New Brunswick, NJ, USA

Scott Dunkley, MD Institute of Haemotology, Royal Prince Alfred Hospital,
Sydney, NSW, Australia

Offer Erez, MD Department of Obstetrics and Gynecology "B", Soroka
University Medical Center, School of Medicine, Faculty of Health Sciences,
Ben Gurion University of the Negev, Beer-Sheva, Israel

Idit Erez-Weiss, Department of Family Medicine, School of Medicine, Faculty of Health Sciences, Ben-Gurion University of the Negev, Beer-Sheva, Israel

Donald Peter Goldstein, MD Department of Obstetrics, Gynecology and Reproductive Biology, Harvard Medical School, Boston, MA, USA; New England Trophoblastic Disease Center, Brigham and Women's Hospital, Boston, MA, USA

Avi Harlev, MD Department of Obstetrics and Gynecology, Faculty of Health Sciences, Soroka University Medical Center, Ben-Gurion University of the Negev, Beer-Sheva, Israel

Gershon Holcberg, MD Departments of Obstetrics and Gynecology, Soroka University Medical Center, Ben-Gurion University of the Negev, Beer-Sheva, Israel

Ashwin R. Jadhav, MD, MS Division of Maternal-Fetal Medicine, Department of Obstetrics and Gynecology, New York University Medical Center, New York, NY, USA

Wendy L. Kinzler, MD Division of Maternal Fetal Medicine, Winthrop University Hospital, Mineola, NY, USA; Department of Obstetrics and Gynecology, SUNY Stony Brook School of Medicine, Stony Brook, NY, USA

Vered Kleitman-Meir, MD Department of Obstetrics and Gynecology, Soroka University Medical Center, School of Medicine, Faculty of Health Sciences, Ben-Gurion University of the Negev, Beer-Sheva, Israel

Moshe Mazor, MD Department of Obstetrics and Gynecology, Soroka University Medical Center, School of Medicine, Faculty of Health Sciences, Ben-Gurion University of the Negev, Beer-Sheva, Israel

Deirdre J. Murphy, MD, MRCOG Department of Obstetrics and Gynaecology, Trinity College Dublin, and Coombe Women and Infants University Hospital, Dublin, Ireland

Iris Ohel, MD Departments of Obstetrics and Gynecology, Soroka University Medical Center, Ben-Gurion University of the Negev, Beer-Sheva, Israel

Yinka Oyelese, MD, MRCOG Division of Maternal Fetal Medicine, Department of Obstetrics and Gynecology, Jersey Shore University Medical Center, Neptune, NJ, USA; UMDNJ-Robert Wood Johnson Medical School, New Brunswick, NJ, USA

Felicity Plaat, BA, MBBS, FRCA Queen Charlotte's and Chelsea Hospital, Department of Anaesthesia, Hammersmith House, Hammersmith Hospital, London, UK

Rachel Pope, MPH Departments of Obstetrics and Gynecology, Soroka University Medical Center, Ben-Gurion University of the Negev, Beer-Sheva, Israel

Sharon R. Sheehan, MD, MRCPI, MRCOG Academic Department
of Obstetrics and Gynaecology, Trinity College Dublin, Coombe Women
and Infants University Hospital, Dublin, Ireland

Eyal Sheiner, MD, PhD Department of Obstetrics and Gynecology, Faculty
of Health Sciences, Soroka University Medical Center, Ben-Gurion University
of the Negev, Beer-Sheva, Israel

Jennifer A. Taylor, MBChB, FANZCA Queen Charlotte's and Chelsea
Hospital, Department of Anaesthesia, Hammersmith House, Hammersmith
Hospital, London, UK

Kristel Van Calsteren, MD, PhD Department of Obstetrics and Gynecology,
University Hospitals of Leuven, Leuven, Belgium

Asnat Walfisch, MD Department of Obstetrics and Gynecology,
Hillel Yaffe Medical Center, Hadera, The "Technion" University Medical School,
Faculty of Health Sciences, Haifa, Israel

Adi Y. Weintraub, MD Department of Obstetrics and Gynecology, Faculty
of Health Sciences, Soroka University Medical Center, Ben-Gurion University
of the Negev, Beer-Sheva, Israel

Arnon Wiznitzer, MD Department of Obstetrics and Gynecology, Faculty
of Health Sciences, Soroka University Medical Center, Ben-Gurion University
of the Negev, Beer-Sheva, Israel

Part I
Introduction to Bleeding During Pregnancy

Chapter 1
Clinical Approach to Pregnancy-Related Bleeding

Nardin Aslih and Asnat Walfisch

Introduction

Vaginal bleeding is a common event during pregnancy. The incidence varies, ranging from 1 to 22% [1–3]. The source of bleeding is mostly maternal. The significance, initial diagnosis, and clinical approach to vaginal bleeding depend on the gestational age and the bleeding characteristics. Vaginal bleeding during early pregnancy is associated with a 1.6-fold increased risk of many adverse outcomes, including preterm labor (PTL) and preterm premature rupture of membranes (PPROM) [3]. As bleeding persists or recurs later in pregnancy, the risk of associated morbidities grows [4]. Although 50% of the women who suffer from vaginal bleeding during early pregnancy go on to have a normal pregnancy [3], vaginal bleeding in the second half of pregnancy is linked to perinatal mortality, disorders of the amniotic fluid, premature rupture of membranes (PROM), preterm deliveries, low birth weight, and low neonatal Apgar scores [1].

We review the general clinical approach to pregnancy-related bleeding. The approach is mainly based on the time of bleeding, including the first or second half of the pregnancy and the postpartum period. Separate detailed chapters are devoted to each of these topics.

Vaginal Bleeding During the First Half of Pregnancy

Vaginal bleeding is common in the first half of pregnancy, occurring in about 20% of pregnancies [5]. The exact etiology of vaginal bleeding often cannot be determined. The importance of the initial evaluation lies in making a definitive diagnosis

A. Walfisch (✉)
High Risk Pregnancy Unit, Department of Obstetrics and Gynecology,
Hillel Yaffe Medical Center, Hadera, Israel; Faculty of Health Sciences,
The Technion University Medical School, Haifa, Israel
e-mail: asnatwalfisch@yahoo.com

E. Sheiner (ed.), *Bleeding During Pregnancy: A Comprehensive Guide*,
DOI 10.1007/978-1-4419-9810-1_1, © Springer Science+Business Media, LLC 2011

when possible but, more importantly, ruling out serious pathology. Figure 1.1 describes the initial clinical approach to first trimester bleeding.

Some studies have found an association between first trimester bleeding and adverse outcomes later in pregnancy such as PTL and PPROM, intrauterine growth

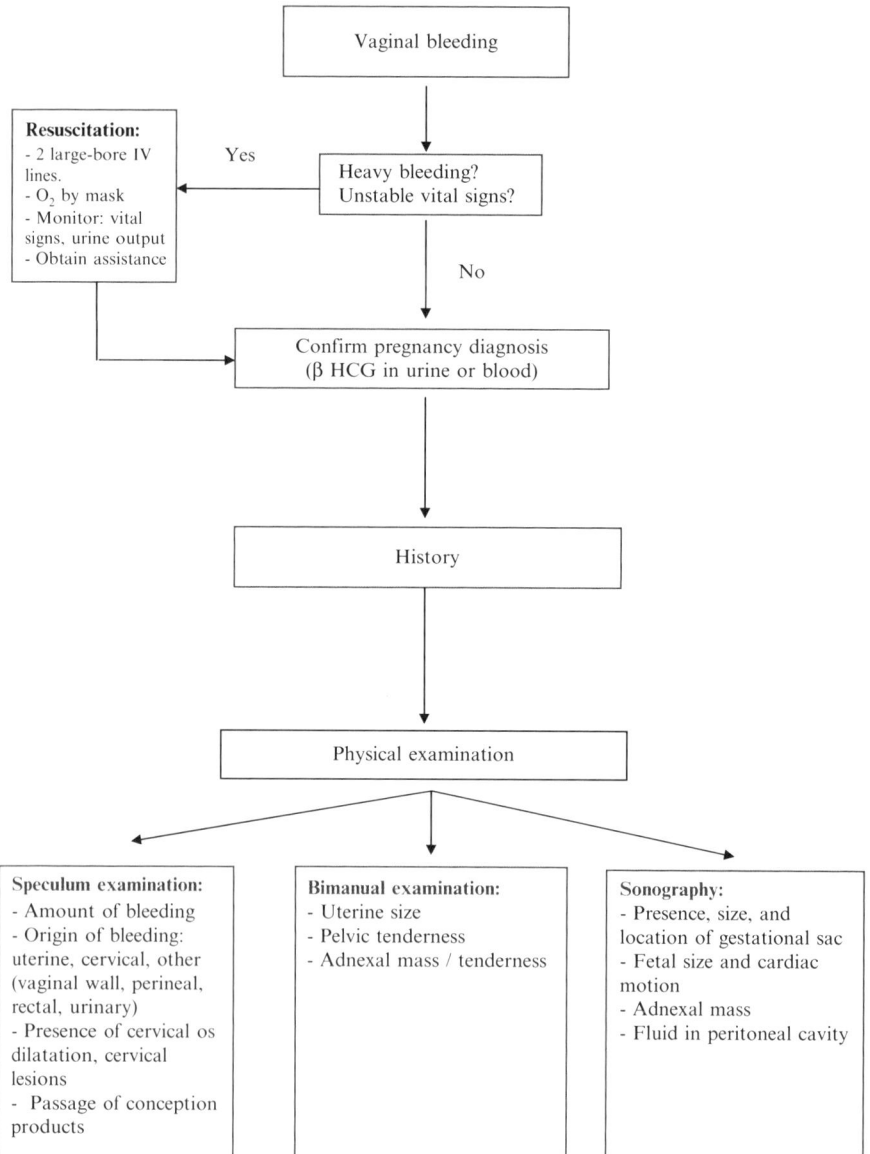

Fig. 1.1 Clinical approach to first trimester bleeding. *β-hCG* β-chorionic gonadotropin, *US* ultrasonography, *EUP* extrauterine pregnancy, *CRL* crown–rump length, *GS* gestational sac

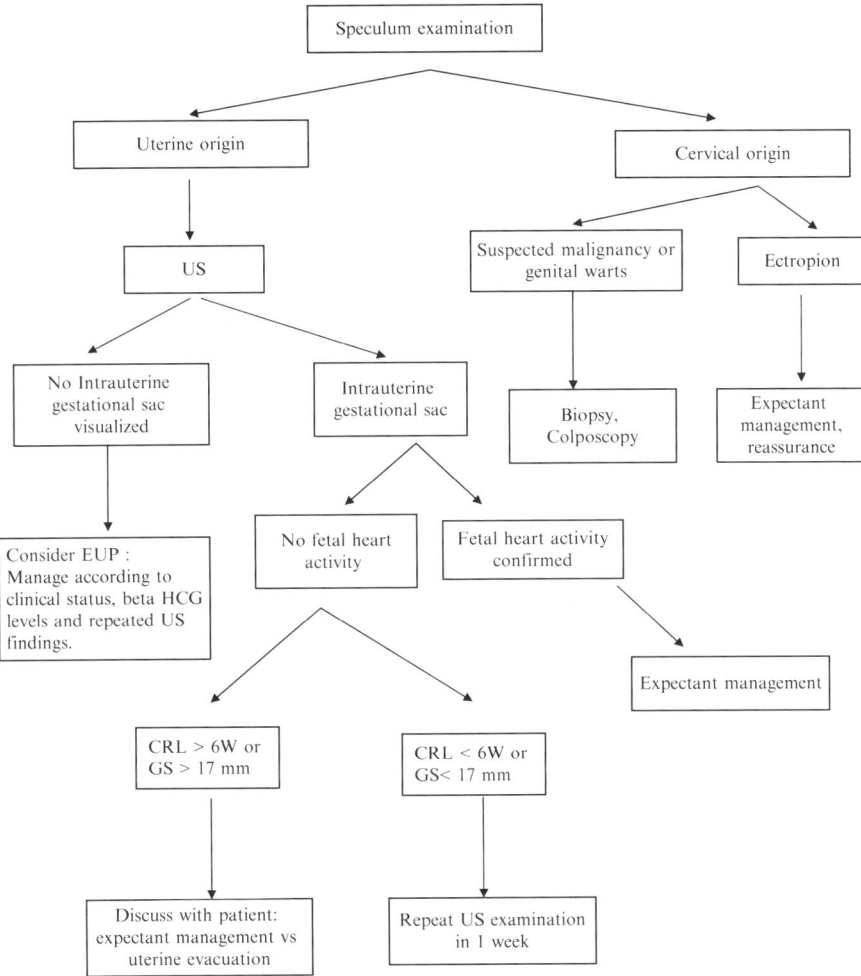

Fig. 1.1 (continued)

restriction (IUGR), and antepartum hemorrhage (APH) [6]. Prognosis is best when the bleeding is light and limited to early pregnancy [7–10]. The risk of a subsequent miscarriage depends on the gestational week and on the sonographic findings (Table 1.1) [11].

Etiology of Vaginal Bleeding

The etiologies of vaginal bleeding during the first half of the pregnancy can be categorized by origin (vaginal, cervical, and uterine) or by cause (threatened abortion,

Table 1.1 Risk of a subsequent miscarriage according to the gestational week and sonographic findings

Sonographic findings	Risk of miscarriage (%)
Gestational sac	12
Yolk sac	8
Fetal pole	
5 mm	7
6–10 mm	3
10 mm	<1

inevitable abortion, spontaneous abortion, implantation bleeding, ectopic pregnancy, hyaditiform mole, and local lesions of the vagina or cervix).

The initial evaluation, as a rule, should always include a detailed history and gynecological examination. Imaging by ultrasonography (US) is an integral part of the initial assessment.

The approach to the maternal history should be consistent. The history must include the following items.

1. Last menstrual period, menstrual regularity, pregnancy diagnosis and confirmation method(s)
2. Characterization and quantification of bleeding
3. Presence of other symptoms (e.g., dizziness, nausea, abdominal pain, passage of "tissue," and shoulder pain)
4. Detailed medical and obstetrical history
5. History of bleeding disorders and clotting abnormalities
6. Use of medications, specifically anticoagulation therapy

The physical examination must include the following inspections.

1. Vital signs
2. Abdominal examination for tenderness, peritoneal signs
3. Inspection of the perineum for amount of bleeding, signs of trauma or lesions
4. Speculum examination to: (a) localize the bleeding origin: vagina, cervix, uterus; (b) quantify the bleeding; (c) inspect the cervix for dilatation of the os, presence of polyps, ulcers or other lesions, passage of tissue
5. Bimanual examination and estimation of uterine size, shape, position, and consistency; examination of the adnexae for masses or tenderness

Imaging with US is the cornerstone of the evaluation of bleeding during early pregnancy. With confirmation of pregnancy, US is used to determine whether pregnancy is intrauterine or extrauterine and if the pregnancy is viable. By the fifth to sixth gestational week and in the presence of β-human chorionic gonadotropin (β-hCG) levels that are >1,000–2,000 mIU/ml, most transvaginal US transducers can demonstrate an intrauterine gestational sac [11–15]. Failure to do so suggests an ectopic pregnancy.

Common Causes of Vaginal Bleeding

The common causes of vaginal bleeding are outlined here. See individual chapters on each topic for more extensive information.

Threatened Abortion

Threatened abortion (see Chap. 2) is defined as the presence of vaginal bleeding while pregnancy is still confined to the uterine cavity and there has been no passage of tissue. Bleeding results from marginal abruption and separation of chorion from the endometrial lining [3]. More than 90% of pregnancies with both fetal cardiac activity and vaginal bleeding at 7–11 weeks of gestation do not miscarry [6–17]. The risk of miscarriage depends on both the gestational week and the sonographic findings, as presented in Table 1.1.

Threatened abortion is usually managed expectantly, and bleeding is light in most cases. Nevertheless, if the maternal hemodynamic status is unstable due to severe bleeding, uterine evacuation is an option.

Inevitable Abortion

Inevitable abortion (see Chap. 2) is defined by the presence of a dilated cervical os, uterine cramps, and bleeding together with an amniotic sac or gestational tissue that are palpated or visualized at the external os. Fetal cardiac activity may be present.

Heavy bleeding with an unstable maternal hemodynamic state is an indication for uterine evacuation. Otherwise, inevitable abortion may be managed either expectantly or by evacuating the uterus while taking into account maternal desire.

Spontaneous Abortion

Spontaneous abortion (see Chap. 2) is defined as a pregnancy that ends unexpectedly at a nonviable gestational age [18]. Diagnosis is made by physical examination and sonography. Fetal chromosomal anomalies are the most frequent cause of spontaneous abortion. The various types of spontaneous abortion include the following.

- Missed abortion: in utero death of the embryo before 20 weeks of gestation. Bleeding may be present but the cervical os is closed [19].
- Blighted ovum, also called "unembryonic pregnancy": This is defined as the presence of a gestational sac with a minimum diameter of 13 mm and no yolk sac or embryonic pole [20–22].

- Incomplete abortion: the presence of bleeding and an open cervical os. US demonstrates retained products of conception with the absence of a gestational sac.
- Complete abortion: the complete expulsion of products of conception, with a closed cervical os. Bleeding is usually light.

Septic Abortion

The presence of maternal fever and foul-smelling vaginal discharge suggests a septic abortion. This type of abortion mandates extended-spectrum antibiotic treatment and evacuation of the uterus. Septic abortion may be a life-threatening event and is a risk factor for Asherman's syndrome and future infertility.

Ectopic Pregnancy

Ectopic pregnancy (extrauterine pregnancy or EUP) (see Chap. 3) is defined as the implantation of gestational products outside the uterine cavity, usually in the fallopian tube. An incidence of 16–19:1,000 pregnancies is reported [20, 23]. The incidence varies depending on the risk factors. The risk factors and their odds ratios are presented in Table 1.2 [24–26].

The classic clinical presentation usually includes amenorrhea, irregular vaginal bleeding, and lower abdominal pain. The diagnosis of ectopic pregnancy is based on the history, physical examination, serial β-hCG measurements, and pelvic US. Failure to diagnose ectopic pregnancy may result in a catastrophic outcome, including rupture of the viscera (usually the fallopian tube), intraperitoneal bleeding, and maternal death.

Treatment includes a spectrum of possibilities ranging from expectant management through medical to surgical interventions. Decisions on the appropriate treatment should take into account the clinical presentation and maternal hemodynamic status, β-hCG levels, and sonographic findings.

Table 1.2 Odds ratios of risk factors for ectopic pregnancy

Risk factors for ectopic pregnancy	Odds ratio
Previous ectopic pregnancy	6.0–11.5
Prior tubal surgery	9.3–47.0
Tubal ligation	3.0–139.0
Tubal pathology	3.5–25.0
In utero DES exposure	2.4–13.0
Current IUD use	1.1–45.0
Infertility	1.1–28.0
History of PID	2.1–3.0
Smoking	2.3–3.9
Pelvic/abdominal surgery	0.93–3.90
Early age at intercourse (<18 years)	1.1–2.5

DES diethylstilbestrol, *IUD* intrauterine device, *PID* pelvic inflammatory disease

Implantation Bleeding

Implantation bleeding is a common cause of first trimester vaginal bleeding and is usually a diagnosis made by exclusion. Implantation bleeding occurs approximately 4 weeks after the last menstrual period. The bleeding is a result of a fertilized egg implanting and invading the endometrial cavity. During this process the blastocyst burrows into the decidua and causes disruption of the endometrial tissue and blood vessels. Bleeding is usually slight and is sometimes believed to be menses by the woman. Implantation bleeding is a benign process [27].

Gestational Trophoblastic Disease

Gestational trophoblastic disease (GTD) (see Chap. 4) refers to a wide spectrum of disorders arising from abnormal proliferation of the trophoblastic tissue. These disorders share certain characteristics with malignant neoplasms. Hydatiform mole (complete or partial), persistent/invasive gestational neoplastic neoplasia, choriocarcinoma, and placental-site trophoblastic tumors are all classified as GTD. Hydatiform mole is the most common type of GTD, comprising 90% of GTD cases [3, 28, 29]. These tumors have different tendencies for invasion and metastatic development.

The incidence of GTD varies widely in different regions of the world [30]. It varies from 66 to 121 per 100,000 pregnancies in North America and Europe to 23–81 per 100,000 pregnancies in Latin America and Asia [30].

The most common clinical feature of GTD is vaginal bleeding, which occurs in 84% of patients [31]. Bleeding results when the tumor separates from the underlying decidua. Other features include uterine enlargement, pelvic pressure or pain, hyperemesis gravidarum, hyperthyroidism, theca lutein ovarian cysts, and anemia.

GTD is suspected when excessive levels of β-hCG levels are encountered together with the typical sonographic appearance of a hypertrophic placenta with anechoic spaces [32, 33]. The final diagnosis is confirmed by histology. The availability of sensitive quantitative measurements of serum β-hCG levels and US has resulted in an earlier diagnosis of GTD.

Treatment depends on the specific diagnosis, presence of metastasis, and patient's age and desired future fertility. With hydatiform mole, for example, treatment is based on evacuating the uterus. Chemotherapy is added if evidence of persistent gestational trophoblastic tumor exists.

Local Lesions

Local lesions (see Chap. 5) include cervical polyps or erosions, cervical neoplasia, and vaginitis, which can present as vaginal bleeding, which is usually postcoital. Cervical infection or inflammation, such as chlamydial infection, can be a cause of vaginal bleeding at any time during pregnancy [20]. It is diagnosed by direct visualization as well as culture or biopsy of a suspicious lesion.

Vaginal Bleeding During the Second Half of Pregnancy

The incidence of vaginal bleeding during the second half of pregnancy ranges from 2 to 5% of all pregnancies [34–36]. Vaginal bleeding, especially if recurrent, is a risk factor for adverse pregnancy outcome. Some of the associated adverse outcomes include a higher perinatal mortality rate, amniotic fluid disorders, PROM and PPROM, recurrent abortion, preterm delivery, low birth weight, and a lower Apgar score [1].

Etiologies of vaginal bleeding during the second half of pregnancy can be divided according to the origin, as follows: uterine (placenta previa, placental abruption, uterine rupture); cervical and vaginal (cervical lesion, "bloody show," vaginal lesions or lacerations); fetal (vasa previa); other (coagulation disorders).

The initial evaluation, history taking, and clinical assessment in women present-ing with vaginal bleeding during the second half of pregnancy are similar to those performed in the case of bleeding during the first half. In contrast to the first half of pregnancy, however, manual digital examination should be deferred until placenta previa is excluded.

What follows in the next sections are brief summaries of items that should be included in the differential diagnosis. See individual chapters on each topic for more extensive information.

Placenta Previa

Placenta previa (see Chap. 8) is defined as the placental implantation over the inter-nal cervical os or within 2 cm of it. Its incidence is increasing and is estimated to be 1 per 200 deliveries [37]. Figure 1.2 shows the frequency of placenta previa during the years 1988–2010 at the Soroka University Medical Center, Beer-Sheva, Israel.

Four types of placenta previa exist.

1. Complete placenta previa: Internal os is covered completely by the placenta.
2. Partial placenta previa: Internal os is partially covered by the placenta.
3. Marginal placenta previa: Placenta lies in proximity to the internal os but does not cover it.
4. Low-lying placenta: Placental edge lies within 2 cm of the internal os.

Risk factors for placenta previa include previous cesarean delivery, high parity, increased maternal age, uterine anomalies, smoking, cocaine abuse, multiple preg-nancy, previous placenta previa, previous termination of pregnancy, intrauterine surgery, and assisted reproductive techniques (ARTs) [38].

The classic presentation is one of painless vaginal bleeding that could be severe and life-threatening. An absence of uterine contractions and normal uterine tone distinguishes placenta previa from placental abruption [36]. It is diagnosed by sono-graphic examination (US is 87.5% sensitive and 98.0% specific) [36]. More than

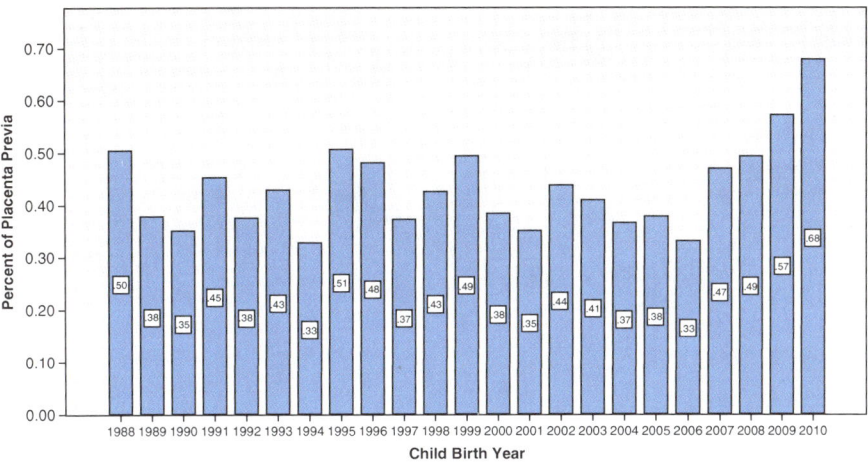

Fig. 1.2 Frequency of placenta previa during the years 1988–2010 at the Soroka University Medical Center, Beer-Sheva, Israel

90% of low-lying placentas diagnosed during early pregnancy migrate away from the lower uterine segment as the pregnancy progresses. Placenta previa diagnosed during later pregnancy has a higher chance of persistence until delivery [36].

Management depends on maternal and fetal status, gestational age at presentation, and bleeding severity. Management options vary from expectant management to urgent cesarean delivery. Some retrospective studies have demonstrated that the use of tocolysis is associated with greater prolongation of pregnancy and higher birth weights [39, 40].

Placental Abruption

Placental abruption (see Chap. 7) is premature separation of the placenta from its implantation site. Its average frequency is 1 in 100 deliveries [36]. The frequency of placental abruption during the years 1988–2010 at the Soroka University Medical Center, Beer-Sheva, Israel is presented in Fig. 1.3. Risk factors include preeclampsia, abdominal trauma, smoking, cocaine use, multiple pregnancy, increasing maternal age and parity, polyhydramnios, and previous abruption [41, 42]. Placental abruption predisposes to stillbirth, adverse perinatal outcome, and preterm delivery.

The clinical presentation is one of vaginal bleeding accompanied by abdominal pain. Hemorrhage from placental abruption may be apparent (70% of cases) or concealed (30%) [36]. Fifty percent of the women are in established labor at the time of presentation. The uterus is usually rigid and tender. There may be signs of acute

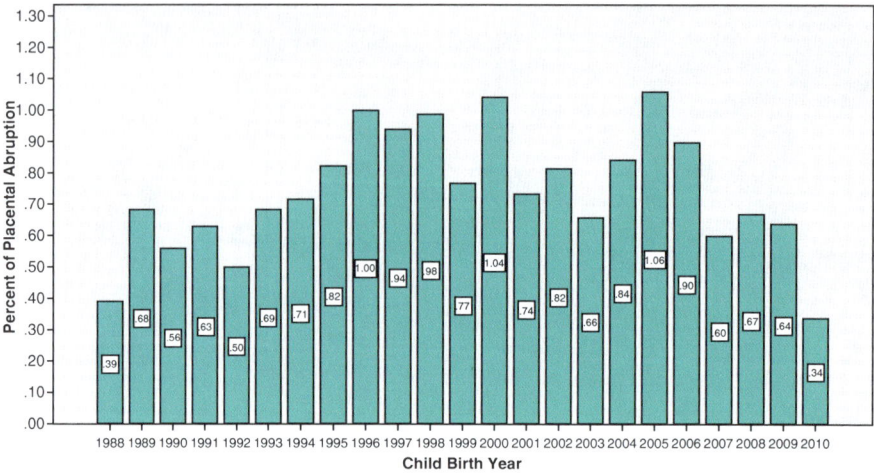

Fig. 1.3 Frequency of placental abruption during the years 1988–2010 at the Soroka University Medical Center, Beer-Sheva, Israel

fetal distress, and abnormal fetal heart rate patterns are detected in up to 70% of cases. In cases where more than 50% of the placenta has separated, fetal demise is common [43, 44].

The clinical approach to patients with suspected placental abruption is similar to the general approach for any APH. It includes assessment of maternal and fetal status and bleeding quantification. A thorough physical examination is carried out focusing on fundal height and uterine tone, a speculum examination to confirm a uterine origin of the bleeding, and US to rule out placenta previa and to assess the fetus. Mild cases of abruption are diagnosed by the presence of some clinical signs and the exclusion of other causes; severe cases can be confirmed by demonstrating a retroplacental hematoma with US, which has sensitivity, specificity, positive and negative predictive values of 24%, 96%, 88%, and 53%, respectively, in regard to detecting placental abruption. Thus, US falls short in diagnosing at least half of abruption cases [45].

Management depends on the maternal and fetal status, gestational age at presentation, and bleeding severity, similar to the management of placenta previa. Options vary from expectant management to urgent cesarean delivery.

Controversy still exists regarding the efficacy and safety of tocolysis in cases of third trimester bleeding in general and of placental abruption specifically [46]. Some authors suggest the use of tocolysis in cases of mild abruption remote from term in an attempt to reduce neonatal morbidity and mortality that are related to prematurity and not to the abruption itself [46, 47]. Others oppose its use because of the general concern regarding usage of tocolytic drugs (especially β-sympathomimetic agents) and the associated tachycardia, which could mask the clinical signs of blood loss [43].

Uterine Rupture

Uterine rupture (see Chap. 10) is a potentially catastrophic obstetrical complication that could arise for various reasons but mostly is due to separation of a previous cesarean scar. The incidence varies according to the presence of risk factors, with a 1:200 chance in women with a trial of labor after a previous cesarean section but only 1:15,000 deliveries in the presence of an intact uterus.

Symptoms and physical findings with uterine rupture can be vague and undefined. The clinical presentation usually consists of nonreassuring fetal heart rate monitoring together with some of the following: vaginal bleeding, signs of maternal hypovolemia (due to intraabdominal hemorrhage), cessation of contractions, and disengagement of the fetal presenting part. A high index of suspicion is the key to early diagnosis of uterine rupture. Management includes immediate laparotomy and maternal hemodynamic stabilization.

Cervical and Vaginal Lesions

Cervical and vaginal lesions (see Chap. 5), including cervical polyps or erosions, cervical neoplasia, and "bloody show," are possible causes of vaginal bleeding from a cervical origin during the second half of pregnancy. Bleeding is usually mild and mostly provoked by minor trauma during digital examination or intercourse. Vaginal lesions or lacerations may also result from neoplasia or trauma. When a speculum examination reveals a cervical or vaginal lesion suggestive of neoplasia, it is mandatory to attain a biopsy specimen for definitive histological confirmation. It is of major importance to have an early diagnosis and treatment of such lesions.

Cervical Dilatation and Labor

The most common cause of bleeding from a cervical origin is the "bloody show" [16]. "Bloody show" is considered an early sign of labor. As the cervix begins to soften and dilate, blood vessels break, which may cause the mucous plug to have a tinge of brown, pink or red. Bleeding is usually light. Passing the mucous plug is typically a sign that labor is imminent during the next few hours or days, although it may be dislodged a few weeks prior to labor due to intercourse or a digital examination. When cervical dilatation and mild bleeding occur before 37 completed weeks of gestation, it may be the first sign of PTL. See Chap. 6 for more complete information.

Vasa Previa

Vasa previa (see Chap. 9), a rare diagnosis, is associated with velamentous insertion of the umbilical cord. Fetal vessels cross or run in close proximity to the inner cervical os. An incidence of 3 per 10,000 deliveries is reported [48]. Fetal hemorrhage is caused by tearing of fetal vessels when the membranes rupture.

The diagnosis is suspected when bleeding starts with membrane rupture followed by an abnormal fetal heart rate, detected by monitoring. Trace abnormalities may be consistent with fetal anemia caused by exsanguination. An antepartum diagnosis is sometimes possible with vaginal sonography combined with color Doppler, which demonstrates fetal vessels overlying or close to the internal os [49]. When the diagnosis is made antepartum, delivery by cesarean section is indicated at 36–37 weeks [36].

No firm diagnosis can be made in as many as half of the patients presenting with second and third trimester bleeding, even following a thorough investigation. If maternal and fetal well-being are established, expectant management is an accepted strategy. If either the mother or the fetus is compromised, prompt delivery should be considered.

Initial management of a significant bleed late in pregnancy is similar, regardless of the etiology. Figure 1.4 indicates the initial clinical approach to bleeding during the second half of pregnancy.

Postpartum Hemorrhage

Postpartum hemorrhage (PPH) (see Chap. 11) is the most common type of obstetrical hemorrhage [50] and one of the leading causes of maternal morbidity and mortality. Its incidence varies but has been reported to be as high as 18% of deliveries [51]. In developing countries, PPH accounts for 25% of maternal mortality. In developed countries, PPH is responsible for about 17% of all maternal deaths [52].

PPH is classically defined as excessive bleeding following delivery, with an estimated blood loss of more than 500 ml following a vaginal delivery and more than 1,000 ml following a cesarean section. This classic definition of PPH is lacking as accurate assessment of blood loss is challenging and often is an underestimation. Other definitions of PPH consider the maternal hemodynamic status or the decline in hemoglobin levels. PPH may be primary (early), occurring within 24 h of delivery, or secondary (late), occurring 24 h to 12 weeks postpartum [53, 54].

Differential Diagnosis

The differential diagnosis for PPH includes the following.

- Bleeding from implantation site due to: (1) uterine atony, with predisposing factors that include an overdistended uterus, infection, prolonged or precipitated labor, multiparity, some drugs, uterine inversion, poorly perfused myometrium,

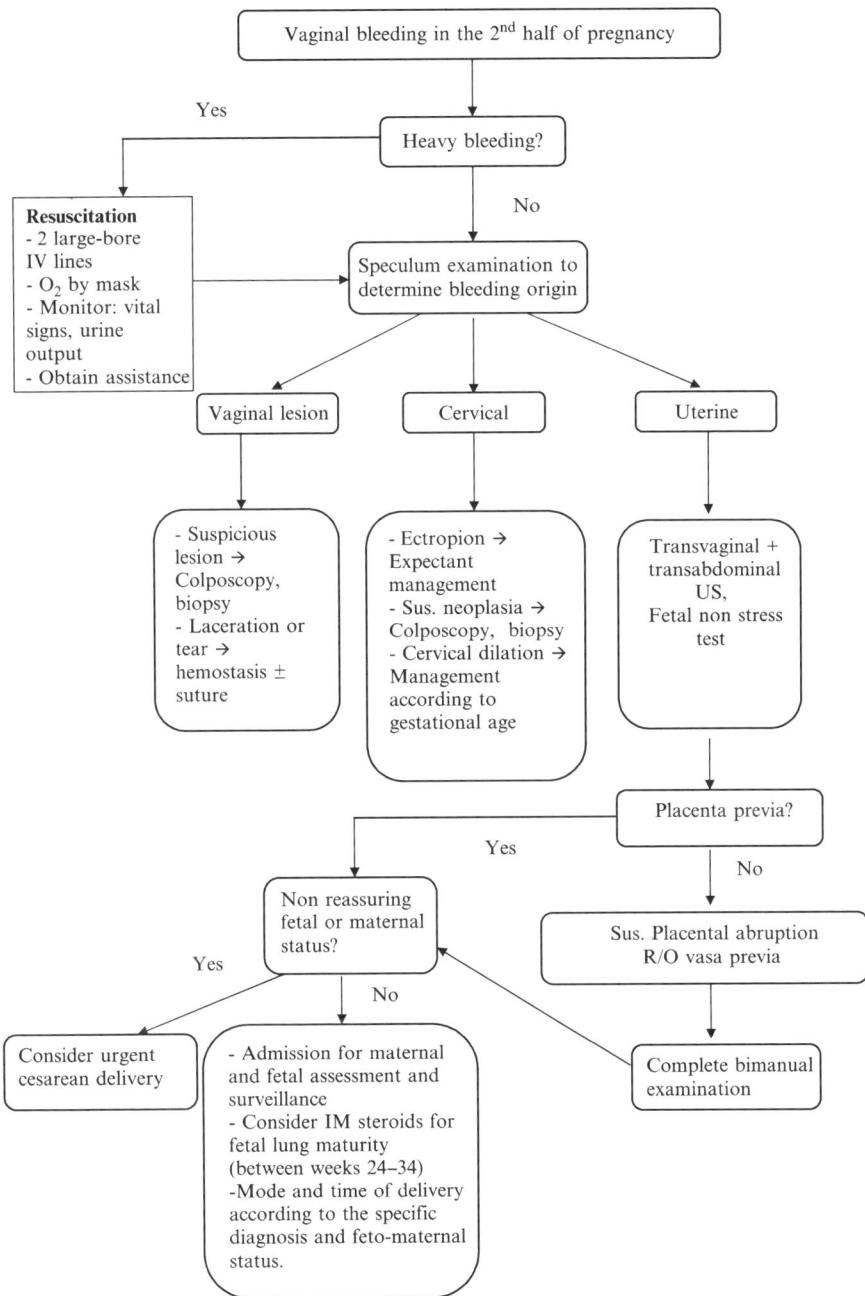

Fig. 1.4 Clinical approach to bleeding during the second half of pregnancy. *Sus.* suspected, *R/O* rule out, *IM* intramuscular

history of uterine atony; (2) retained placental tissue (e.g., cotyledon, accessory or succentriate lobe) or due to abnormal placentation (accrete, increta, percreta)
- Trauma to the genital tract due to: uterine rupture, cervical tears, vaginal and perineal lacerations and hematomas, episiotomy
- Coagulation disorders

Recognition of excessive bleeding following delivery should alert the physician of the possibility of PPH, keeping in mind that blood loss is usually underestimated. This possibility mandates a prompt investigation to determine the possible etiology while simultaneously providing the patient with standard maternal resuscitation measures.

Etiology

Uterine Atony

Uterine contraction is essential for hemostasis and placental separation. Uterine atony is the most common cause of PPH, accounting for 70% of cases [51]. Treatment of uterine atony consists of uterine massage and uterotonic drugs, including oxytocin, ergot alkaloids, and prostaglandins.

Trauma

Vaginal delivery can result in vaginal and perineal lacerations of varying severity. These lacerations can result in significant but unnoticed blood loss. Immediate recognition, treatment, and suture of lacerations and tears can help decrease the blood loss. Avoidance of episiotomy – unless urgent delivery is necessary and in cases in which the perineum is believed to be a limiting factor – can help decrease blood loss and reduce perineal trauma. Vaginal lacerations can result in concealed retroperitoneal or suprafascial hematomas that may lead to significant blood loss. Symptoms usually include pain and deteriorating vital signs disproportionate to the amount of the apparent bleeding.

Uterine rupture is another form of birth trauma that could result in life-threatening PPH. It is a rare obstetrical complication, with an incidence of approximately 0.6–0.7% in cases of a trial of vaginal birth after a cesarean section. As mentioned previously, intrapartum signs of rupture include nonreassuring fetal heart rate monitoring among other, less consistent signs. Uterine rupture can become symptomatic during the postpartum period, manifesting as abdominal tenderness and maternal hemodynamic collapse. This catastrophic event necessitates urgent laparotomy for hemostasis and attempting to repair the uterus, although hysterectomy is unavoidable in many cases.

Retained Placenta

The mean duration of the third stage of labor is 8–9 min [54]. Longer intervals are associated with an increased risk of PPH, with double the rate after 10 min. Retained placental parts interfere with uterine contractions and may cause early or late PPH. Removal of large retained placental segments is necessary for effective uterine involution and bleeding control. These women should be followed for signs of late sequelae, including infection and late PPH [55, 56].

Coagulopathies

Coagulation disorders (see Chap. 12) are a rare cause of PPH, accounting for 1% of cases [51]. Failure of PPH to respond to standard measures of treatment should raise the suspicion of such a possibility. The more common disorders include idiopathic thrombocytopenic purpura, thrombotic thrombocytopenic purpura, Von Willebrand's disease, hemophilias, and disseminated intravascular coagulation. Congenital clotting factor deficiencies can also manifest as PPH. These disorders are rare, and there is little literature on the subject.

Initial evaluation should include a complete blood count with a platelet count and measurement of the prothrombin time, partial thromboplastin time, and fibrinogen level. Management includes standard resuscitation methods and replacement of clotting factors with various blood products, as required [57].

Approach to PPH

Recognition of PPH requires immediate action that combines diagnostic measures with standard maternal resuscitation efforts (see Chap. 13). Effective, successful treatment requires an interdisciplinary team approach that could be lifesaving. For women who desire to preserve fertility, uterine-sparing procedures may be attempted, including uterine packing or tamponade, B-Lynch sutures, and ligation or embolization of the feeding artery [39]. Figure 1.5 describes the initial clinical approach to PPH.

Summary

Pregnancy-related hemorrhage remains a leading cause of maternal mortality despite modern improvement in practice and transfusion services. The fact that two patients are involved – mother and fetus – adds to the complexity of the event. The key to successful treatment of obstetrical hemorrhage is early recognition and rapid

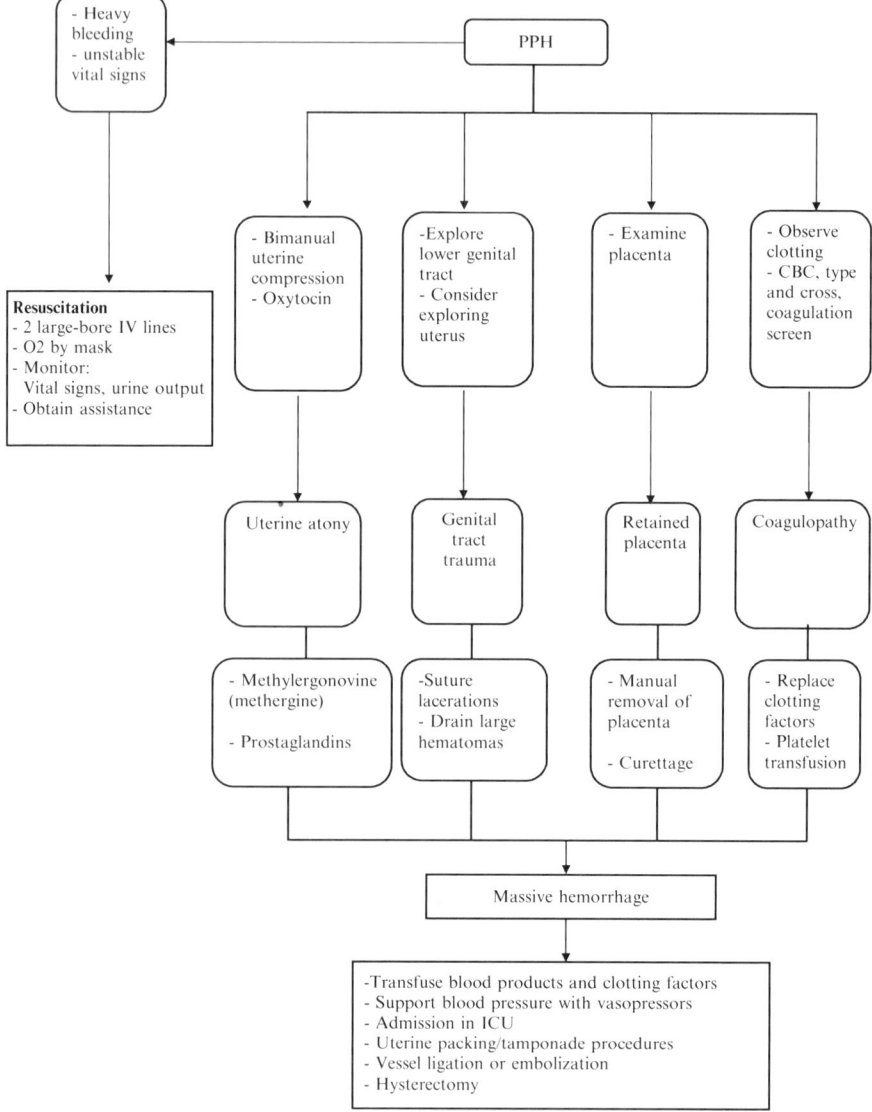

Fig. 1.5 Clinical approach to postpartum hemorrhage (PPH). *CBC* complete blood count, *ICU* intensive care unit

response to life-threatening events for both mother and fetus. Early resuscitation with fluids and blood products can be lifesaving. Successful treatment of hemorrhage in a gravid woman involves full awareness to the normal physiological hemodynamic changes during pregnancy.

The key principles in the diagnosis and management of pregnancy-related hemorrhage include (1) assessment of maternal and fetal well-being; (2) quick action and fetomaternal resuscitation in parallel with the investigation; (3) careful physical examination to determine the origin of the bleeding; (4) treatment approach and decision making based on a presumed diagnosis and the clinical status.

References

1. Koifman A, Levy A, Zaulan Y, Harlev A, Mazor M, Wiznitzer A, et al. The clinical significance of bleeding during the second trimester of pregnancy. Arch Gynecol Obstet. 2008;278:47–51.
2. Harlev A, Levy A, Zaulan Y, Koifman A, Mazor M, Wiznitzer A, et al. Idiopathic bleeding during the second half of pregnancy as a risk factor for adverse perinatal outcome. J Matern Fetal Neonatal Med. 2008;21(5):331–5.
3. Snell BJ. Assessment and management of bleeding in the first trimester of pregnancy. J Midwifery Womens Health. 2009;54:483–91.
4. Hossain R, Harris T, Lohsoonthorn V, Williams MA. Risk of preterm delivery in relation to vaginal bleeding in early pregnancy. Eur J Obstet Gynecol Reprod Biol. 2007;135: 158–63.
5. Everett C. Incidence and outcome of bleeding before the 20th week of pregnancy: prospective study from general practice. BMJ. 1997;315:32–4.
6. Saraswat L, Bhattacharya S, Maheshwari A, Bhattacharya S. Maternal and perinatal outcome in women with threatened miscarriage in the first trimester: a systemic review. BJOG. 2010; 117:245–57.
7. Promislow JHE, Baird DD, Wilcox AJ, Weinberg CR. Bleeding following pregnancy loss before 6 weeks' gestation. Hum Reprod. 2007;22(3):853–7.
8. Rai R, Regan L. Recurrent miscarriage. Lancet. 2006;368:601–11.
9. Andersen AMN, Wohlfahrt J, Christens P, Olsen J, Melbye M. Maternal age and fetal loss: population based register linkage study. BMJ. 2000;320:1708–12.
10. Regan L, Braude PR, Trembath PL. Influence of past reproductive performance on the risk of spontaneous abortion. BMJ. 1989;299:541–5.
11. Goldstein SR. Embryonic death in early pregnancy: a new look at the first trimester. Obstet Gynecol. 1994;84(2):294–7.
12. Abramovici H, Auslender R, Lewin A, Faktor JH. Gestational-pseudogestational sac: a new ultrasonic criterion for differential diagnosis. Am J Obstet Gynecol. 1983;145:377–9.
13. Bree RL, Edwards M, Bohm VM, et al. Transvaginal sonography in the evaluation of normal early pregnancy: correlation with HCG level. AJR Am J Roentgenol. 1989;53:75–9.
14. Nyberg DA, Mack LA, Laing FC, Jeffrey RB. Early pregnancy complications: endovaginal sonographic findings correlated with human chorionic gonadotropin levels. Radiology. 1988;167:619–22.
15. Bernaschek G, Rudelstorfer R, Csaicsich P. Vaginal sonography versus serum human chorionic gonadotropin in early detection of pregnancy. Am J Obstet Gynecol. 1988;158:608–12.
16. Tongsong T, Srisomboon J, Wanapirak C, Sirichotiyakul S, Pongsatha S, Polsrisuthikul T. Pregnancy outcome of threatened abortion with demonstrable fetal cardiac activity: a cohort study. J Obstet Gynaecol. 1995;21:331–5.
17. Tannirandorm Y, Sangsawang S, Manotaya S, Uerpairojkit B, Samritpradit P, Charoenvidhya D. Fetal loss in threatened abortion after embryonic/fetal heart activity. Int J Gynaecol Obstet. 2003;81:263–6.
18. Regan L, Rai R. Epidemiology and the medical causes of miscarriage. Baillieres Best Pract Res Clin Obstet Gynecol. 2000;14:839–54.
19. Zeqiri F, Paçarada M, Kongjeli N, Zeqiri V, Kongjeli G. Missed abortion and application of misoprostol. Med Arh. 2010;64(3):151–3.
20. McKennett M, Fullerton JT. Vaginal bleeding in pregnancy. Am Fam Physician. 1995;51(3): 639–46.

21. Rowling SE, Langer JE, Coleman BG, Nisenbaum HL, Horii SC, Arger PH. Sonography during early pregnancy: dependence of threshold and discriminatory values on transvaginal transducer frequency. Am J Roentgenol. 1999;172:983–8.
22. Tongsong T, Wanapirak C, Srisomboon J, Sirichotiyakul S, Polsrisuthikul T, Pongsatha S. Transvaginal ultrasound in threatened abortions with empty gestational sacs. Int J Gynaecol Obstet. 1994;46:297–301.
23. Centers for Disease Control and Prevention. Ectopic pregnancy–United States, 1990–1992. MMWR Morb Mortal Wkly Rep. 1995;44:46–468.
24. Ankum WM, Mol BW, Van der Veen F, Bossuyt PM. Risk factors for ectopic pregnancy: a meta-analysis. Fertil Steril. 1996;65(6):1093–9.
25. Murray H, Baakdah H, Bardell T, Tulandi T. Diagnosis and treatment of ectopic pregnancy. CMAJ. 2005;173(8):905–12.
26. Bouyer J, Coste J, Shojaei l T, Pouly JL, Fernandez H, Gerbaud L, et al. Risk factors for ectopic pregnancy: a comprehensive analysis based on a large case-control, population-based study in France. Am J Epidemiol. 2003;157:185–94.
27. Promes SB, Nobay F. Pitfalls in first-trimester bleeding. Emerg Med Clin N Am. 2010;28:219–34.
28. Berkowitz RS, Goldstein DP. Chorionic tumors. N Engl J Med. 1996;335:1740.
29. Soto-Wright V, Bernstein M, Goldstein DP, Berkowitz RS. The changing clinical presentation of complete molar pregnancy. Obstet Gynecol. 1995;86:775–9.
30. Altieri A, Franceschi S, Ferlay J, Smith J, Vecchia C. Epidemiology of gestational trophoblastic diseases. Lancet Oncol. 2003;4:670–8.
31. Goldstein DP, Berkowitz RS. Current management of complete and partial molar pregnancy. J Reprod Med. 1994;39:139–46.
32. Wagner BJ, Woodward PJ, Dickey GE. From the archives of the AFIP. Gestational trophoblastic disease: radiologic-pathologic correlation. Radiographics. 1996;16:131–48.
33. Fine C, Bundy AL, Berkowitz RS, Boswell SB, Berezin AF, Doubilet PM. Sonographic diagnosis of partial hydatidiform mole. Obstet Gynecol. 1989;73:414–8.
34. Mukherjee S, Bhide A. Antepartum haemorrhage. Obstet Gynaecol Rep Med. 2008;18(12):335–9.
35. Paintin DB. The epidemiology of ante-partum haemorrhage: a study of all Births in a Community. BJOG. 1962;69:614–24.
36. Sinha P, Kuruba N. Ante-partum haemorrhage: an update. J Obstet Gynaecol. 2008;28(4):377–81.
37. Ananth CV, Smulian JC, Vintzileos AM. Incidence of placental abruption in relation to cigarette smoking and hypertensive disorders during pregnancy: a meta-analysis of observational studies. Obstet Gynecol. 1999;93:622–8.
38. Ananth CV, Wilcox AJ, Savitz DA, Bowes WA, Luther ER. Effect of maternal age and parity on the risk of uteroplacental bleeding disorders in pregnancy. Obstet Gynecol. 1996;88:511–6.
39. Sharma A, Suri V, Gupta I. Tocolytic therapy in conservative management of symptomatic placenta previa. Int J Gynaecol Obstet. 2004;84:109–13.
40. Besinger RE, Moniak CW, Paskiewicz LS, Fisher SG, Tomich PG. The effect of tocolytic use in the management of symptomatic placenta previa. Am J Obstet Gynecol. 1995;172:1770–8.
41. Ananth CV, Berkowitz GS, Savitz DA, Lapinski RH. Placental abruption and adverse perinatal outcomes. JAMA. 1999;282:1646–51.
42. Kramer MS, Usher RH, Pollack R, Boyd M, Usher S. Etiologic determinants of abruptio placentae. Obstet Gynecol. 1997;89:221–6.
43. Oyelese Y, Ananth CV. Placental abruption. Obstet Gynecol. 2006;108(4):1005–16.
44. Tikkanen M, Nuutila M, Hiilesmaa V, Paavonen J, Ylikorkala O. Clinical presentation and risk factors of placental abruption. Acta Obstet Gynecol Scand. 2006;85(6):700–5.
45. Glantz C, Purnell L. Clinical utility of sonography in the diagnosis and treatment of placental abruption. J Ultrasound Med. 2002;21:837–40.

46. Towers CV, Pircon RA, Hepprad M. Is tocolysis safe in the management of third-trimester bleeding? Am J Obstet Gynecol. 1999;180:1572–8.
47. Bond AL, Edersheim TG, Curry L, Druzin ML, Hutson JM. Expectant management of abruptio placentae before 35 weeks gestation. Am J Perinatol. 1989;6:121–3.
48. Oyelese KO, Turner M, Lees C, Campbell S. Vasa pervia: an avoidable obstetric tragedy. Obstet Gynecol Surv. 1999;54:138–45.
49. Lee W, Lee V, Kirk JS, Sloan CT, Smith RS, Comstock CH. Vasa previa: prenatal diagnosis, natural evolution and clinical outcome. Obstet Gynecol. 2000;95:572–6.
50. Tsu VD, Langer A, Aldrich T. Postpartum hemorrhage in developing countries: is the public health community using the right tools? Int J Gynaecol Obstet. 2004;85:S42–51.
51. Anderson JM, Etches D. Prevention and management of postpartum hemorrhage. Am Fam Physician. 2007;75:875–82.
52. Statistics from EUPHIN network database: http://www.euphin.dk/hfa/Phfa.asp. Accessed 28 Mar 2002.
53. King PA, Duthie SJ, Ven D, Dong ZG, Ma HK. Secondary postpartum haemorrhage. Aust N Z J Obstet Gynecol. 1989;29:394–8.
54. Magann EF, Evans S, Chauhan SP, Lanneau G, Fisk AD, Morrison JC. The length of the third stage of labor and the risk of postpartum hemorrhage. Obstet Gynecol. 2005;105:290–3.
55. Mussalli GM, Shah J, Berck DJ, Elimian A, Tejani N, Manning FA. Placenta accrete and methotrexate therapy: three case reports. J Perinatol. 2000;20:331–4.
56. O'Brien JM, Barton JR, Donaldson ES. The management of placenta percreta: conservative and operative strategies. Am J Obstet Gynecol. 1996;175:1632–8.
57. Kadir R, Chi C, Bolton-Maggs P. Pregnancy and rare bleeding disorders. Haemophilia. 2009;15:990–1005.

Part II
Bleeding During Early Pregnancy

Chapter 2
Early Pregnancy Loss

Adi Y. Weintraub and Eyal Sheiner

Introduction

Pregnancy is a significant event in a woman's life, and emotional attachment to the pregnancy and developing baby may begin early in the first trimester. For most women, experiencing a first trimester loss is a difficult and vulnerable time. When it occurs, the grief can be as profound as for any perinatal or other major loss [1]. Spontaneous abortion (a pregnancy that ends spontaneously before the fetus has reached a viable gestational age) is among the most common complications of pregnancy. Approximately 12–15% of recognized pregnancies and 17–22% of all pregnancies end in spontaneous abortion [2, 3].

The best-documented risk factors for spontaneous abortion are advanced maternal age, a previous spontaneous abortion, and maternal smoking. Most spontaneous abortions are attributed to structural or chromosomal abnormalities in the embryo.

Stages and Types of Spontaneous Abortions

There are various stages and types of spontaneous abortions (threatened, inevitable, incomplete and complete abortions, missed abortion, and fetal/embryonic demise). These types are clearly defined.

A.Y. Weintraub (✉)
Department of Obstetrics and Gynecology, Faculty of Health Sciences,
Soroka University Medical Center, Ben-Gurion University of the Negev,
P.O. Box 151, Beer-Sheva, Israel
e-mail: adiyehud@bgu.ac.il

E. Sheiner (ed.), *Bleeding During Pregnancy: A Comprehensive Guide*,
DOI 10.1007/978-1-4419-9810-1_2, © Springer Science+Business Media, LLC 2011

- *Spontaneous abortion/miscarriage*: A pregnancy that ends spontaneously before the fetus has reached a viable gestational age. The World Health Organization defines it as expulsion or extraction of an embryo or fetus weighing ≤500 g (typically corresponds to a gestational age of ≤22 weeks).
- *Threatened abortion*: Bleeding through a closed cervical os during the first half of pregnancy. The bleeding is often painless, although it may be accompanied by mild suprapubic pain. On examination, the uterine size is appropriate for gestational age, and the cervix is long and closed. Fetal cardiac activity can be detectable if the gestation is sufficiently advanced.
- *Inevitable abortion*: When abortion is pending, there may be increased bleeding, intensely painful uterine cramps, and a dilated cervix. The gestational tissue can often be felt or visualized through the internal cervical os.
- *Incomplete abortion*: When the fetus is passed, but significant amounts of placental tissue may be retained, also called an abortion with retained products of conception (RPOC) (commonly occurs after 12 weeks' gestation). On examination, the cervical os is open, gestational tissue may be observed in the vagina/cervix, and the uterus is smaller than expected for gestational age but not well contracted. The amount of bleeding varies but can be severe enough to cause hypovolemic shock. Painful cramps are often present.
- *Complete abortion*: When an abortion occurs (usually before 12 weeks of gestation) and the entire contents of the uterus are expelled. More than one-third of all cases are complete abortions. If a complete abortion has occurred, the uterus is small and well contracted with a closed cervix; slight vaginal bleeding and mild cramping can be present.
- *Missed abortion*: Refers to in utero death of the embryo or fetus prior to the 20th week of gestation, with prolonged retention of the pregnancy (4–8 weeks). Vaginal bleeding may occur, and the cervix is usually closed.
- *Septic abortion*: An abortion accompanied by fever, chills, malaise, abdominal pain, vaginal bleeding, and frequently purulent discharge. Physical examination may reveal tachycardia, tachypnea, lower abdominal tenderness, and a tender uterus with dilated cervix. Infection is usually due to *Staphylococcus aureus*, Gram-negative bacilli, or some Gram-positive cocci. Mixed infections (anaerobic organisms and fungi) can also be encountered. The infection may spread, leading to salpingitis, generalized peritonitis, and septicemia.

Caution Box

- In a patient who presents with vaginal bleeding and abdominal or pelvic pain, although normal and abnormal intrauterine pregnancies are more common, ectopic pregnancy and gestational trophoblastic disease should always be ruled out.

Women with an active spontaneous abortion usually present with a history of amenorrhea, vaginal bleeding, and pelvic pain. The differential diagnosis includes bleeding related to implantation (physiological bleeding), ectopic pregnancy, gestational trophoblastic disease, and cervical, vaginal, or uterine pathology (see the relevant chapters). In addition to the physical examination, ultrasonography is the most useful test for diagnosing and evaluating women suspected of having a spontaneous abortion.

Etiology and Risk Factors

Many factors have been implicated as etiological or risk factors for spontaneous abortions. The most common cause is a genetic abnormality in the fetus, accounting for 50–76% of cases [4, 5]. Yet, a large proportion of spontaneous abortions can be explained by several other etiologies [6], including genetic, placental, and host factors.

In healthy women, maternal age is the most important risk factor for spontaneous abortion. In a large population-based study aimed to estimate the association between maternal age and fetal death (spontaneous abortion, ectopic pregnancy, stillbirth), 13.5% of pregnancies ended with fetal loss. At age 42 years, more than half of the pregnancies resulted in fetal loss. The risk of a spontaneous abortion was 8.9% among women aged 20–24 years and 74.7% among those aged ≥45 years. High maternal age was a significant risk factor for spontaneous abortion irrespective of the number of previous miscarriages, parity, or calendar period [7].

Chromosomal abnormalities account for more than 50% of spontaneous abortions. Most of these abnormalities are aneuploidies. Other abnormalities, such as structural abnormalities, mosaicism, and single gene defects, are responsible for relatively few abortions. The earlier the gestational age at the time of abortion, the incidence of cytogenic defects is higher.

Placental anatomical abnormalities are found in as many as two-thirds of early pregnancy failures. Anatomical evidence of defective placentation is characterized by a thin and fragmented trophoblast shell and reduced cytotrophoblast invasion of the lumen at the tips of the spiral arteries [8]. In most cases of miscarriage, these features are associated with premature maternal circulation throughout the placenta [9–11]. These findings are similar in euploid and most aneuploid abortions but are most profound in hydatiform moles.

Pregnancy losses may be related to the host environment. Congenital or acquired cervical and uterine abnormalities, infections, maternal endocrinopathies and a hypercoagulable state are some factors that have been implicated in the occurrence of spontaneous abortion.

- *Congenital or acquired uterine abnormalities* (i.e., septated uterus, submucosal myomas, intrauterine adhesions) can interfere with implantation and growth. In a recent review of the literature regarding fibroids and their effect on reproductive performance, the authors suggested that the best available evidence indicates that submucous myomas decrease fertility and increase the spontaneous abortion rate.

Myomectomy is likely to be of value. This may be true for intramural myomas as well [12].

- *Acute maternal infection* could lead to abortion due to fetal or placental involvement. Infections are an accepted cause of late fetal demise; therefore, it is logical that they are responsible for early fetal losses as well. A large number of organisms have been reported to be associated with spontaneous abortions including, among others, *Listeria monocytogenes*, *Parvovirus B19*, *Rubella*, *Herpes simplex*, *Toxoplasma gondii*, *Mycoplasma hominis*, *Chlamydia trachomatis*, and *Ureaplasma urealyticum*. However, evidence of this relation has not been extensively conformed [13].
- *Maternal endocrinopathies* such as poorly controlled diabetes mellitus [14] and thyroid dysfunction [15, 16] can contribute to a suboptimal host environment. Luteal phase defect is another condition that has been suggested to be associated with spontaneous miscarriage. A successful pregnancy is dependent on sufficient progesterone support. Before the placenta takes over progesterone production, the progesterone produced by the corpus luteum provides the necessary support of early pregnancy. A defect in corpus luteum function is associated not only with implantation failure but with miscarriage. However, the association between corpus luteum defects and miscarriage is controversial. Vitzthum et al. [17] showed that maternal serum progesterone levels around the time of implantation were similar for subsequently lost and ongoing pregnancies.
- *Hypercoagulable state* due to inherited or acquired thrombophilia and abnormalities of the immune system (i.e., systemic lupus erythematosus, antiphospholipid antibody syndrome) may lead to immunological rejection or placental damage and are accepted causes of miscarriage [18].
- *Additional factors* that are considered possible causes of spontaneous abortion include trauma; alloimmune disease; exposure to drugs, substance use, and environmental contaminants; some maternal illnesses; and psychological factors.

When the etiology of abortion in chromosomally and structurally normal embryos of women that are apparently healthy remains unclear, it is considered unexplained. A list of possible causes and risk factors for spontaneous abortions are presented in Table 2.1.

Diagnosis

Women with an active spontaneous abortion usually present with a history of amenorrhea, vaginal bleeding, and pelvic pain. On examination, the cervix is open, and the products of conception can be visualized in the vagina or cervical os if they have not already been passed.

An accurate diagnosis of early pregnancy loss is paramount for appropriately counseling patients about their pregnancy management options. Laboratory and ultrasonographic (US) evaluations are frequently used to diagnose early pregnancy loss.

Table 2.1 Possible causes and risk factors for spontaneous abortion

Embryonic/fetal factors

  Chromosomal abnormalities

  Other genetic abnormalities: mosaicism, single gene defects

  Structural/morphological abnormalities

Placental factors

  Placental anatomical abnormalities

  Abnormal placentation

Uterine/cervical factors

  Cervical os incompetence

  Mullerian uterine abnormalities: septated uterus, unicoruate uterus, bicornuate uterus, uterus didelphys

  Asherman's syndrome

  Endometriosis

  Fibroids: submucous and intramural

Maternal factors

  Demographic factors: advanced maternal age, two or more previous miscarriages

  Maternal illnesses: Wilson's disease, phenylketonuria, cyanotic heart disease, hemoglobin-opathies, inflammatory bowel disease

  Endocrinopathies: uncontrolled diabetes mellitus, abnormal thyroid function, luteal phase defect

  Infection (maternal fever): colonization with *Listeria monocytogenes*, *parvovirus B19*, *rubella*, *herpes simplex*, *Toxoplasma gondii*, *Mycoplasma hominis*, *Chlamydia trachomatis*, *Ureaplasma urealyticum*, and others

  Hypercoagulable state, abnormalities of the immune system: inherited or acquired thrombo-philia, APLA syndrome. systemic lupus erythematosus, alloimmune disease

Exposures

  Substance use: caffeine, cigarette smoking, alcohol, cocaine

  Drugs: NSAIDs, anesthetic gases

  Environmental contaminants: lead, formaldehyde, herbicides, solvents, radiation

Other factors

  Catastrophic physical trauma

  Conception with an IUD

  Psychological factors

Unexplained

APLA antiphospholipid antibodies, *NSAIDs* nonsteroidal antiinflammatory drugs, *IUD* intrauterine device

Common indications for US examinations during early pregnancy include vaginal bleeding, pelvic pain, and determination of gestational age [19].

In a patient who presents with vaginal bleeding and abdominal or pelvic pain, although normal and abnormal intrauterine pregnancies are more common, ectopic pregnancy should always be ruled out. Transvaginal (TV)US and measurement of quantitative β-human chorionic gonadotropin (β-hCG) are important for differentiating these diagnoses [19]. The discriminatory level is the level of β-hCG at which a normal intrauterine pregnancy should be visualized. Most commonly, a gestational sac should be visualized in a normal pregnancy via TVUS with a β-hCG level of > 2,000 mIU/ml [20] or via transabdominal US with a β-hCG level of >6,500 mIU/ml [21]. However, with a β-hCG level >2,000 mIU/ml and no visible intrauterine pregnancy, the possibility of a multiple gestation should be considered.

Barnhart et al. [22] analyzed serum hCG values from 287 subjects who presented during early pregnancy with pain or bleeding and were eventually diagnosed with a viable intrauterine pregnancy. The main purpose of the study was to determine the lower limits of β-hCG increase for viable intrauterine pregnancies to be able to avoid unnecessary interruptions of viable pregnancies. The lowest 99% confidence interval (CI) for serum hCG change was 24% at 1 day and 53% at 2 days. It should be noted that a normal rise in β-hCG levels does not exclude an abnormal intrauterine pregnancy or an ectopic pregnancy; and an abnormal rise in β-hCG levels cannot distinguish between an abnormal intrauterine pregnancy and an ectopic pregnancy. A pseudosac, which consists of blood or fluid within the uterine cavity, is seen in some ectopic pregnancies. Distinguishing between a pseudosac and a gestational sac is important in the diagnosis of early pregnancy. A pseudosac can only be excluded with visualization of a yolk sac or embryo within the gestational sac [23].

The US examination has become the mainstay of early pregnancy diagnosis. It provides a safe, noninvasive diagnosis of normal and abnormal early pregnancy. Table 2.2 summarizes chronological landmarks and sonographic features of normal embryonic development. The safety of US has been investigated with epidemiological studies, looking at markers of normal child development plus childhood cancers in women who have had routine US scans. No woman or baby was shown to be directly affected by the use of diagnostic US [24].

Traditionally, an early pregnancy scan was performed with a transabdominal transducer, but this method was found to be inadequate in up to 42% of women [25]. Transvaginal sonography provides better images owing to the proximity to the pelvic organs. Additionally, a transvaginal scan can be used at an earlier gestational age [26], it gives clearer images, and it can be performed instantly, as the patient needs an empty bladder. Cullen et al. [27] found that vaginal sonography was superior to abdominal sonography for gestations ≤10 weeks, obese patients, and patients with a retroverted uterus [27]. The limitations of vaginal sonography include limited maneuverability. Some women feel it is invasive or are concerned about the safety of their pregnancy and refuse a transvaginal scan.

An intrauterine pregnancy can be diagnosed earliest by sonographic visualization of a gestational sac. Gestational age can be estimated by measuring the mean sac diameter (MSD) – averaging the length, width, and depth of the gestational sac – or the embryonic pole/crown–rump length. A true "crown" and "rump" should be visible at an MSD of 18 mm; before that time, US evaluations include only identification of an embryonic pole (the long axis of the embryo) [23]. When using TVUS, a yolk sac should be visualized when the MSD is ≥8 mm. Similarly, an embryonic pole should be visualized with a MSD of 16 mm [28, 29]. Rowling et al. [30], however, reported that 22% of 135 patients without a yolk sac of 8 mm MSD developed live embryos. Similarly, 8% of 59 patients with a MSD of 16 mm and no visible

Table 2.2 Chronological landmarks and sonographic features of normal embryonic development

Time from last menstrual period	Sonographic features of embryonic development	Clinical recommendation
4^{+3}–5^{+0}	Small gestation sac (2–5 mm) is seen in the endometrium. Sac is spherical; it has a regular outline and is eccentrically located toward the fundus. It is implanted below the surface of the endometrium and is surrounded by echogenic trophoblast	In symptomatic patients, the scan should be repeated in a week, when a yolk sac should be visible
5^{+1}–5^{+5}	Yolk sac becomes visible within the chorionic cavity when the gestational sac diameter is >12 mm	If it is not seen, early embryonic demise is likely; and the scan should be repeated a week later to confirm it
5^{+6}–6^{+0}	Embryonic pole measuring 2–4 mm in length is visible. Heart action could be detected. An embryo is usually visible with a mean gestational sac diameter of >20 mm	If this is not the case, the pregnancy is likely to be abnormal; and another scan should be organized a week later
6^{+1}–6^{+6}	Embryo is kidney bean-shaped, with the yolk sac separated from it by the vitelline duct. Crown–rump length measures 4–10 mm	If the heart rate is not detectable, early embryonic demise is almost certain
7^{+0}–7^{+6}	Crown–rump length measures 11–16 mm. Rhombencephalon becomes distinguishable as a diamond-shaped cavity, enabling distinction of cephalad and caudal. Spine is seen as double echogenic parallel lines. Amniotic membrane becomes visible, defining the amniotic cavity from the chorionic cavity. Umbilical cord can be seen	
8^{+0}–8^{+6}	Crown–rump length is 17–23 mm. Forebrain, midbrain, hindbrain, and skull are distinguishable. Limb buds are visible. Midgut hernia is present. Amniotic cavity expands, and umbilical cord and vitelline duct lengthen	
9^{+0}–10^{+0}	Crown–rump length is 23–32 mm. Limbs lengthen, and hands and feet are seen. Embryonic heart rate peaks at 170–180 bpm	

embryonic pole later developed live embryos. Thus, in patients with borderline US findings and a desired pregnancy, close follow-up with a repeat US examination is necessary before diagnosing an early pregnancy loss [30]. Nyberg et al. [31] used a threshold of 20 mm MSD without a yolk sac or 25 mm without an embryo via abdominal US to diagnosis anembryonic gestations. They study found that an

Table 2.3 Discrimination for β-HCG levels

Sonographic findings	Gestational age (weeks)	β-hCG (mIU/ml)
Gestational sac detection (MSD 2–3 mm)	4.5	1,000 by TVS, 1,800 by TAS
Yolk sac identification (MSD 5–6 mm)	5.0	1,000–7,200
Fetal pole identification	5–7	7,200–10,800
Cardiac activity identification	6–7	>10,800

β-hCG β-human chorionic gonadotropin, *MSD* mean sac diameter, *TVUS* transvaginal ultrasonography, *TAUS* transabdominal ultrasonography

increase in the gestational sac MSD of <3 mm over 5 days or <4 mm over 7 days can also be used to diagnose early pregnancy loss [31]. Gestational cardiac activity should be present by day 35 from the last menstrual period (day 21 from conception) and can be visualized when the embryonic pole is as small as 2 mm. However, lack of detectable cardiac activity in embryos <3 mm is associated with a 41% continuation rate [32]. To diagnose embryonic demise, an embryonic pole should measure >5 mm with no evidence of gestational cardiac activity [32, 33].

Pregnancy viability can be determined using a combination of quantitative β-hCG and US assessments. After implantation of the blastocyst, as early as 8–9 days after ovulation or day 23 of a 28-day cycle, β-hCG is detectable because it is produced in the placenta by the syncytiotrophoblast. The level of β-hCG approximately doubles every 48 h during early pregnancy and is an indicator of normal gestational development [34].

Levels of β-hCG have been correlated with the sonographic findings during early pregnancy [29]. β-hCG levels can assist with the interpretation of the US findings and help distinguish normal from abnormal conditions. When β-hCG is above a specified discriminatory level, structures identifying a normal pregnancy are present [35]. Discriminatory levels for β-hCG that correlate with normal pregnancy development are listed in Table 2.3.

The β-hCG levels are important for both initial and follow-up management of women presenting with first trimester bleeding to confirm and identify normal vs. abnormal development of a pregnancy. β-hCG levels can be used to follow an early pregnancy when US is not available or until US would be of value (e.g., once β-hCG levels reach 1,000 mIU/ml for detection using transvaginal sonography or β-hCG levels of 1,800 mIU/ml for detection using transabdominal sonography). These values may vary based on the institution's US equipment, experience, and analysis.

Management

Different types of early pregnancy loss are managed differently. Standard management of early pregnancy loss has been to perform suction dilatation and curettage to evacuate the uterus. This is due to the historical management that was based on the high prevalence of illegal abortions that were a frequent cause of vaginal bleeding and cramping. When women presented with such symptoms, surgical evacuation was performed to reduce rates of sepsis and hemorrhage [19]. However, other safe options exist for management of early pregnancy loss, including medical and expectant management.

The qualities of the studies on expectant and medical management vary, making them difficult to compare. The studies vary by inclusion criteria (which are often poorly defined) and exclusion criteria; and medical management varies with the dosing regimens and routes of administration, the length of time before considering a treatment successful or unsuccessful, and the definition of success [19].

Moreover, one of the more common criteria used for defining success in early studies of expectant and medical management was a sonographic measurement of the anteroposterior endometrial thickness, with a threshold of <15 mm as diagnostic of RPOC. This was determined to be the lower limit in one study because <15 mm dilatation and curettage would not be performed at the institution where this study took place. Unfortunately, this threshold criterion has been propagated in many studies since then [36]. This 15-mm sonographic criterion for establishing the need for treatment has proven to be misleading and inexact in clinical trials. Accordingly, most of the previously published literature on expectant and medical management is confusing and inaccurate by current standards [19].

Threatened Abortion

Women with a threatened abortion should be managed expectantly until their symptoms resolve, a nonviable pregnancy is definitively diagnosed, or there is progression to an inevitable, incomplete, or complete abortion.

There are no therapeutic interventions that prevent first trimester pregnancy loss. Occasionally, upon sonographic examination of a patient presenting with first trimester vaginal bleeding, a subchorionic hematoma can be seen (Fig. 2.1). Bed rest and abstinence from sexual intercourse are commonly recommended, although there is no evidence that they are beneficial [37]. Administration of progesterone has not been proven effective for preventing early pregnancy loss [38]. A proposed flowchart for the management of first trimester vaginal bleeding is presented in Fig. 2.2.

Septic Abortion

Suspected septic abortion with RPOC is a medical emergency, and management should be immediate. The uterus should be evacuated promptly after initiating antibiotics and stabilizing the patient in cases of suspected septic abortion or RPOC as delay may be fatal [39, 40]. Suction curettage is less traumatic than sharp curettage. If the patient fails to respond to uterine evacuation and antibiotics, a pelvic abscess or clostridial

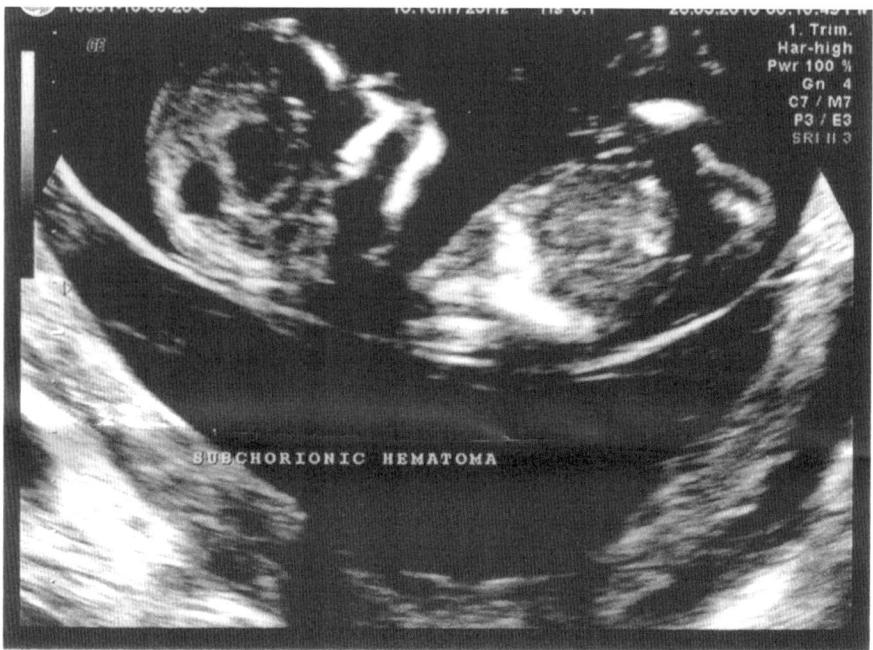

Fig. 2.1 Two-dimensional ultrasonography scan of a subchorionic hematoma in a patient who presented with first trimester vaginal bleeding

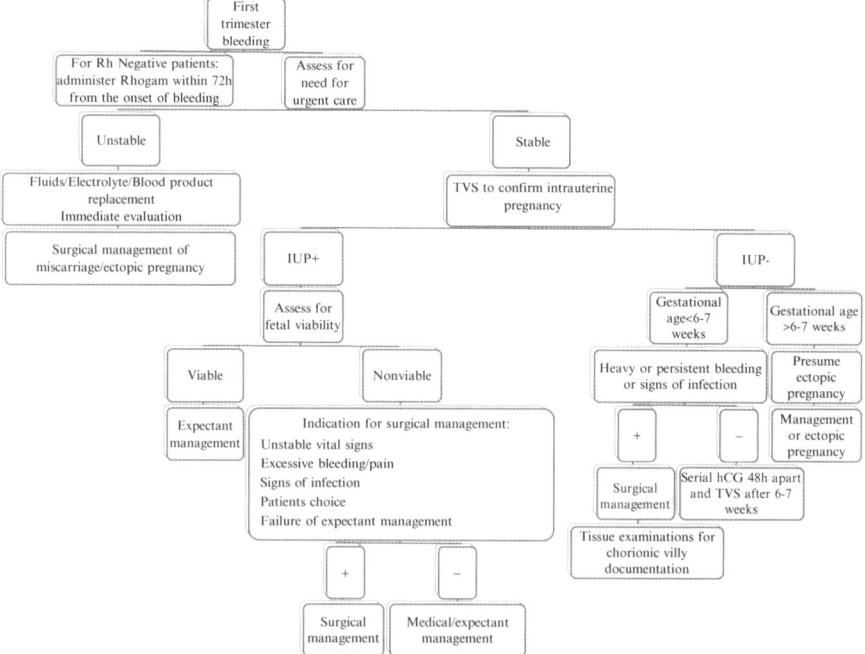

Fig. 2.2 Proposed flowchart for the management of first trimester vaginal bleeding. IUP= intra-uterine pregnancy

necrotizing myonecrosis (gas gangrene), although rare, should be suspected. In such cases, laparotomy and possible hysterectomy might be considered.

Caution Box

- In cases of suspected septic abortion or related products of conception evacuation of the uterus should begin promptly after initiating antibiotics and stabilizing the patient.

Complete Abortion

Passage of an intact gestational sac or contractions with scant uterine bleeding and diminishing uterine cramps suggests that a complete abortion has occurred. Tissue that passed should undergo pathological examination to confirm the presence of products of conception. US examination may be useful for confirming the absence of significant amounts of retained intrauterine tissue, but there are no universally defined criteria for an empty uterus.

Complete abortions do not require therapy, it is difficult to reliably distinguish them clinically or sonographically from incomplete abortions. Although, it is clear that surgery is necessary for women with excessive bleeding, unstable vital signs, or obvious signs of infection [41], some clinicians recommend suction curettage for all patients with complete abortions. However, if US shows an empty uterus and the bleeding is minimal, it is reasonable to take no further actions. Serum β-hCG levels should be measured and followed until they are undetected.

Caution Box

- In cases with complete abortion tissue that passed should undergo pathological examination in order to confirm the presence of products of conception.

Inevitable and Incomplete Abortion, Missed Abortion, Embryonic/Fetal Demise (Dead Fetus)

Women with inevitable or incomplete abortion, missed abortion, or embryonic/fetal demise (dead fetus) can be managed surgically, medically, or expectantly.

Surgical Management

The conventional treatment of first or early second trimester pregnancy loss is dilatation and curettage (D&C) or dilatation and evacuation (D&E) to prevent potential hemorrhagic and infectious complications from the RPOC. The benefits of surgical management include convenient timing for the patient and high success rates, ranging from 93 to 100%, with most studies reporting success rates at or above 98% [19]. Surgical risks include infection, uterine perforation, cervical trauma, and uterine adhesions, which might lead to subsequent infertility or ectopic pregnancy [42]. These complications are relatively rare. Anesthetic risks vary depending on the type of anesthesia used (general anesthesia, intravenous sedation, and local anesthesia). Uterine evacuation can be performed safely and effectively even as an office procedure [43].

Surgical management is appropriate for women with heavy bleeding or sepsis in whom delaying therapy could be harmful as well as for women who do not want to wait for spontaneous or medically induced evacuation of the uterus. Suction curettage is preferable to sharp curettage, which is associated with greater morbidity [44, 45].

Based on a meta-analysis that found women given periabortal antibiotics had a 42% lower risk of infection, some authors recommend antimicrobial administration to reduce the risk of postabortal sepsis (doxycycline 100 mg orally for two doses 12 h apart on the day of the surgical procedure) [46]. However, a single randomized study of intravenous doxycycline at time of curettage for incomplete abortion did not decrease the risk of postoperative febrile morbidity when compared with placebo [47].

In many trials, suction curettage was performed in an operating room. However, given that 93% of induced abortions in the USA in 2000 were performed at an outpatient clinic [48], it seems reasonable that surgical treatment of early pregnancy loss can also be an outpatient procedure. Manual vacuum aspiration consists of a 60-ml syringe attached to a cannula, which provides suction force equal to that of electric vacuum aspiration. Performing D&Cs in a clinic setting rather than in the operating room has decreased overall hospital costs by 41% [49].

Medical Treatment

The availability of effective medical therapies for inducing abortion has created new options for women who want to avoid surgery or when surgical intervention needs to be avoided. With medical management, medications are used to induce expulsion of the products of conception from the uterus. Regimens have typically included a prostaglandin analog (most commonly misoprostol) or a combination of mifepristone or methotrexate with misoprostol [19]. Unfortunately, many studies that have compared medical management with expectant management or surgical management are limited by having different inclusion criteria and patient populations, the inappropriate use of a US diagnosis of failed management, and different follow-up periods before surgical intervention [19].

Misoprostol, a prostaglandin E_1 analog, has been approved by the US Food and Drug Administration (FDA) for the prevention of gastric ulcers. Off-label it has also been used for a variety of obstetrical and gynecological indications, including induction of labor, cervical ripening, and medical abortion. It is the most commonly used agent for medical abortions. Its safety and effectiveness have been established by multiple randomized controlled trials (RCTs) [50, 51]. The advantages of misoprostol are its low cost [52], it can be administered via several routes (oral, buccal, sublingual, vaginal, and rectal), there is a low incidence of side effects when given intravaginally, it is stable at room temperature, and it is readily available. The risk of a major complication is rare.

Zhang et al. [53] investigated the efficacy of misoprostol for medical management of pregnancy failure during the first trimester. They conducted a large, well-designed trial in which women with missed, incomplete, or inevitable abortion were randomly assigned to receive misoprostol intravaginally or undergo vacuum aspiration. Complete expulsion occurred in 71–84% of medically managed patients. Pregnancy duration did not affect the rate of successful expulsion, but successful expulsion was at a lower percentage with missed abortion compared with incomplete or inevitable abortion (81% vs. 93%). Both medical and surgical therapies were safe, effective, and acceptable to patients [53].

Several trials investigated dosing regimens and routes of administration of misoprostol [54–60]. However, there is no consensus on the optimal choice for either. Success rates for misoprostol ranged from 25% for oral misoprostol in a small study to as high as 95% for oral, sublingual, or vaginal misoprostol in other studies. The oral and sublingual routes seemed to be associated with more side effects, such as diarrhea, nausea, and vomiting when compared with the vaginal route. Repeated dosing does not seem to improve the success rate and results in more side effects [58–60].

A combination of a progesterone antagonist (mifepristone) with misoprostol has also been used. However, the value of adding a progesterone antagonist is questionable and expensive. It has been reported that misoprostol alone or a combination of misoprostol and mifepristone had similar success rates in the treatment of early pregnancy failure [61, 62].

Patients who are treated medically are instructed to go to the emergency department if they develop excessive bleeding. Tissues that are passed vaginally at home should be placed in a container and brought to the hospital for analysis.

Expectant Management

Expectant management is an alternative for women with early pregnancy failure at less than 13 weeks of gestation who have stable vital signs and no evidence of infection. Expectant management allows spontaneous passage of the products of conception, allows women to avoid surgical and anesthesia risks, and may be perceived as a "more natural" option. Risks and side effects include an unpredictable duration of time until resolution, the possibility of increased pain and bleeding, and the potential need for emergent surgical evacuation [19].

A systematic Cochrane database review that included five randomized trials concluded that compared to surgical management expectant management was associated with a higher risk of incomplete abortions, the need for unplanned surgical evacuation of the uterus, and bleeding; however, it was also concluded that it was not an unreasonable approach if the woman preferred nonintervention [63]. Randomized trials comparing medical with expectant management have reported similar rates of successful evacuation [64, 65]. Differences in success rates could be attributed to the length of expectant management, the medical regimen used, and the type of early pregnancy failure (incomplete abortion vs. missed abortion or fetal demise). With expectant management, most expulsions occur during the first 2 weeks after diagnosis, although the duration may extend to 3–4 weeks. Incomplete miscarriage is more likely than a missed abortion to proceed to expulsion within 2 weeks [66, 67].

Medical or surgical treatment should be offered if spontaneous expulsion does not occur. Following spontaneous or medically induced expulsion, the uterine cavity should undergo US evaluation when RPOC are suspected. Some physicians perform this examination routinely.

Postabortion Care

After surgical evacuation or if medical management or expectant management is planned, women who are Rh(D)-negative and unsensitized should receive Rh(D)-immune globulin. A dose of 50 µg is effective through the 12th week of gestation due to the small volume of red blood cells in the fetoplacental circulation, although the more readily available 300 µg dose is normally given.

Women are advised to refrain from coitus and the use of tampons for at least 2 weeks after evacuation of the uterus. Postponing pregnancy for 2–3 months is usually advised, although there seems to be no greater risk of adverse outcomes with a shorter interpregnancy interval [68]. Any type of contraception, including placement of an intrauterine device [69], may be started immediately.

Caution Box

- Mild vaginal bleeding can persist for a couple of weeks after the abortion. If heavy bleeding, fever, or abdominal pain develops patients should be referred without delay for a medical examination.
- Women who are Rh(D)-negative and unsensitized should receive Rh(D)-immune globulin, after surgical evacuation or at the time of diagnosis of early pregnancy failure if medical management or expectant management is planned.

Mild vaginal bleeding can persist for a couple of weeks after the abortion. If heavy bleeding, fever, or abdominal pain develops, patients should be referred without delay for a medical examination. Menses typically resumes within 6 weeks.

If normal menses does not resume, the presence of a new pregnancy or gestational trophoblastic disease should be considered. On rare occasions, intrauterine adhesions (Asherman's syndrome) occur after surgical evacuation of the uterus. Serum hCG levels normally return to normal within 2 weeks after an abortion [22]. Follow-up hCG testing is unnecessary if the normal menstrual cycle resumes.

It is important to acknowledge the patient's (and partner's) grief and provide empathy and support as well as a referral to professional counseling in some cases. Risk factors for abnormal grief following a miscarriage include a history of or current depression, anxiety, or other psychiatric disorder; neurotic personality traits; and lack of social support [70]. If the etiology of the loss is known or suspected, the couple should be informed and counseled about recurrence risks. If the etiology is not known, it is important to reassure the patient and alleviate any feelings of guilt or blame.

Prognosis

Many women may feel anxiety and have concerns regarding the possibility of another loss in a future pregnancy. Women could be reassured that one previous miscarriage does not necessarily increase the risk of another one. Nevertheless, the overall risk of another miscarriage is not insignificant [71].

The overall risk of miscarriage in a future pregnancy is approximately 20% after one miscarriage, 28% after two miscarriages, and 43% after three or more miscarriages [72]. There also appears to be an increased risk of preterm delivery of subsequent pregnancies [73]. Second trimester pregnancy loss is significantly associated with recurrent second-trimester loss and future spontaneous preterm birth. After a second trimester pregnancy loss, one study reported that 39% of women had a preterm delivery in their next pregnancy, 5% had a stillbirth, and 6% had a neonatal death [74]. Interestingly, three more recent studies reported that an initial miscarriage is associated with a higher risk of obstetrical complications in the following pregnancy [75–77]. Nevertheless, the long-term conception rate and pregnancy outcome are similar for women who underwent medical or surgical evacuation for early pregnancy loss [78].

Summary

Spontaneous abortions are among the most common complications of pregnancy. Many risk factors for spontaneous abortion, including advanced maternal age and a previous spontaneous abortion, have been reported. Most spontaneous abortions are attributed to structural or chromosomal abnormalities in the embryo.

There are various stages and types of spontaneous abortions. Women usually present with a history of amenorrhea, vaginal bleeding, and pelvic pain. Ultrasonography is the most useful test for diagnosing and evaluating women suspected of having a spontaneous abortion.

There are no useful interventions to prevent first trimester pregnancy loss. In most patients, surgical, medical, and expectant management ultimately result in evacuation of the products of conception. Surgical evacuation seems more successful than medical or expectant management. The success of medical and expectant management depends on the length of time allowed before a secondary surgical intervention and on the type of nonviable pregnancy. Postabortal infection rates are similar for all three strategies, and the frequency of other complications is low. The choice of treatment should take into account the patient's preferences.

Women who are unstable because of bleeding or infection and women who want an immediate, definitive treatment should undergo surgical management. Of women undergoing medical management, 70–90% have a successful outcome. This strategy is preferable for women who want to avoid a surgical procedure but do not want to wait for a spontaneous abortion to occur. Women who are stable hemodynamically, who do not want a medical or surgical intervention, and who are willing to wait days to weeks for expulsion to occur may choose expectant management. Bleeding and cramping may be prolonged, and surgical evacuation may still be required; but as many as 80% of women have a successful outcome with expectant management alone. Expectant management for 1 month appears to be a safe, effective alternative to immediate surgical evacuation. In addition, sonographic classification of the miscarriage at presentation appears to be predictive of successful outcome without surgical intervention.

The long-term conception rate and pregnancy outcome are similar for women who undergo medical or surgical evacuation for early pregnancy loss. Although there are several treatment options available to women who are diagnosed with early pregnancy failure, counseling needs to be individualized to patient expectations and preferences.

With a thorough understanding of the experience and process of first trimester loss, and appreciation of its emotional impact and significance, and making an educated choice of management physicians can provide sensitive and complete care to women at this important time.

References

1. Brier N. Grief following miscarriage: a comprehensive review of the literature. J Womens Health (Larchmt). 2008;17:451–64.
2. Zinaman MJ, Clegg ED, Brown CC, O'Connor J, Selevan SG. Estimates of human fertility and pregnancy loss. Fertil Steril. 1996;65:503–9.
3. Ellish NJ, Saboda K, O'Connor J, Nasca PC, Stanek EJ, Boyle C. A prospective study of early pregnancy loss. Hum Reprod. 1996;11:406–12.
4. Guerneri S, Bettio D, Simoni G, Brambati B, Lanzani A, Fraccaro M. Prevalence and distribution of chromosome abnormalities in a sample of first trimester internal abortions. Hum Reprod. 1987;2:735–9.
5. Ohno M, Maeda T, Matsunobu A. A cytogenetic study of spontaneous abortions with direct analysis of chorionic villi. Obstet Gynecol. 1991;77:394–8.

6. Gracia CR, Sammel MD, Chittams J, Hummel AC, Shaunik A, Barnhart KT. Risk factors for spontaneous abortion in early symptomatic first-trimester pregnancies. Obstet Gynecol. 2005;106:993–9.

7. Nybo Andersen AM, Wohlfahrt J, Christens P, Olsen J, Melbye M. Maternal age and fetal loss: population based register linkage study. BMJ. 2000;320:1708–12.

8. Hustin J, Jauniaux E, Schaaps JP. Histological study of the materno-embryonic interface in spontaneous abortion. Placenta. 1990;11:477–86.

9. Jauniaux E, Gulbis B, Burton GJ. The human first trimester gestational sac limits rather than facilitates oxygen transfer to the foetus – a review. Placenta. 2003;24:S86–93.

10. Jauniaux E, Zaidi J, Jurkovic D, Campbell S, Hustin J. Comparison of colour Doppler features and pathological findings in complicated early pregnancy. Hum Reprod. 1994;9:2432–7.

11. Jauniaux E, Greenwold N, Hempstock J, Burton GJ. Comparison of ultrasonographic and Doppler mapping of the intervillous circulation in normal and abnormal early pregnancies. Fertil Steril. 2003;79:100–6.

12. Olive DL, Pritts EA. Fibroids and reproduction. Semin Reprod Med. 2010;28:218–27.

13. Matovina M, Husnjak K, Milutin N, Ciglar S, Grce M. Possible role of bacterial and viral infections in miscarriages. Fertil Steril. 2004;81:662–9.

14. Mills JL, Simpson JL, Driscoll SG, Jovanovic-Peterson L, Van Allen M, Aarons JH, et al. Incidence of spontaneous abortion among normal women and insulin-dependent diabetic women whose pregnancies were identified within 21 days of conception. N Engl J Med. 1988;319:1617–23.

15. Anselmo J, Cao D, Karrison T, Weiss RE, Refetoff S. Fetal loss associated with excess thyroid hormone exposure. JAMA. 2004;292:691–5.

16. Ashoor G, Maiz N, Rotas M, Jawdat F, Nicolaides KH. Maternal thyroid function at 11 to 13 weeks of gestation and subsequent fetal death. Thyroid. 2010;20:989–93.

17. Vitzthum VJ, Spielvogel H, Thornburg J, West B. A prospective study of early pregnancy loss in humans. Fertil Steril. 2006;86:373–9.

18. Sarig G, Younis JS, Hoffman R, Lanir N, Blumenfeld Z, Brenner B. Thrombophilia is common in women with idiopathic pregnancy loss and is associated with late pregnancy wastage. Fertil Steril. 2002;77:342–7.

19. Chen BA, Creinin MD. Contemporary management of early pregnancy failure. Clin Obstet Gynecol. 2007;50:67–88.

20. Bateman BG, Nunley Jr WC, Kolp LA, Kitchin 3rd JD, Felder R. Vaginal sonography findings and hCG dynamics of early intrauterine and tubal pregnancies. Obstet Gynecol. 1990;75:421–7.

21. Kadar N, DeVore G, Romero R. Discriminatory hCG zone: its use in the sonographic evaluation for ectopic pregnancy. Obstet Gynecol. 1981;58:156–61.

22. Barnhart KT, Sammel MD, Rinaudo PF, Zhou L, Hummel AC, Guo W. Symptomatic patients with an early viable intrauterine pregnancy: HCG curves redefined. Obstet Gynecol. 2004;104:50–5.

23. Goldstein SR. Sonography in early pregnancy failure. Clin Obstet Gynecol. 1994;37:681–92.

24. Sawyer E, Jurkovic D. Ultrasonography in the diagnosis and management of abnormal early pregnancy. Clin Obstet Gynecol. 2007;50:31–54.

25. Shillito J, Walker JJ. Early pregnancy assessment units. Br J Hosp Med. 1997;58:505–9.

26. Fossum GT, Davajan V, Kletzky OA. Early detection of pregnancy with transvaginal ultrasound. Fertil Steril. 1988;49:788–91.

27. Cullen MT, Green JJ, Reece EA, Hobbins JC. A comparison of transvaginal and abdominal ultrasound in visualizing the first trimester conceptus. J Ultrasound Med. 1989;8:565–9.

28. Levi CS, Lyons EA, Lindsay DJ. Early diagnosis of nonviable pregnancy with endovaginal US. Radiology. 1988;167:383–5.

29. Dighe M, Cuevas C, Moshiri M, Dubinsky T, Dogra VS. Sonography in first trimester bleeding. J Clin Ultrasound. 2008;36:352–66.

30. Rowling SE, Coleman BG, Langer JE, Arger PH, Nisenbaum HL, Horii SC. First-trimester US parameters of failed pregnancy. Radiology. 1997;203:211–7.

31. Nyberg DA, Mack LA, Laing FC, Patten RM. Distinguishing normal from abnormal gestational sac growth in early pregnancy. J Ultrasound Med. 1987;6:23–7.

32. Goldstein SR. Significance of cardiac activity on endovaginal ultrasound in very early embryos. Obstet Gynecol. 1992;80:670–2.

33. Brown DL, Emerson DS, Felker RE, Cartier MS, Smith WC. Diagnosis of early embryonic demise by endovaginal sonography. J Ultrasound Med. 1990;9:631–6.

34. Snell BJ. Assessment and management of bleeding in the first trimester of pregnancy. J Midwifery Womens Health. 2009;54:483–91.

35. Peisner DB, Timor-Tritsch IE. The discriminatory zone of beta-hCG for vaginal probes. J Clin Ultrasound. 1990;18:280–5.

36. Nielsen S, Hahlin M. Expectant management of first-trimester spontaneous abortion. Lancet. 1995;345:84–6.

37. Aleman A, Althabe F, Belizán J, Bergel E. Bed rest during pregnancy for preventing miscarriage. Cochrane Database Syst Rev. 2005;CD003576.

38. Wahabi HA, Abed Althagafi NF, Elawad M. Progestogen for treating threatened miscarriage. Cochrane Database Syst Rev. 2007;CD005943.

39. Stubblefield PG, Grimes DA. Septic abortion. N Engl J Med. 1994;331:310–4.

40. Finkielman JD, De Feo FD, Heller PG, Afessa B. The clinical course of patients with septic abortion admitted to an intensive care unit. Intensive Care Med. 2004;30:1097–102.

41. Forna F, Gülmezoglu AM. Surgical procedures to evacuate incomplete abortion. Cochrane Database Syst Rev. 2001;CD001993.

42. Demetroulis C, Saridogan E, Kunde D, Naftalin AA. A prospective randomized control trial comparing medical and surgical treatment for early pregnancy failure. Hum Reprod. 2001;16:365–9.

43. Harris LH, Dalton VK, Johnson TR. Surgical management of early pregnancy failure: history, politics, and safe, cost-effective care. Am J Obstet Gynecol. 2007;196:445.e1–5.

44. Grimes DA. Unsafe abortion: the silent scourge. Br Med Bull. 2003;67:99–113.

45. Grimes DA, Benson J, Singh S, Romero M, Ganatra B, Okonofua FE, et al. Unsafe abortion: the preventable pandemic. Lancet. 2006;368:1908–19.

46. Sawaya GF, Grady D, Kerlikowske K, Grimes DA. Antibiotics at the time of induced abortion: the case for universal prophylaxis based on a meta-analysis. Obstet Gynecol. 1996;87: 884–90.

47. Prieto JA, Eriksen NL, Blanco JD. A randomized trial of prophylactic doxycycline for curettage in incomplete abortion. Obstet Gynecol. 1995;85:692–6.

48. Finer LB, Henshaw SK. Abortion incidence and services in the United States in 2000. Perspect Sex Reprod Health. 2003;35:6–15.

49. Blumenthal PD, Remsburg RE. A time and cost analysis of the management of incomplete abortion with manual vacuum aspiration. Int J Gynaecol Obstet. 1994;45:261–7.

50. Neilson JP, Hickey M, Vazquez J. Medical treatment for early fetal death (less than 24 weeks). Cochrane Database Syst Rev. 2006;3:CD002253.

51. Blum J, Winikoff B, Gemzell-Danielsson K, Ho PC, Schiavon R, Weeks A. Treatment of incomplete abortion and miscarriage with misoprostol. Int J Gynaecol Obstet. 2007;99: S186–9.

52. Graziosi GC, van der Steeg JW, Reuwer PH, Drogtrop AP, Bruinse HW, Mol BW. Economic evaluation of misoprostol in the treatment of early pregnancy failure compared to curettage after an expectant management. Hum Reprod. 2005;20:1067–71.

53. Zhang J, Gilles JM, Barnhart K, Creinin MD, Westhoff C, Frederick MM. National Institute of Child Health Human Development (NICHD) Management of Early Pregnancy Failure Trial. A comparison of medical management with misoprostol and surgical management for early pregnancy failure. N Engl J Med. 2005;353:761–9.

54. Creinin MD, Moyer R, Guido R. Misoprostol for medical evacuation of early pregnancy failure. Obstet Gynecol. 1997;89:768–72.

55. Ngoc NT, Blum J, Westheimer E, Quan TT, Winikoff B. Medical treatment of missed abortion using misoprostol. Int J Gynaecol Obstet. 2004;87:138–42.

56. Gilles JM, Creinin MD, Barnhart K, Westhoff C, Frederick MM. National Institute of Child Health and Human Development Management of Early Pregnancy Failure Trial. A randomized

trial of saline solution-moistened misoprostol versus dry misoprostol for first-trimester pregnancy failure. Am J Obstet Gynecol. 2004;190:389–94.

57. Tang OS, Chan CC, Ng EH, Lee SW, Ho PC. A prospective, randomized, placebo-controlled trial on the use of mifepristone with sublingual or vaginal misoprostol for medical abortions of less than 9 weeks gestation. Hum Reprod. 2003;18:2315–8.

58. Tang OS, Ong CY, Tse KY, Ng EH, Lee SW, Ho PC. A randomized trial to compare the use of sublingual misoprostol with or without an additional 1 week course for the management of first trimester silent miscarriage. Hum Reprod. 2006;21:189–92.

59. Phupong V, Taneepanichskul S, Kriengsinyot R, Sriyirojana N, Blanchard K, Winikoff B. Comparative study between single dose 600 microg and repeated dose of oral misoprostol for treatment of incomplete abortion. Contraception. 2004;70:307–11.

60. Nguyen TN, Blum J, Durocher J, Quan TT, Winikoff B. A randomized controlled study comparing 600 versus 1,200 microg oral misoprostol for medical management of incomplete abortion. Contraception. 2005;72:438–42.

61. Grønlund A, Grønlund L, Clevin L, Andersen B, Palmgren N, Lidegaard Ø. Management of missed abortion: comparison of medical treatment with either mifepristone + misoprostol or misoprostol alone with surgical evacuation. A multi-center trial in Copenhagen county, Denmark. Acta Obstet Gynecol Scand. 2002;81:1060–5.

62. Stockheim D, Machtinger R, Wiser A, Dulitzky M, Soriano D, Goldenberg M, et al. A randomized prospective study of misoprostol or mifepristone followed by misoprostol when needed for the treatment of women with early pregnancy failure. Fertil Steril. 2006;86:956–60.

63. Nanda K, Peloggia A, Grimes D, Lopez L, Nanda G. Expectant care versus surgical treatment for miscarriage. Cochrane Database Syst Rev. 2006;CD003518.

64. Nielsen S, Hahlin M, Platz-Christensen J. Randomised trial comparing expectant with medical management for first trimester miscarriages. Br J Obstet Gynaecol. 1999;106:804–7.

65. Shelley JM, Healy D, Grover S. A randomised trial of surgical, medical and expectant management of first trimester spontaneous miscarriage. Aust N Z J Obstet Gynaecol. 2005;45:122–7.

66. Casikar I, Bignardi T, Riemke J, Alhamdan D, Condous G. Expectant management of spontaneous first-trimester miscarriage: prospective validation of the '2-week rule'. Ultrasound Obstet Gynecol. 2010;35:223–7.

67. Luise C, Jermy K, May C, Costello G, Collins WP, Bourne TH. Outcome of expectant management of spontaneous first trimester miscarriage: observational study. BMJ. 2002;324:873–5.

68. Goldstein RR, Croughan MS, Robertson PA. Neonatal outcomes in immediate versus delayed conceptions after spontaneous abortion: a retrospective case series. Am J Obstet Gynecol. 2002;186:1230–4.

69. Grimes D, Schulz K, Stanwood N. Immediate postabortal insertion of intrauterine devices. Cochrane Database Syst Rev. 2002;CD001777.

70. Stratton K, Lloyd L. Hospital-based interventions at and following miscarriage: literature to inform a research-practice initiative. Aust N Z J Obstet Gynaecol. 2008;48:5–11.

71. Thorstensen KA. Midwifery management of first trimester bleeding and early pregnancy loss. J Midwifery Womens Health. 2000;45:481–97.

72. Regan L, Braude PR, Trembath PL. Influence of past reproductive performance on risk of spontaneous abortion. BMJ. 1989;299:541–5.

73. Swingle HM, Colaizy TT, Zimmerman MB, Morriss Jr FH. Abortion and the risk of subsequent preterm birth: a systematic review with meta-analyses. J Reprod Med. 2009;54:95–108.

74. Edlow AG, Srinivas SK, Elovitz MA. Second-trimester loss and subsequent pregnancy outcomes: what is the real risk? Am J Obstet Gynecol. 2007;197:581.e1–6.

75. Kashanian M, Akbarian AR, Baradaran H, Shabandoust SH. Pregnancy outcome following a previous spontaneous abortion (miscarriage). Gynecol Obstet Invest. 2006;61:167–70.

76. Bhattacharya S, Townend J, Shetty A, Campbell D, Bhattacharya S. Does miscarriage in an initial pregnancy lead to adverse obstetric and perinatal outcomes in the next continuing pregnancy? BJOG. 2008;115:1623–9.

77. Weintraub AY, Sergienko R, Harlev A, Holcberg G, Mazor M, Wiznitzer A, et al. An initial miscarriage is associated with an increased rate of adverse pregnancy outcomes in the following pregnancy. Presented at the 31st Annual Meeting of the Society of Maternal Fetal Medicine (SMFM). San Francisco, CA, USA, 7–12 February 2011.
78. Tam WH, Tsui MH, Lok IH, Yip SK, Yuen PM, Chung TK. Long-term reproductive outcome subsequent to medical versus surgical treatment for miscarriage. Hum Reprod. 2005;20: 3355–9.

Chapter 3
Ectopic Pregnancy

Avi Harlev, Arnon Wiznitzer, and Eyal Sheiner

Introduction

Ectopic pregnancy is defined as an implantation of a fertilized ovum at a site other than within the endometrium. Ectopic pregnancies are responsible for approximately 10% of all maternal mortality and are the leading cause of pregnancy-related death during the first trimester [1], mainly related to hemorrhage [2]. In addition to maternal mortality and ectopic pregnancy-related complications, ectopic pregnancy is an economic burden. The total cost associated with ectopic pregnancy in the USA in 1990 was estimated at $1.1 billion [3].

Incidence

The reported number of hospitalizations due to ectopic pregnancies increased dramatically from 17,800 in 1970 to 88,400 in 1989, with an incidence of 16:1,000 in 1989 – a fivefold increase of ectopic pregnancies [1]. This rise might be explained by the general increase in risk factors. Moreover, there has been more early detection of ectopic pregnancies owing to technological improvements, such as higher-resolution ultrasonography (US) scanners and sensitive human chorionic gonadotropin (hCG) hormone test kits, which have diagnosed cases of ectopic pregnancy that previously resolved spontaneously [4, 5].

The exact incidence of ectopic pregnancy over the last few decades is debatable. Some studies reported that the incidence slowed or declined [6–8], a difference that

A. Harlev (✉)
Department of Obstetrics and Gynecology, Faculty of Health Sciences,
Soroka University Medical Center, Ben-Gurion University of the Negev,
P.O. Box 151, Beer-Sheva, Israel
e-mail: harlev@bgu.ac.il

E. Sheiner (ed.), *Bleeding During Pregnancy: A Comprehensive Guide*,
DOI 10.1007/978-1-4419-9810-1_3, © Springer Science+Business Media, LLC 2011

could be due to underestimating the incidence of ectopic pregnancy. There are two main advances that have changed the diagnosis and treatment of ectopic pregnancy. The first was the appearance of technological advances that permitted early, accurate diagnosis of ectopic pregnancy, including highly sensitive home pregnancy tests, high-resolution transvaginal US (TVUS), and quantitative measurement of the β subunit of hCG (β-hCG). The second advance was the progress achieved in treatment modalities since 1987, including outpatient management of ectopic pregnancy with use of methotrexate (MTX) injection, expectant management, and laparoscopic surgery [9]. The advent of managed care on a large scale during this period contributed to a shift away from inpatient hospitalization to control costs. Therefore, the decline in reported cases could be due to the lowered rates of inpatient registration and not an actual decline in incidence [10].

Etiology and Risk Factors

The increased awareness and knowledge of risk factors enables an early, accurate diagnosis of ectopic pregnancy [11]. A damaged fallopian tube, which impairs migration of the fertilized ovum to the uterus, has a strong association with ectopic pregnancy. Current evidence supports the hypothesis that tubal ectopic pregnancy is caused by a combination of retention of the embryo in the fallopian tube due to impaired embryo–tubal transport and alterations in the tubal environment, allowing early implantation to occur [12].

Ankum and colleagues reported in a meta-analysis that reviewed 36 studies in which the following conditions were thought to impede migration of the fertilized ovum to the uterus: prior pelvic inflammatory disease (PID), history of ectopic pregnancy, and previous tubal ligation [13]. The strongest risk factor for ectopic pregnancy was previous ectopic pregnancy, with an odds ratio of 6.6 [95% confidence interval (CI) 5.2–8.4] [13, 14]. Moreover, previous ectopic pregnancy was significantly associated with the risk of a tubal ectopic pregnancy to rupture [15].

Another possible etiologic factor is a reduction in the peristaltic movement of the fallopian tube [16]. Myoelectrical activity is responsible for the peristaltic activity in the fallopian tube and is hormonally controlled. Estrogen is known to increase smooth muscle activity, and progesterone decreases it. Aging results in decreased myoelectrical activity of the fallopian tube, perhaps accounting for the increased rate of ectopic tubal pregnancies in perimenopausal women. Furthermore, hormonal control of the muscular activity in the fallopian tube may explain the increased incidence of ectopic pregnancy associated with failures of the progesterone-only contraceptive pills, progesterone-containing intrauterine devices (IUDs), and ovulation induction [16].

Combination oral contraception does not increase the risk of ectopic pregnancy [17]. However, conceiving while using oral or subdermal progesterone-only contraceptives increases the risk of the pregnancy being extrauterine [18, 19]. Likewise, women who become pregnant while using an IUD (Fig. 3.1) have an increased risk to have an ectopic pregnancy compared to women not using an IUD. A progesterone-coated IUD imposes a greater risk than a copper IUD (17% vs. 4%) [20].

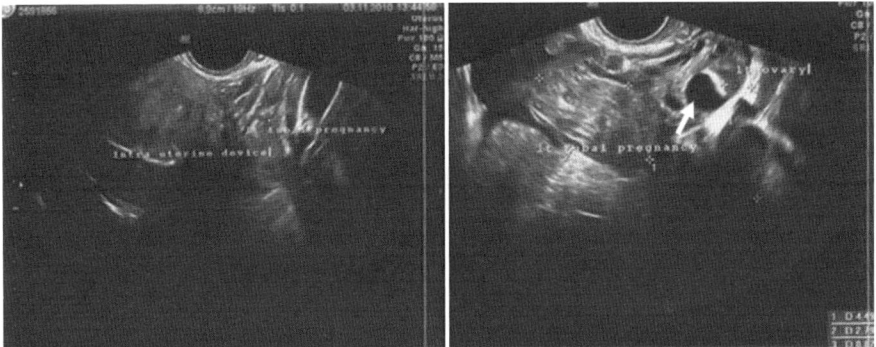

Fig. 3.1 Ectopic pregnancy in the presence of an intrauterine device (*arrow*)

Cigarette smoking is a well-documented risk factor for ectopic pregnancy. It is probably due to a toxic effect of the nicotine on tubal or ciliary movement [12, 21, 22]. The risk is dose-dependent and increases the relative risk to 2.5 when smoking more than 20 cigarettes a day when compared to nonsmokers [21].

Assisted reproductive technology (ART), specifically in vitro fertilization (IVF), increases the risk of ectopic pregnancy. The risk is elevated for women whose infertility is due to a mechanical factor (e.g., tubal disease). In addition to an underlying tubal disease, hormone alterations during ovulation induction can cause alterations in tubal function and peristalsis [23]. Another potential mechanism is placement of the embryo high in the uterine cavity during embryo transfer, causing fluid reflux into the tubes [24].

Salpingitis isthmica nodosa is an anatomical thickening of the fallopian tube with epithelium. This condition leads to multiple luminal diverticula, which may also increase the risk of ectopic pregnancy [25].

Assessing the risk factors for tubal rupture, Job-Spira et al. analyzed 849 tubal ectopic pregnancies. The rate of rupture for this population was 18%. Four factors were identified that increased the risk of rupture: never having used contraception, a history of tubal damage together with infertility, induction of ovulation, and a high level of β-HDG (at least 10,000 IU/l) upon admission. They also concluded that tubal rupture seriously affects the immediate health of the woman concerned, but it appears to have no independent effect on subsequent fertility [26].

Approach to the Diagnosis

History

Clinical manifestation of an ectopic pregnancy varies widely, from hemodynamic instability and shock to an asymptomatic patient. This wide spectrum of clinical presentations makes diagnosing ectopic pregnancy complicated. The classic symptom triad of ectopic pregnancy [27] comprises abdominal pain, amenorrhea, and vaginal bleeding. Nonetheless, this triad is present in only about 50% of patients. Reviewing 147 cases of ectopic pregnancy, Alsuleiman and Grimes reported the appearance of abdominal pain (98.6%), amenorrhea (74.1%), and irregular vaginal bleeding (56.4%) as the most common presenting symptoms [28]. Although severe abdominal pain is the most common complaint, the severity and the nature of the pain differ widely.

Caution Box

The classic symptom triad of ectopic pregnancy [27] – abdominal pain, amenorrhea, vaginal bleeding – is present in only about 50% of patients. Vital signs of hypotension and tachycardia along with rebound tenderness and guarding on abdominal examination should alert the clinician to a probable tubal rupture necessitating immediate surgical intervention.

Physical Examination

Vital signs of hypotension and tachycardia along with rebound tenderness and guarding on abdominal examination should alert the clinician to a probable tubal rupture necessitating immediate surgical intervention. However, most patients present with less severe symptoms and more subtle signs on examination [29].

The signs and symptoms of amenorrhea, nonspecific lower abdominal pain, and vaginal bleeding are also associated with spontaneous miscarriage, cervical irritation or trauma, and infection. Hence, patients may delay reporting these symptoms to their physicians; and even after they have been reported, the diagnosis may be delayed [30]. Differentiating unruptured ectopic pregnancy from early intrauterine pregnancy is difficult and requires further evaluation and diagnostic measures. Although history and physical examination findings may raise the suspicion of ectopic pregnancy, there is no constellation of findings that could confirm or exclude this diagnosis with a high degree of reliability [31]. Therefore, TVUS and a serum β-hCG measurement are the next diagnostic steps. The sensitivity and specificity of combining these tests has been reported to range from 93 to 100% [27, 32].

Transvaginal Ultrasonography

A TVUS examination specifically to gestations older than 5.5 weeks should identify an intrauterine pregnancy with almost 100% accuracy [33, 34]. Structures become visible by TVUS, including the gestational sac ("double decidual sign") at 4.5–5.0 weeks after the last menstrual period, the yolk sac at 5 weeks, and the fetal

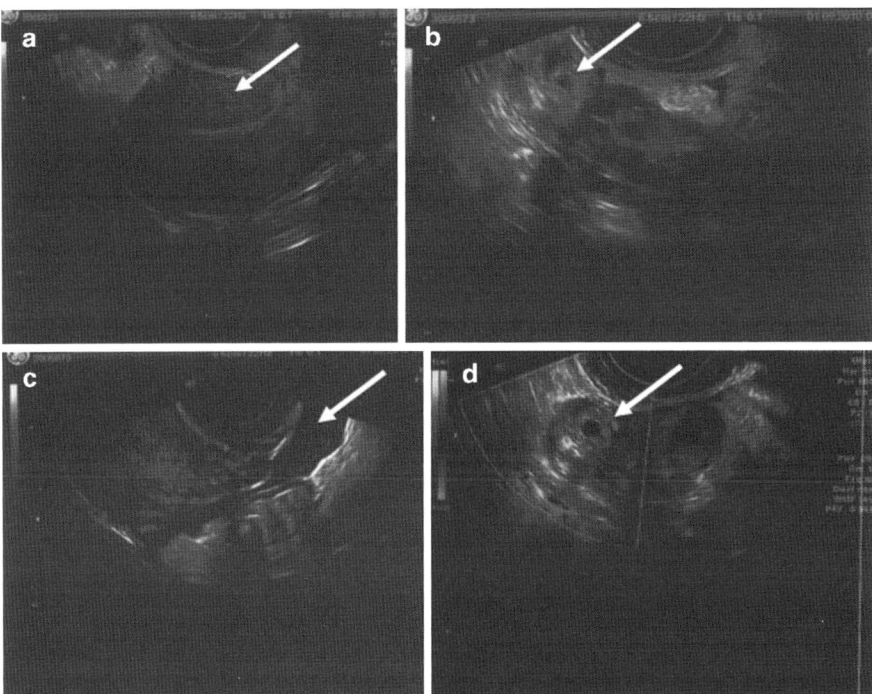

Fig. 3.2 Common sonographic findings in ectopic pregnancies. (**a**) Empty uterine cavity with thickened endometrium (*arrow*). (**b**) Normal ovary with a separated adnexrl mass next to it (*arrow*). (**c**) Free fluid in the pelvis (*arrow*). (**d**) "Ring of fire sign" (*arrow*) demonstrated in a Doppler study

pole with subsequent cardiac motion at 5.5–6.0 weeks. An adnexal mass separated from the ovary is the most common finding of a tubal pregnancy, visualized in up to 89–100% of patients [35] (Fig. 3.1). The tubal ring sign, the second most common sign of a tubal pregnancy, is a hyperechoic ring surrounding an extrauterine gestational sac [36]. A trilaminar endometrium is formed during the late proliferative phase of the normal menstrual cycle. When an abnormal pregnancy is suspected, the absence of a true gestational sac in the presence of a trilaminar endometrium on US images is highly suggestive of an ectopic pregnancy [36, 37]. Cardiac activity in the ectopic pregnancy may be detected after the fifth gestational week, usually excluding the patient from medical pharmacological treatment of the ectopic pregnancy (Figs. 3.2 and 3.3). A pseudosac is a collection of fluid in the endometrial cavity that occurs due to bleeding from the decidualized endometrium when an extrauterine gestation is present [29].

Identifying an intrauterine pregnancy rules out ectopic pregnancy unless a heterotopic pregnancy is present [38]. Heterotopic pregnancy is rare in women with normal spontaneous fertilization. In women with IVF pregnancies, the combination of an ectopic implantation along with an intrauterine pregnancy ranges from 1 to 3% [39].

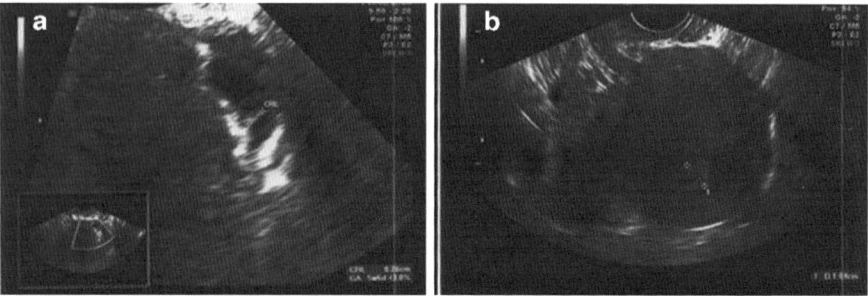

Fig. 3.3 Cardiac motion in ectopic pregnancy. (**a**) Tubal ectopic pregnancy with a crown–rump length (CRL) of 5 weeks and 6 days' gestation. (**b**) Empty uterine cavity with thickened endometrium

---

Caution Box

Identifying an intrauterine pregnancy rules out ectopic pregnancy unless a heterotopic pregnancy is present. Heterotopic pregnancy is rare in women with spontaneous fertilization. In women with IVF pregnancies, the incidence ranges from 1 to 3%.

Human Chorionic Gonadotropin

A positive hCG immunoassay confirms that the patient is pregnant. Therefore, urinary hCG should be measured for every patient suspected of having an ectopic pregnancy; the test is positive in nearly all ectopic pregnancy cases [40].

For those cases in which TVUS cannot establish the location of the pregnancy, serial hCG assays are necessary for the diagnostic workup [41, 42]. In a viable intrauterine pregnancy, the hCG level is anticipated to double every 2 days [43, 44]. This pattern is referred to as the "doubling time"; thus, the minimal hCG rate of increase for a normal intrauterine pregnancy is 24% at 1 day and 53% at 2 days [40]. It is well established that for a viable intrauterine pregnancy the expected rise in serial hCG measurements is different from the slow rise or plateau of an ectopic pregnancy [40, 45–47].

However, analyzing 200 cases of ectopic pregnancy, Silva et al. concluded that there is no single way to characterize the hCG pattern for ectopic pregnancy. The number of women with an ectopic pregnancy who experience an increase in hCG values is approximately equal to the number of those who experience a decrease. The hCG profile in women with an ectopic pregnancy can mimic that of an intrauterine pregnancy or a completed spontaneous abortion in approximately 29% of cases [48]. Furthermore, in 2004, Barnhart et al. reported that the slowest increase associated with viability is 53% after 2 days [45]. An uncharacteristic pattern of a rising hCG level is suggestive of an abnormal pregnancy, although it cannot differentiate an ectopic pregnancy from an intrauterine pregnancy abortion. However, when decreasing hCG levels are observed, the presence of an ectopic pregnancy should be highly suspected over a spontaneous abortion (for which the hCG levels do not fall by 21–35% in 2 days) [45].

The discriminatory zone is defined as the hCG level that distinguishes patients with intrauterine pregnancies in whom a gestational sac can be seen from those in whom it cannot be seen [49]. An intrauterine sac associated with hCG levels above the discriminatory zone reliably indicates an intrauterine pregnancy, whereas hCG values below the zone suggest an abnormal pregnancy – an abortion or an ectopic gestation. An intrauterine gestation is usually visible on a transvaginal scan at an hCG concentration of ≥ 1,500 IU/l or one of 6,500 IU/l with transabdominal US [41].

Serum Progesterone

Serum progesterone has been suggested as a diagnostic tool in the evaluation of a possible ectopic pregnancy. Serum progesterone levels of >20 ng/ml indicate an intrauterine viable pregnancy [50]. Serum progesterone values of <5 nmol/l represent spontaneous abortions in 85% of the cases; 14% of the cases are ectopic pregnancies [51]. The accuracy of a single progesterone measurement for the diagnosis of ectopic pregnancy was investigated in a meta-analysis by Mol et al., who reviewed 26 eligible studies [52]. They concluded that a single serum progesterone measurement could not discriminate between ectopic pregnancy and nonectopic pregnancy. Nevertheless, the serum progesterone measurement can identify patients at risk for ectopic pregnancy and who need further evaluation, although its discriminative capacity is insufficient to diagnose ectopic pregnancy with certainty [52, 53].

Dilatation and Curettage

In cases of a slow rise or fall of the hCG levels without identification of the gestational sac, dilatation and curettage (D&C) is advised as part of the diagnostic workup [29]. D&C is necessary to differentiate an ectopic pregnancy from a miscarriage before a woman is presumptively treated with methotrexate (MTX) [54]. The presence of villi in the tissue sample obtained by the curettage confirms the diagnosis of intrauterine abnormal pregnancy. After performing curettage, decreasing hCG levels of ≥15% during the following 12 h indicates a complete abortion. A plateau or rise in the hCG levels is diagnostic of an ectopic pregnancy, and medical or surgical treatment for ectopic pregnancy is obligatory [54, 55].

Laparoscopy is considered a good modality for the diagnosis of ectopic pregnancy. Generally, the fallopian tubes are easily visualized and evaluated, although

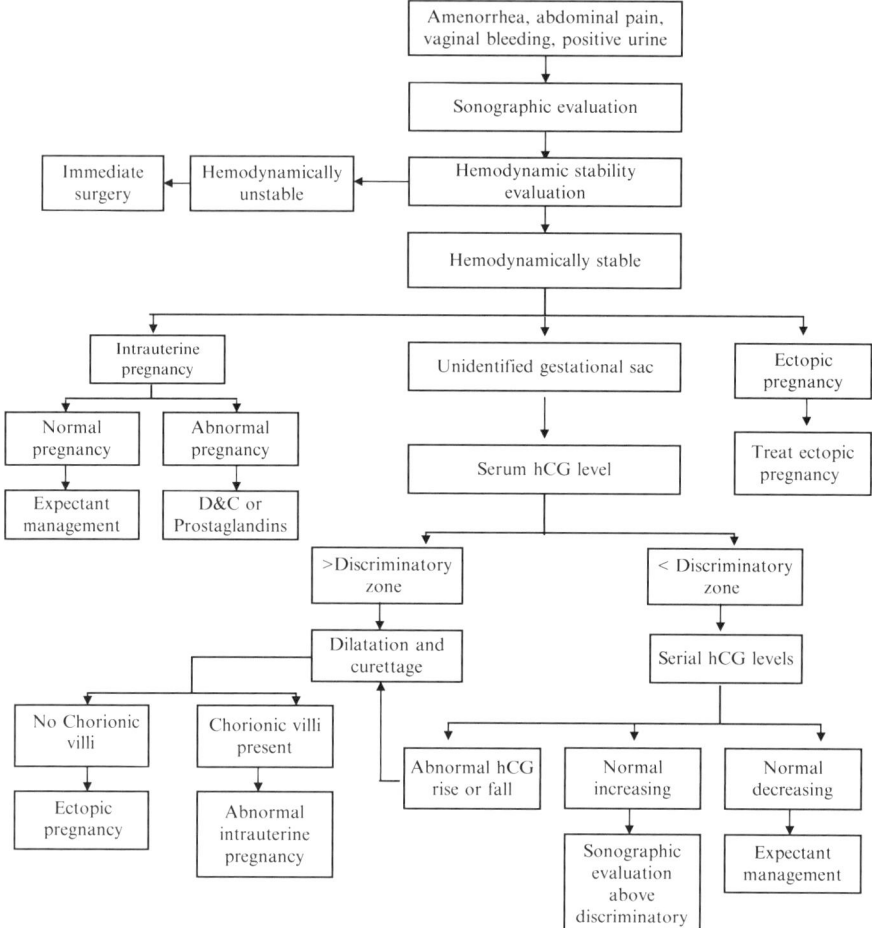

Fig. 3.4 Ectopic pregnancy – a suggested diagnostic approach

the diagnosis of ectopic pregnancy is missed in 3–4% of patients who have very small ectopic gestations [56].

A suggested diagnostic approach is summarized in Fig. 3.4.

Treatment of Tubal Ectopic Pregnancy

After diagnosing the ectopic pregnancy, the therapeutic options for women with a tubal ectopic pregnancy are surgery, medical treatment, or expectant management. Obviously, medical treatment and expectant management can be considered only for hemodynamically stable patients [29].

Expectant Management

The natural history of an untreated ectopic pregnancy takes one of three courses: (1) spontaneous resolution; (2) tubal abortion; (3) rupture of the ectopic pregnancy. The result of a ruptured ectopic pregnancy may be fatal owing to hemorrhage. Ruptured ectopic pregnancy is the leading cause of pregnancy-related maternal death during the first trimester [57]. Comparing pharmacological treatment with MTX to expectant management of ectopic pregnancy, Korhonen et al. concluded that oral MTX, 2.5 mg for 5 days, does not appear to be more effective than placebo in the treatment of ectopic pregnancy in women eligible for expectant management [58]. Candidates for expectant management are hemodynamically stable patients with an initial hCG titer <1,000 mIU/ml [59, 60]. Assessing the clinical and sonographic predictors for the spontaneous resolution of ectopic pregnancies, Atri et al. reported that longer times from the last menstrual period, low β-hCG levels, absence of gestational sacs, and high resistive indexes of ectopic pregnancy at the time of presentation appear to be independent predictors of a spontaneous resolution of ectopic pregnancy [61].

Surgical Treatment

Surgical treatment is mandatory whenever ectopic pregnancy is suspected and the patient is unstable. In a hemodynamically stable patient, surgical treatment is offered to patients who do not meet the criteria for medical treatment. After deciding to operate on the patient, two questions arise: (1) the type of surgery to be selected (i.e., laparotomy vs. laparoscopy) and (2) fallopian tube preservation (i.e., salpingectomy vs. salpingostomy).

Laparotomy vs. Laparoscopy

Laparotomy is still the mainstay of therapy for hemodynamically unstable patients with a high suspicion of tubal rupture. In these cases, quick, good visualization is the most important factor; hence, laparotomy is required. Medical advances now allow earlier diagnosis of ectopic pregnancy, along with the minimally invasive procedure of laparoscopy. In fact, laparoscopy has become the favored treatment of ectopic pregnancy [29].

In a meta-analysis, Mol et al. compared the various treatment modalities for tubal ectopic pregnancy, including medical, surgical, and expectant management. They concluded that laparoscopy is the treatment of choice as it is less costly than the open surgical approach [62]. Indeed, laparoscopy is the preferable surgical technique in a hemodynamically stable patient. The advantages of laparoscopy include decreased surgical blood loss, decreased amount of analgesia, and shorter postoperative hospital stay [63–65]. In a randomized trial, Lundorff et al.

evaluated fertility outcome after surgical treatment of ectopic pregnancy. They randomized patients with tubal ectopic pregnancy to salpingostomy by either laparoscopy or laparotomy. There was no difference between the two groups in regard to the overall fertility outcome. A substantially higher proportion of patients in the laparotomy group were subjected to adhesiolysis performed at a second-look laparoscopy [66].

Salpingectomy vs. Salpingostomy

Salpingostomy is removal of the ectopic pregnancy through an incision in the fallopian tube. This method is considered when preservation of the fallopian tube is required for future fertility. The main disadvantage of this procedure is incomplete removal of trophoblastic tissue, resulting in rising or plateauing serum hCG concentrations (persistent trophoblast) [67]. In this condition, clinical symptoms may proceed, and further treatment might be required. The possible advantages of removing the tube completely include almost entirely eliminating the risk of persistent trophoblast and a subsequent ectopic pregnancy, whereas the possible advantage of conserving the fallopian tube is that future fertility is preserved [41].

No randomized controlled trials have compared salpingectomy to salpingostomy. In a recently published review of the literature, the risk of normal pregnancy or ectopic recurrence is similar between salpingotomy and salpingectomy when the contralateral tube is normal. Conversely, in the case of an altered tube, the fertility appears higher after conservative treatment [68]. Still, most caregivers consider laparoscopic salpingectomy to be the surgical treatment of choice [64].

Assessing the predictors to succeed in laparoscopic salpingostomy, Rabischong et al. found that an hCG level of at least 1,960 IU/l is the only factor related to treatment failure. However, the prognostic value of this cutoff is low and with limited clinical relevance [69]. Interestingly, after presenting the dilemma to decide between preserving the tube (which increases the chance of persistent trophoblast and a higher chance of a recurrent ectopic pregnancy) vs. removing the tube (which reduces the fertile capacity) women preferred to avoid a repeat ectopic pregnancy to gaining a higher chance of a spontaneous intrauterine pregnancy [70].

Medical Therapy

A folic acid antagonist, MTX is the most commonly used drug for the treatment of ectopic pregnancy. MTX inhibits dehydrofolate reductase and thereby prevents the synthesis of DNA. MTX acts on the rapidly dividing trophoblast cells of an ectopic pregnancy [71]. The classic candidates for medical therapy of ectopic pregnancy are hemodynamically stable patients with an unruptured ectopic pregnancy [72]. Table 3.1 lists the commonly used selection criteria for determining the eligibility of a patient to be treated with MTX.

Table 3.1 Commonly used selection criteria for eligible patients to be treated by methotrexate

1. Hemodynamic stability
2. Ability and willingness of the patient to comply with posttreatment monitoring
3. Pretreatment serum β-hCG concentration <5,000 IU/l
4. Ectopic pregnancy mass of ≤4.0 cm without cardiac activity
5. Ectopic pregnancy mass of ≤3.5 cm when cardiac activity is visualized
6. No signs of impending or ongoing ectopic mass rupture
7. No important abnormalities in baseline hematological, renal, or hepatic laboratory values
8. No immunodeficiency, active pulmonary disease, peptic ulcer disease

Two main MTX treatment protocols are used: single-dose and the multiple-dose regimens. The multiple-dose regimen includes MTX 1 mg/kg intramuscularly alternating with leucovorin 0.1 mg/kg intramuscularly for up to four daily doses of each drug. The single-dose MTX regimen is based on body surface area (at 50 mg/m^2) and does not require leucovorin rescue [73]. It is more frequently used for treating hemodynamically stable patients with small ectopic pregnancies. The MTX treatment, in addition to being more convenient to the patient and the physician, was also determined to be more cost-effective compared to laparoscopy [74]. No evidence of a difference was found comparing systemic MTX in different dosages: a single-dose regimen vs. the fixed multiple-dose regimen and a lower dose (25 mg/m^2) vs. the standard dose of 50 mg/m^2 [75].

The preferred MTX treatment approach between the single-dose and the multiple-dose regimens is debatable. In a prospective cohort of 120 hemodynamically stable women with an ectopic pregnancy, Stovall and Ling concluded that the single-dose protocol should be the regimen of choice for medical treatment of unruptured ectopic pregnancy [76]. Barnhart et al. performed a meta-analysis comparing 1,067 women treated with a single-dose regimen and 260 women treated with a multiple-dose regimen. The crude overall success rate for women managed with the single-dose therapy was 88.1% as compared to 92.7% success rate with the multiple-dose protocol ($P = 0.035$). The mean hCG value for those treated with a single-dose regimen was significantly lower than that of those on the multidose regimen. Controlling for confounding factors, all demonstrate a statistically greater failure rate for treatment with single-dose therapy. Nevertheless, women treated with the single-dose regimen had significantly fewer side effects. The authors concluded that the success of using MTX to treat an ectopic pregnancy medically is high (89%). Side effects, though prevalent, are relatively minor and self-limited, although failed medical management is nearly five times as likely with the single-dose regimen [73].

A contrasting study by Lipscomb et al. compared multiple-dose and single-dose MTX protocols for the treatment of ectopic pregnancy and concluded that single-dose MTX therapy is as effective as multiple-dose MTX therapy for the treatment of ectopic pregnancy [77]. Furthermore, a prospective, randomized clinical trial on 108 women with ectopic pregnancy reported that single-dose treatment with MTX could be as successful as multiple doses. The incidence of complications did not differ between the two groups. It appears that single-dose treatment could be the first line of treatment in selected patients [78]. A meta-analysis in 2008 verified that when comparing single- vs. multiple-dose MTX, there was no significant difference in treatment success [relative risk (RR) 0.99, 95% CI 0.89–1.10] [62]. Moreover, a randomized trial by Guvendag Guven et al. confirmed that multiple doses of MTX for the treatment of unruptured tubal ectopic pregnancy are no more effective than a single dose. In addition, multiple doses may cause more side effects, but the time for hCG levels to fall below 5 mU/ml is shorter [79].

Trying to predict a successful treatment with MTX, Nowak-Markwitz et al. reported that when the initial hCG level is > 1,790 mIU/ml, the MTX treatment of ectopic pregnancy is at risk of failure. However, the initial β-hCG titer is not a predictor of the number of MTX cycles that can guarantee a successful outcome [80].

Assessing the predictors of MTX treatment failure in ectopic pregnancy, Dilbaz et al. found that the presence of an embryo [odds ratio (OR) 24, CI 2.1–269, $P=0.01$] and a day 1 serum β-hCG level ≥3,000 mIU/ml (OR 27.1, CI 2.1–342.5, $P=0.01$) were the main predictors of treatment failure. They concluded that TVUS findings are as important as the serum hCG level on the first day of MTX treatment. In unruptured cases, the day 3 serum hCG level is important to reevaluate the decision to continue follow-up or perform early surgery for increased risk of treatment failure [81]. In addition to hCG levels, the presence of a yolk sac was found to be a reliable predictor of treatment failure after single-dose MTX treatment of ectopic pregnancy [82].

Side Effects

The most common side effects of MTX are gastrointestinal, including nausea, vomiting, and stomatitis. The side effects are usually self-limited. The severity of the side effects is correlated with duration and dosage of the drug. Abdominal pain 2–3 days after administration, apparently from the cytotoxic effect of the drug on the trophoblast tissue, is common. In the absence of signs of tubal rupture, abdominal pain can be managed expectantly [83].

Liver enzyme elevation may be elevated, especially with multiple-dose regimens, and resolves after MTX cessation or by increasing the rescue dose of folinic acid. Therefore, blood tests to examine the liver enzymes prior to the initiation of medical treatment is advised. The patient should be advised during therapy not to use folic acid supplements, nonsteroidal antiinflammatory drugs (NSAIDs), or alcohol; to avoid sunlight exposure; and to abstain from sexual intercourse or vigorous physical activity [84].

Follow-Up

The follow-up of a patient after medical treatment with MTX or after preserving the infected tube during laparoscopy includes serial hCG levels until disappearance. In addition, tubal patency testing by hysterosalpingography is indicated. Early (5–7 weeks' gestation) TVUS during every future pregnancy should be advised [85].

Nontubal Ectopic Pregnancies

Most ectopic pregnancies are tubal (up to 95%), 2% are interstitial or corneal, 2% are ovarian, and the remainder are cervical or abdominal [41].

- *Cervical pregnancy*: A rare life-threatening form of ectopic pregnancy, cervical pregnancy occurs in 1 per 8,628 deliveries. Obligatory sonographic criteria of acervical pregnancy include endocervical localization of the gestational sac [86, 87]. Cervical pregnancy is diagnosed when the entire gestational sac, having a well-formed shape, is demonstrated in the dilated cervix. The sac may contain a yolk sac and embryo, with or without cardiac activity, located below the level of the internal os. Except in the case of heterotopic pregnancy, the endometrial stripe is visualized, and an hourglass shape of the uterus is evident. With true cervical pregnancy, Doppler studies show characteristic patterns of trophoblast with high flow velocity and low impedance, whereas with a miscarriage the sac is mobile with no Doppler evidence of blood flow [88]. Nonsurgical treatment, including intraamniotic and systemic MTX administration, has been used successfully [87, 89, 90].
- *Ovarian pregnancy*: A pregnancy confined to the ovary represents 0.5–1.0% of all ectopic pregnancies; it is the most common type of nontubal ectopic pregnancy [56]. Unlike tubal gestation, ovarian pregnancy is associated with neither PID nor infertility. The only risk factor associated with the development of an ovarian pregnancy is the current use of an IUD [56]. Ovarian pregnancies usually appear on or within the ovary as a cyst with a wide echogenic outside ring. A yolk sac or embryo is less commonly seen. The sonographic appearance of the contents usually lags in comparison with the gestational age [91]. Ovarian laparoscopic cystectomy is the preferred treatment [92, 93]. Treatment with MTX or prostaglandin injection has also been reported.
- *Interstitial pregnancy*: Interstitial pregnancy accounts for up to 1–3% of ectopic pregnancies. Cornual resection and abdominal hysterectomy are optional treatments (Fig. 3.5). Prior to rupture, the cornual ectopic can be managed by laparoscopic resection of the pregnancy [94]. However, it should no longer be the first line of treatment for a hemodynamically stable patient with an interstitial pregnancy. In selected cases, MTX and laparoscopy can be used successfully to treat early interstitial pregnancy [95, 96].
- *Abdominal pregnancy*: Abdominal pregnancies are classified as primary and secondary. Commonly, secondary abdominal pregnancies result from tubal abortion or rupture [56]. Ectopic abdominal pregnancies may be undetected until an advanced age and often result in severe hemorrhage [97]. The Studdiford criteria for diagnosing primary abdominal pregnancy include (1) the presence of normal tubes and ovaries with no evidence of a recent or past pregnancy, (2) no evidence of a uteroplacental fistula, and (3) the presence of a pregnancy related exclusively to the peritoneal surface and early enough to eliminate the possibility of secondary implantation after primary tubal nidation [56]. Surgical intervention is recommended when an abdominal pregnancy is diagnosed.

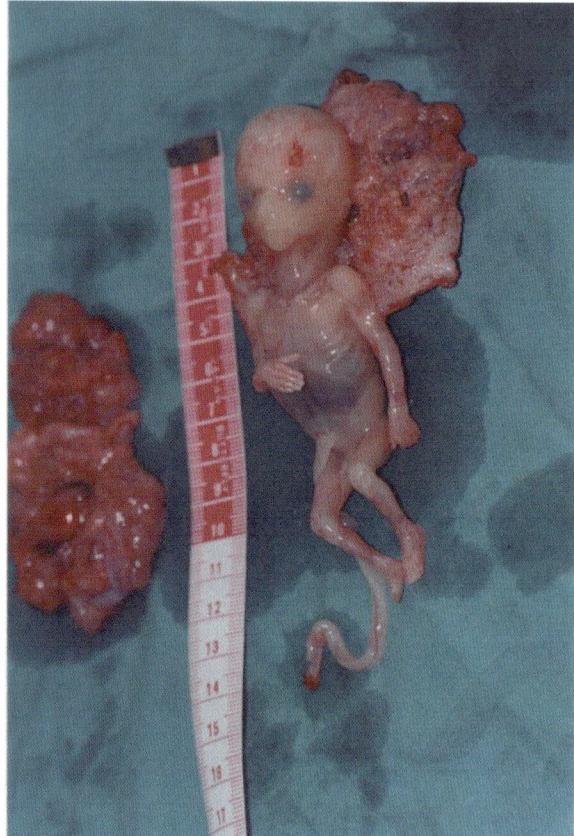

Fig. 3.5 Interstitial (corneal) 15-week pregnancy after resection

- *Pregnancy in a previous uterine scar*: Embryo implantation in a previous cesarean scar resulting in a cesarean scar pregnancy is a rare but potentially catastrophic complication of a prior cesarean birth [98]. The diagnosis is usually established by TVUS along with color flow Doppler. There is no consensus on the preferred mode of treatment. Systemic or local administration of MTX is commonly used [98].

Summary

Ectopic pregnancy refers to implantation of a fertilized ovum outside the uterus. The most common site is the fallopian tubes, accounting for about 98% of all ectopic pregnancies. In rare cases, implantation can occur in other ectopic sites including the ovary, uterine cervix (i.e., cervical pregnancy), and abdomen. A coexistent intrauterine or extrauterine pregnancy is referred as a heterotopic pregnancy. Clinical manifestations are varied and depend on whether rupture has occurred. The most common symptoms are abdominal or pelvic pain accompanied by vaginal bleeding and amenorrhea. The first stage in the evaluation of women with a suspected EP is to determine if the patient is pregnant. The hCG enzyme immunoassay is positive in virtually all cases. The best diagnosis of ectopic pregnancy is based on the positive US visualization of an extrauterine pregnancy, although it is not seen in all cases. A small number of patients with an ectopic pregnancy present with a surgical abdomen and signs of hypovolemia and shock. They require immediate operation. Most of the other cases can be treated by medical (MTX), surgical (laparoscopy or laparotomy), or expectant management alone. The choice depends on the medical conditions, available resources, and the site involved.

References

1. Goldner TE, Lawson HW, Xia Z, Atrash HK. Surveillance for ectopic pregnancy–United States, 1970–1989. MMWR CDC Surveill Summ. 1993;42(6):73–85.
2. Dorfman SF, Grimes DA, Cates Jr W, Binkin NJ, Kafrissen ME, O'Reilly KR. Ectopic pregnancy mortality, United States, 1979 to 1980: clinical aspects. Obstet Gynecol. 1984;64(3): 386–90.
3. Washington AE, Katz P. Ectopic pregnancy in the United States: economic consequences and payment source trends. Obstet Gynecol. 1993;81(2):287–92.
4. Centers for Disease Control and Prevention (CDC). Ectopic pregnancy–United States, 1990–1992. MMWR Morb Mortal Wkly Rep. 1995;44:46–8. http://www.ncbi.nlm.nih.gov/pubmed/7823895.
5. Coste J, Bouyer J, Job-Spira N. [Epidemiology of ectopic pregnancy: incidence and risk factors]. Contracept Fertil Sex. 1996;24(2):135–9.
6. Cooper GM, Lewis G, Neilson J. Confidential enquiries into maternal deaths, 1997–1999. Br J Anaesth. 2002;89(3):369–72.
7. Ory SJ. New options for diagnosis and treatment of ectopic pregnancy. JAMA. 1992;267(4): 534–7.
8. Kamwendo F, Forslin L, Bodin L, Danielsson D. Epidemiology of ectopic pregnancy during a 28 year period and the role of pelvic inflammatory disease. Sex Transm Infect. 2000;76(1): 28–32.
9. Ankum WM, Hajenius PJ, Schrevel LS, Van der Veen F. Management of suspected ectopic pregnancy. Impact of new diagnostic tools in 686 consecutive cases. J Reprod Med. 1996; 41(10):724–8.
10. Zane SB, Kieke Jr BA, Kendrick JS, Bruce C. Surveillance in a time of changing health care practices: estimating ectopic pregnancy incidence in the United States. Matern Child Health J. 2002;6(4):227–36.
11. Karaer A, Avsar FA, Batioglu S. Risk factors for ectopic pregnancy: a case-control study. Aust N Z J Obstet Gynaecol. 2006;46(6):521–7.
12. Shaw JL, Dey SK, Critchley HO, Horne AW. Current knowledge of the aetiology of human tubal ectopic pregnancy. Hum Reprod Update. 2010;16(4):432–44.
13. Ankum WM, Mol BW, Van der Veen F, Bossuyt PM. Risk factors for ectopic pregnancy: a meta-analysis. Fertil Steril. 1996;65(6):1093–9.
14. Barnhart KT, Sammel MD, Gracia CR, Chittams J, Hummel AC, Shaunik A. Risk factors for ectopic pregnancy in women with symptomatic first-trimester pregnancies. Fertil Steril. 2006;86(1):36–43.

15. Sindos M, Togia A, Sergentanis TN, et al. Ruptured ectopic pregnancy: risk factors for a life-threatening condition. Arch Gynecol Obstet. 2009;279(5):621–3.
16. Pulkkinen MO, Talo A. Tubal physiologic consideration in ectopic pregnancy. Clin Obstet Gynecol. 1987;30(1):164–72.
17. A Multinational Case-Control Study of Ectopic Pregnancy. The World Health Organization's Special Programme of Research, Development and Research Training in Human Reproduction: Task Force on Intrauterine Devices for Fertility Regulation. Clin Reprod Fertil. 1985;3(2): 131–43.
18. Liukko P, Erkkola R, Laakso L. Ectopic pregnancies during use of low-dose progestogens for oral contraception. Contraception. 1977;16(6):575–80.
19. Sivin I. International experience with NORPLANT and NORPLANT-2 contraceptives. Stud Fam Plann. 1988;19(2):81–94.
20. Sivin I. Dose- and age-dependent ectopic pregnancy risks with intrauterine contraception. Obstet Gynecol. 1991;78(2):291–8.
21. Coste J, Job-Spira N, Fernandez H. Increased risk of ectopic pregnancy with maternal cigarette smoking. Am J Public Health. 1991;81(2):199–201.
22. Handler A, Davis F, Ferre C, Yeko T. The relationship of smoking and ectopic pregnancy. Am J Public Health. 1989;79(9):1239–42.
23. Karande VC, Flood JT, Heard N, Veeck L, Muasher SJ. Analysis of ectopic pregnancies resulting from in-vitro fertilization and embryo transfer. Hum Reprod. 1991;6(3):446–9.
24. Nazari A, Askari HA, Check JH, O'Shaughnessy A. Embryo transfer technique as a cause of ectopic pregnancy in in vitro fertilization. Fertil Steril. 1993;60(5):919–21.
25. Homm RJ, Holtz G, Garvin AJ. Isthmic ectopic pregnancy and salpingitis isthmica nodosa. Fertil Steril. 1987;48(5):756–60.
26. Job-Spira N, Fernandez H, Bouyer J, Pouly JL, Germain E, Coste J. Ruptured tubal ectopic pregnancy: risk factors and reproductive outcome: results of a population-based study in France. Am J Obstet Gynecol. 1999;180(4):938–44.
27. Weckstein LN, Boucher AR, Tucker H, Gibson D, Rettenmaier MA. Accurate diagnosis of early ectopic pregnancy. Obstet Gynecol. 1985;65(3):393–7.
28. Alsuleiman SA, Grimes EM. Ectopic pregnancy: a review of 147 cases. J Reprod Med. 1982;27(2):101–6.
29. Seeber BE, Barnhart KT. Suspected ectopic pregnancy. Obstet Gynecol. 2006;107(2 Pt 1): 399–413.
30. Della-Giustina D, Denny M. Ectopic pregnancy. Emerg Med Clin North Am. 2003;21(3): 565–84.
31. Dart RG, Kaplan B, Varaklis K. Predictive value of history and physical examination in patients with suspected ectopic pregnancy. Ann Emerg Med. 1999;33(3):283–90.
32. Aleem FA, DeFazio M, Gintautas J. Endovaginal sonography for the early diagnosis of intra-uterine and ectopic pregnancies. Hum Reprod. 1990;5(6):755–8.
33. Shalev E, Yarom I, Bustan M, Weiner E, Ben-Shlomo I. Transvaginal sonography as the ultimate diagnostic tool for the management of ectopic pregnancy: experience with 840 cases. Fertil Steril. 1998;69(1):62–5.
34. Barnhart K, Mennuti MT, Benjamin I, Jacobson S, Goodman D, Coutifaris C. Prompt diagnosis of ectopic pregnancy in an emergency department setting. Obstet Gynecol. 1994;84(6): 1010–5.
35. Atri M, Leduc C, Gillett P, et al. Role of endovaginal sonography in the diagnosis and management of ectopic pregnancy. Radiographics. 1996;16(4):755–74. discussion 75.
36. Lin EP, Bhatt S, Dogra VS. Diagnostic clues to ectopic pregnancy. Radiographics. 2008;28(6):1661–71.
37. Hammoud AO, Hammoud I, Bujold E, Gonik B, Diamond MP, Johnson SC. The role of sonographic endometrial patterns and endometrial thickness in the differential diagnosis of ectopic pregnancy. Am J Obstet Gynecol. 2005;192(5):1370–5.
38. Fernandez H, Gervaise A. Ectopic pregnancies after infertility treatment: modern diagnosis and therapeutic strategy. Hum Reprod Update. 2004;10(6):503–13.

39. Goldman GA, Fisch B, Ovadia J, Tadir Y. Heterotopic pregnancy after assisted reproductive technologies. Obstet Gynecol Surv. 1992;47(4):217–21.
40. Kadar N, Caldwell BV, Romero R. A method of screening for ectopic pregnancy and its indications. Obstet Gynecol. 1981;58(2):162–6.
41. Farquhar CM. Ectopic pregnancy. Lancet. 2005;366(9485):583–91.
42. Chung K, Allen R. The use of serial human chorionic gonadotropin levels to establish a viable or a nonviable pregnancy. Semin Reprod Med. 2008;26(5):383–90.
43. Pittaway DE, Reish RL, Wentz AC. Doubling times of human chorionic gonadotropin increase in early viable intrauterine pregnancies. Am J Obstet Gynecol. 1985;152(3):299–302.
44. Braunstein GD, Rasor J, Danzer H, Adler D, Wade ME. Serum human chorionic gonadotropin levels throughout normal pregnancy. Am J Obstet Gynecol. 1976;126(6):678–81.
45. Barnhart KT, Sammel MD, Rinaudo PF, Zhou L, Hummel AC, Guo W. Symptomatic patients with an early viable intrauterine pregnancy: HCG curves redefined. Obstet Gynecol. 2004;104(1):50–5.
46. Kadar N, Freedman M, Zacher M. Further observations on the doubling time of human chorionic gonadotropin in early asymptomatic pregnancies. Fertil Steril. 1990;54(5):783–7.
47. Romero R, Kadar N, Copel JA, Jeanty P, DeCherney AH, Hobbins JC. The value of serial human chorionic gonadotropin testing as a diagnostic tool in ectopic pregnancy. Am J Obstet Gynecol. 1986;155(2):392–4.
48. Silva C, Sammel MD, Zhou L, Gracia C, Hummel AC, Barnhart K. Human chorionic gonadotropin profile for women with ectopic pregnancy. Obstet Gynecol. 2006;107(3):605–10.
49. Kadar N, Romero R. Sonographic evaluation of ectopic pregnancy. Am J Obstet Gynecol. 1981;141(4):473–5.
50. Stovall TG, Ling FW, Andersen RN, Buster JE. Improved sensitivity and specificity of a single measurement of serum progesterone over serial quantitative beta-human chorionic gonadotrophin in screening for ectopic pregnancy. Hum Reprod. 1992;7(5):723–5.
51. McCord ML, Muram D, Buster JE, Arheart KL, Stovall TG, Carson SA. Single serum progesterone as a screen for ectopic pregnancy: exchanging specificity and sensitivity to obtain optimal test performance. Fertil Steril. 1996;66(4):513–6.
52. Mol BW, Lijmer JG, Ankum WM, van der Veen F, Bossuyt PM. The accuracy of single serum progesterone measurement in the diagnosis of ectopic pregnancy: a meta-analysis. Hum Reprod. 1998;13(11):3220–7.
53. Stovall TG, Ling FW, Carson SA, Buster JE. Serum progesterone and uterine curettage in differential diagnosis of ectopic pregnancy. Fertil Steril. 1992;57(2):456–7.
54. Barnhart KT, Katz I, Hummel A, Gracia CR. Presumed diagnosis of ectopic pregnancy. Obstet Gynecol. 2002;100(3):505–10.
55. Kaplan BC, Dart RG, Moskos M, et al. Ectopic pregnancy: prospective study with improved diagnostic accuracy. Ann Emerg Med. 1996;28(1):10–7.
56. Stovall T. Early pregnancy loss and ectopic pregnancy. In: Berek JS, editor. Berek & Novak's gynecology. 14th ed. Philadelphia: Lippincott William & Wilkins; 2006. p. 882–931.
57. Anderson FW, Hogan JG, Ansbacher R. Sudden death: ectopic pregnancy mortality. Obstet Gynecol. 2004;103(6):1218–23.
58. Korhonen J, Stenman UH, Ylostalo P. Low-dose oral methotrexate with expectant management of ectopic pregnancy. Obstet Gynecol. 1996;88(5):775–8.
59. Trio D, Strobelt N, Picciolo C, Lapinski RH, Ghidini A. Prognostic factors for successful expectant management of ectopic pregnancy. Fertil Steril. 1995;63(3):469–72.
60. Shalev E, Peleg D, Tsabari A, Romano S, Bustan M. Spontaneous resolution of ectopic tubal pregnancy: natural history. Fertil Steril. 1995;63(1):15–9.
61. Atri M, Chow CM, Kintzen G, et al. Expectant treatment of ectopic pregnancies: clinical and sonographic predictors. AJR Am J Roentgenol. 2001;176(1):123–7.
62. Mol F, Mol BW, Ankum WM, van der Veen F, Hajenius PJ. Current evidence on surgery, systemic methotrexate and expectant management in the treatment of tubal ectopic pregnancy: a systematic review and meta-analysis. Hum Reprod Update. 2008;14(4):309–19.
63. Tintara H, Choobun T. Laparoscopic adnexectomy for benign tubo-ovarian disease using abdominal wall lift: a comparison to laparotomy. Int J Gynaecol Obstet. 2004;84(2):147–55.

64. Tulandi T, Saleh A. Surgical management of ectopic pregnancy. Clin Obstet Gynecol. 1999;42(1):31–8. quiz 55–6.
65. Yao M, Tulandi T. Surgical and medical management of tubal and non-tubal ectopic pregnancies. Curr Opin Obstet Gynecol. 1998;10(5):371–4.
66. Lundorff P, Thorburn J, Lindblom B. Fertility outcome after conservative surgical treatment of ectopic pregnancy evaluated in a randomized trial. Fertil Steril. 1992;57(5):998–1002.
67. Seifer DB, Gutmann JN, Doyle MB, Jones EE, Diamond MP, DeCherney AH. Persistent ectopic pregnancy following laparoscopic linear salpingostomy. Obstet Gynecol. 1990;76(6): 1121–5.
68. Desroque D, Capmas P, Legendre G, Bouyer J, Fernandez H. [Fertility after ectopic pregnancy]. J Gynecol Obstet Biol Reprod (Paris). 2010;39(5):395–400.
69. Rabischong B, Larrain D, Pouly JL, Jaffeux P, Aublet-Cuvelier B, Fernandez H. Predicting success of laparoscopic salpingostomy for ectopic pregnancy. Obstet Gynecol. 2010;116(3): 701–7.
70. van Mello NM, Mol F, Opmeer BC, et al. Salpingotomy or salpingectomy in tubal ectopic pregnancy: what do women prefer? Reprod Biomed Online. 2010;21(5):687–93.
71. Berlin NI, Rall D, Mead JA, et al. Folic acid antagonist. Effects on the cell and the patient. Combined clinical staff conference at the National Institutes of Health. Ann Intern Med. 1963;59:931–56.
72. Murray H, Baakdah H, Bardell T, Tulandi T. Diagnosis and treatment of ectopic pregnancy. CMAJ. 2005;173(8):905–12.
73. Barnhart KT, Gosman G, Ashby R, Sammel M. The medical management of ectopic pregnancy: a meta-analysis comparing "single dose" and "multidose" regimens. Obstet Gynecol. 2003;101(4):778–84.
74. Alexander JM, Rouse DJ, Varner E, Austin Jr JM. Treatment of the small unruptured ectopic pregnancy: a cost analysis of methotrexate versus laparoscopy. Obstet Gynecol. 1996;88(1):123–7.
75. Hajenius PJ, Mol F, Mol BW, Bossuyt PM, Ankum WM, van der Veen F. Interventions for tubal ectopic pregnancy. Cochrane Database Syst Rev 2007;(1):CD000324.
76. Stovall TG, Ling FW. Single-dose methotrexate: an expanded clinical trial. Am J Obstet Gynecol. 1993;168(6 Pt 1):1759–62. discussion 62–5.
77. Lipscomb GH, Givens VM, Meyer NL, Bran D. Comparison of multidose and single-dose methotrexate protocols for the treatment of ectopic pregnancy. Am J Obstet Gynecol. 2005;192(6):1844–7. discussion 7–8.
78. Alleyassin A, Khademi A, Aghahosseini M, Safdarian L, Badenoosh B, Hamed EA. Comparison of success rates in the medical management of ectopic pregnancy with single-dose and multiple-dose administration of methotrexate: a prospective, randomized clinical trial. Fertil Steril. 2006;85(6):1661–6.
79. Guvendag Guven ES, Dilbaz S, Dilbaz B, Aykan Yildirim B, Akdag D, Haberal A. Comparison of single and multiple dose methotrexate therapy for unruptured tubal ectopic pregnancy: a prospective randomized study. Acta Obstet Gynecol Scand. 2010;89(7):889–95.
80. Nowak-Markwitz E, Michalak M, Olejnik M, Spaczynski M. Cutoff value of human chorionic gonadotropin in relation to the number of methotrexate cycles in the successful treatment of ectopic pregnancy. Fertil Steril. 2009;92(4):1203–7.
81. Dilbaz S, Caliskan E, Dilbaz B, Degirmenci O, Haberal A. Predictors of methotrexate treatment failure in ectopic pregnancy. J Reprod Med. 2006;51(2):87–93.
82. Bixby S, Tello R, Kuligowska E. Presence of a yolk sac on transvaginal sonography is the most reliable predictor of single-dose methotrexate treatment failure in ectopic pregnancy. J Ultrasound Med. 2005;24(5):591–8.
83. ACOG Practice Bulletin No. 94. Medical management of ectopic pregnancy. Obstet Gynecol 2008;111(6):1479–85.
84. Pisarska MD, Carson SA, Buster JE. Ectopic pregnancy. Lancet. 1998;351(9109):1115–20.
85. Nama V, Manyonda I. Tubal ectopic pregnancy: diagnosis and management. Arch Gynecol Obstet. 2009;279(4):443–53.

86. Ushakov FB, Elchalal U, Aceman PJ, Schenker JG. Cervical pregnancy: past and future. Obstet Gynecol Surv. 1997;52(1):45–59.
87. Sheiner E, Yohai D, Katz M. Cervical pregnancy with placenta accreta. Int J Gynaecol Obstet. 1999;65(2):211–2.
88. Valsky DV, Yagel S. Ectopic pregnancies of unusual location: management dilemmas. Ultrasound Obstet Gynecol. 2008;31(3):245–51.
89. Stovall TG, Ling FW, Smith WC, Felker R, Rasco BJ, Buster JE. Successful nonsurgical treatment of cervical pregnancy with methotrexate. Fertil Steril. 1988;50(4):672–4.
90. Tang PP, Liu XY, Chen N, et al. Diagnosis and treatment of cervical ectopic pregnancy. Zhongguo Yi Xue Ke Xue Yuan Xue Bao. 2010;32(5):497–500.
91. Comstock C, Huston K, Lee W. The ultrasonographic appearance of ovarian ectopic pregnancies. Obstet Gynecol. 2005;105(1):42–5.
92. Van Coevering 2 RJ, Fisher JE. Laparoscopic management of ovarian pregnancy. A case report. J Reprod Med. 1988;33(9):774–6.
93. Odejinmi F, Rizzuto MI, Macrae R, Olowu O, Hussain M. Diagnosis and laparoscopic management of 12 consecutive cases of ovarian pregnancy and review of literature. J Minim Invasive Gynecol. 2009;16(3):354–9.
94. Walid MS, Heaton RL. Diagnosis and laparoscopic treatment of cornual ectopic pregnancy. Ger Med Sci 2010;8. http://www.ncbi.nlm.nih.gov/pubmed?term=Heaton%20RL.%20 Diagnosis%20and%20laparoscopic%20treatment%20of%20cornual%20ectopic%20 pregnancy.
95. Lau S, Tulandi T. Conservative medical and surgical management of interstitial ectopic pregnancy. Fertil Steril. 1999;72(2):207–15.
96. Dilbaz S, Katas B, Demir B, Dilbaz B. Treating cornual pregnancy with a single methotrexate injection: a report of 3 cases. J Reprod Med. 2005;50(2):141–4.
97. Worley KC, Hnat MD, Cunningham FG. Advanced extrauterine pregnancy: diagnostic and therapeutic challenges. Am J Obstet Gynecol. 2008;198(3):297.e1–7.
98. Ash A, Smith A, Maxwell D. Caesarean scar pregnancy. Br J Obstet Gynaecol. 2007;114(3): 253–63.

Chapter 4
Vaginal Bleeding and Gestational Trophoblastic Disease

Lisa M. Barroilhet, Donald Peter Goldstein, and Ross S. Berkowitz

Introduction

Molar pregnancy and gestational trophoblastic neoplasia (GTN) comprise a group of interrelated diseases, including complete and partial molar pregnancy, placental-site trophoblastic tumor (PSTT), and choriocarcinoma, that have varying propensities for local invasion and distal spread. Vaginal bleeding is a common presenting sign, seen in as many as 97% of women with a complete molar pregnancy; it is also a frequent symptom of all types of GTN [1].

Molar Pregnancies

Molar pregnancies are classified as either partial or complete on the basis of their cytogenetic, histopathological, and morphological characteristics. The distinctive features of these two entities are outlined in Table 4.1. Despite clinical and pathological differences, the management of patients with partial and complete hydatidiform moles (CHMs) is generally the same.

CHMs usually have a chromosomal complement derived from the paternal genome. There is no identifiable fetal or embryonic tissue. The 46XX genotype is most common, typically representing reduplication of the haploid genome of the sperm [1]. Fewer molar pregnancies have a 46XY karyotype consistent with dispermic fertilization [2]. Pathological characteristics include diffuse trophoblastic hyperplasia, diffuse swollen villi, and marked atypia at the site of molar implantation [3].

R.S. Berkowitz (✉)
Brigham and Women's Hospital, New England Trophoblastic Disease Center,
75 Francis Street, Boston, MA 02115, USA
e-mail: rberkowitz@partners.org

E. Sheiner (ed.), *Bleeding During Pregnancy: A Comprehensive Guide*,
DOI 10.1007/978-1-4419-9810-1_4, © Springer Science+Business Media, LLC 2011

Table 4.1 Features of complete and partial molar pregnancies

Feature	Complete mole	Partial mole
Fetal (or embryonic) tissue	Absent	Present
Hydropic swelling of villi	Diffuse	Focal
Trophoblastic hyperplasia	Diffuse	Focal
Implantation-site trophoblast	Marked atypia	Mild atypia
Karyotype	Diploid	Triploid
	46,XX (mainly)	
	46,XY (rarely)	

Partial molar pregnancies typically have a complement of 69 chromosomes derived from the two paternal and one maternal haploid set of chromosomes. The triploid genotype is derived from a haploid ovum fertilized by two single sperm. Histopathological features show mild trophoblastic atypia and hyperplasia, focal chorionic swelling, and often the presence of embryonic tissue [4].

Postmolar persistent GTN occurs in 15–20% of patients with complete molar pregnancies but in only 1–4% of patients with a partial mole. GTN may occur after any type of pregnancy, but it most commonly follows a molar pregnancy [5].

Diagnosis

The widespread use of ultrasonography (US) during the first trimester of pregnancy has revolutionized the diagnosis of molar pregnancies. Complete molar pregnancies produce a characteristic vesicular pattern due to generalized swelling of the chorionic villi (Fig. 4.1). Most first trimester complete moles have a typical US appearance: a complex, echogenic intrauterine mass containing many small cystic spaces [6]. Among 24 cases of first trimester complete moles (mean gestational age 8.7 weeks), the initial sonographic interpretation was a complete mole in 17 (71%) cases. Those that were not correctly identified were classified as missed abortions. The specificity of the sonographic findings in a complete molar pregnancy may be increased by correlation with the serum human chorionic gonadotropin (hCG) level [7].

The hyperplastic trophoblastic cells characteristic of molar pregnancy produce markedly elevated hCG levels. Genest et al. reviewed the clinical and pathological characteristics of 153 cases of complete mole managed at the New England Trophoblastic Disease Center (NETDC) between 1980 and 1990 [8]. Preevacuation hCG levels were >100,000 U/l in 46% of the patients. Similarly, Menczer et al. reported that 30 (41%) of 74 patients with molar pregnancy had preevacuation hCG values >100,000 U/l [9]. The measurement of a high hCG level (>100,000 U/l) suggests the diagnosis of a complete molar pregnancy, particularly when associated with vaginal bleeding, uterine enlargement, and abnormal US findings.

In contrast, the PHM is less commonly associated with markedly elevated hCG values. Only 2 (6%) of 30 patients with a PHM at our center had preevacuation hCG

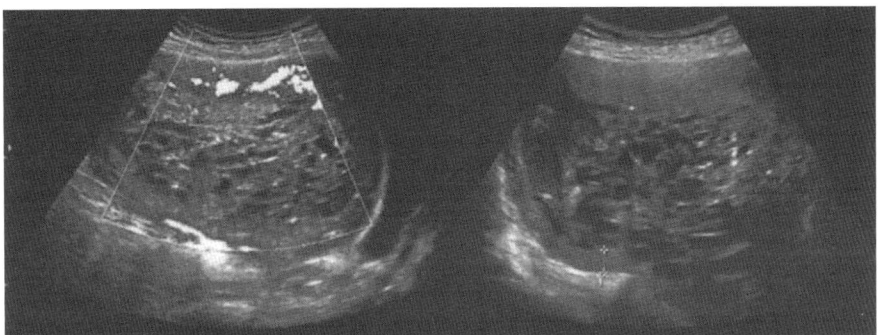

Fig. 4.1 Ultrasonographic image of a complete molar pregnancy with a complex, echogenic intrauterine mass containing many small cystic spaces. Image reprinted with the permission of Dr. Kevin Elias, Brigham and Women's Hospital

levels >100,000 U/l [1]. Because of earlier diagnosis and evacuation, the pathological interpretation of the chorionic material has been made more difficult and may require additional techniques (e.g., cytometry) to determine ploidy and biomarkers of paternally imprinted and maternally expressed gene products [10]. A partial molar pregnancy is often diagnosed by the pathologist after histological review of the curettage specimen and confirmation by either flow cytometry or immunohistochemistry of maternally expressed gene products.

Preevacuation Vaginal Bleeding

Vaginal bleeding is the most common presenting symptom in patients with complete mole, occurring in 89–97% of cases in early series [11, 12]. Although vaginal bleeding continues to be the most common presenting symptom, it occurs in fewer (84% vs. 97%) of our current patients, which is likely related to an earlier diagnosis, before the symptoms manifest [13]. Molar chorionic villi disrupt maternal vessels by separating from the decidua and may result in distention of the endometrial cavity by large volumes of retained blood.

Women with complete molar pregnancies may present with the complaint of scant vaginal spotting or, more dramatically, with acute hemorrhage from the uterus. Because bleeding may be prolonged and occult, 54% of our previous patients were anemic at presentation (hemoglobin <10 g/dl). More recent data show a dramatic decrease in the prevalence of anemia in this population, with only 5% of our current patients with complete mole being anemic at presentation [13].

Partial molar pregnancies often do not present with the same symptoms associated with complete molar pregnancies. Instead, they more typically present as missed or incomplete abortions, with a combination of vaginal bleeding and absent fetal heart tones. Vaginal bleeding occurred in 59 of 81 (72.8%) of the patients ultimately diagnosed with a partial molar pregnancy at our center [14]; uterine enlargement, preeclampsia, and the other classic signs of a complete molar pregnancy were typically absent. The hCG level is uncommonly markedly elevated. US scans of PHM are not as diagnostic as those in CHM patients, although distinct US features have been described [15]. Characteristic US findings in partial molar pregnancies include focal cystic changes in the placenta, an increased transverse diameter of the gestational sac, and the presence of embryonic tissue.

Other Symptoms

Other traditional symptoms are seen less frequently now that earlier detection of complete molar pregnancies has become commonplace. Patients who are not diagnosed until the second trimester more commonly experience excessive uterine enlargement, hyperemesis gravidarum, hyperthyroidism, theca lutein ovarian cysts, preeclampsia, and respiratory insufficiency. Theca lutein cysts are a result of hyperstimulation of the ovaries by extremely high circulating levels of hCG [16]. Hyperthyroidism has become a rare presenting sign of complete molar pregnancies with the earlier diagnosis. Hyperthyroidism is more commonly seen when hCG values exceed 1,000,000 μl/ml. Laboratory evidence of hyperthyroidism was once commonly present in patients with complete moles. Patients with poorly controlled or untreated hyperthyroidism may develop thyroid storm at the time of anesthesia induction and evacuation and thus warrant preoperative β-blockade.

Vaginal Bleeding During Molar Evacuation

When a diagnosis of complete or partial molar pregnancy is suspected, the patient should be evaluated for the presence of medical complications, including anemia, preeclampsia, and hyperthyroidism. All patients should have baseline serum hCG and thyroid function tests performed in addition to a complete blood count with platelets, blood type, and antigen screen. In anticipation of the possible need for chemoprophylaxis, it is reasonable to obtain a creatinine level and liver function tests. Chest radiography may be helpful, primarily to identify preexisting lung disease that may later be misinterpreted as metastases.

After the patient has been medically evaluated and stabilized, a decision must be made concerning the most appropriate method of evacuation. In patients who wish to retain fertility, suction curettage is preferred for evacuation regardless of uterine size [17, 18]. An oxytocin infusion should be started before anesthesia induction to minimize intraoperative bleeding. The cervix is dilated to accommodate a cannula large enough to remove the volume of trophoblastic tissue present. A 12-mm cannula is generally satisfactory because it allows rapid evacuation and subsequent involution of the uterus. During dilatation, brisk bleeding may be encountered owing to passage of blood that had been retained in the endometrial cavity. Despite the potential for prominent blood loss, it is best to proceed promptly with uterine evacuation. After the initiation of suction evacuation, the uterus generally shrinks rapidly, and bleeding is well controlled. If the uterus is larger than 14 weeks' size, one hand may be placed on top of the fundus to monitor uterine size and to massage the uterus. When suction evacuation is thought to be complete, sharp curettage should be performed to remove any residual chorionic tissue.

In women who have completed childbearing, hysterectomy may be an appropriate treatment option. Recent data particularly supports this approach in women >50 years of age, where the risk of persistent or invasive disease was as high as 60% at our center. None of the patients in our series who underwent primary hysterectomy went on to develop GTN [19]. Evacuation of the uterine cavity prior to hysterectomy is not required. The adnexae may be preserved, even in the presence of theca lutein cysts, which typically resolve as hCG levels decline postoperatively. It is important to counsel patients that whereas hysterectomy may prevent local invasion it does not prevent the occurrence of metastases. Postoperative hCG levels must be followed for at least 6 months after normalization.

The RhD antigen is present in trophoblastic cells, and therefore Rh-negative patients with a diagnosis of molar pregnancy should receive Rh immunoglobulin. General anesthesia is preferred for molar evacuation given the possibility of significant blood loss and intraoperative complications. Pulmonary complications, including respiratory failure, are for the most part limited to patients who exhibit the classic signs of CHM (a larger-than-dates uterus, high hCG levels); they generally develop during or after evacuation [20]. Hyperthyroidism and preeclampsia also tend to develop in patients with the classic signs and usually resolve after evacuation. Theca lutein cysts due to high hCG levels may take months to resolve and require decompression only if symptomatic.

High-Risk CHM vs. Low-Risk CHM

Patients with CHM are categorized as having either high-risk or low-risk disease based on their risk of developing postmolar GTN. Patients with signs and symptoms of marked trophoblastic overgrowth, such as markedly elevated hCG levels and excessive uterine enlargement, are at an increased risk of developing GTN and are considered to be at high risk. Among 352 patients with high-risk CHM at our center, 109 (31%) developed nonmetastatic GTN, and 31 (8.8%) developed metastatic GTN. In contrast, among 506 patients with low-risk CHM, only 17 (3.4%) developed nonmetastatic GTN and 3 (0.6%) developed metastatic GTN [1].

It is the policy at the NETDC to consider adjunctive chemotherapy at the time of evacuation in patients with high-risk complete moles when hCG follow-up is not feasible. The goal of prophylactic chemotherapy is to reduce the likelihood that these women will require subsequent treatment [21]. A randomized study by Kim et al. showed a lower incidence of persistent trophoblastic disease among high-risk patients in the group who received prophylactic methotrexate chemotherapy compared to those who did not (14.3% vs. 47.4%) [22]. Similar results were noted with the use of actinomycin-D chemoprophylaxis [23]. Although prophylactic chemotherapy has been shown to decrease the incidence of postmolar GTN in patients with high-risk complete molar pregnancy, it is not routinely recommended. The low morbidity of serial hCG determinations vs. the small but real risk of complications associated with chemotherapy justifies this approach. For patients with a rise or plateau in hCG levels, repeat curettage has been reported to induce remission without the need for chemotherapy [24–26]. In most cases of postmolar GTN, however, the persistent disease is intramyometrial and requires cytotoxic agents. The policy at the NETDC is to perform repeat curettage in conjunction with the first course of chemotherapy if there is residual tissue in the endometrial cavity or persistent bleeding.

Postsurgical Follow-Up

After evacuation (or hysterectomy), all patients require careful monitoring of postoperative hCG levels to facilitate the early diagnosis and treatment of GTN. Although hysterectomy eliminates the risk of nonmetastatic disease, the chance of metastases remains approximately 3–5% [11]. Therefore, it is essential to follow these patients in a manner similar to that used for those who undergo evacuation by suction. Serum hCG levels should be determined every week until undetectable for three consecutive weeks and then monthly for 6 months. A shorter follow-up may become the standard of care as recent data has shown that the risk of relapse is less than 1% after achieving a serum hCG level of <5 mIU/ml [27, 28].

The Cancer Committee of the International Federation of Gynecology and Obstetrics (FIGO) has established the following guidelines for the diagnosis of postmolar GTN: (1) four or more hCG values that have plateaued over at least 3 weeks; (2) a rise in hCG of ≥10% for three or more values over at least 2 weeks; (3) the presence of histological choriocarcinoma; and (4) persistence of hCG 5 months after molar evacuation [29].

Effective contraceptive during this time period is imperative, as the normal rise of hCG in a new gestation may be indistinguishable from neoplasia. Although data from the UK suggest that the use of oral contraceptives after molar evacuation is associated with developing GTN [30], multiple other series indicate that oral contraceptives may be safely prescribed without increasing the risk of subsequent neoplasia [31–33]. The use of intrauterine devices (IUDs) does not confer an increased risk of persistent disease [34]; however it is best to avoid their use when viable tumor may be still be present in the uterine cavity. Patients with a molar pregnancy can expect normal future reproductive function but should be counseled that they have a tenfold increased risk (1–2% incidence) of a second mole during subsequent pregnancies [35]. Subsequent pregnancies should be evaluated with US early in their course.

Gestational Trophoblastic Neoplasia

Gestational trophoblastic neoplasia (GTN) may occur after any gestational event and is diagnosed by the presence of persistently elevated hCG levels following a pregnancy. Nonmetastatic GTN occurs in about 15% of patients with CHM and in 1–4% of patients following PHM. It is distinguished from a molar pregnancy by the presence of invasion into the myometrium. Metastatic GTN develops after CHM in about 4% of patients and occurs infrequently after other pregnancies. The most common sites of metastases in GTN include the lung (80%), vagina (30%), brain (10%), and liver (10%) [17].

Metastatic GTN can have the histological pattern of molar tissue or choriocarcinoma (CCA). GTN occurring after nonmolar pregnancies displays the histological features of CCA, which is characterized by sheets of anaplastic syncytiotrophoblasts and cytotrophoblasts and has a propensity for early vascular invasion. CCA occurs in approximately 1/20,000–40,000 pregnancies. Approximately 50% of gestational CCAs develop after molar pregnancies, with 25% following term deliveries and 25% following other gestations [4]. Gestational CCA tends to metastasize early via the hematogenous route to the lungs, vagina, brain, liver, kidneys, gastrointestinal tract, and other distant organs. All patients with a diagnosis of CCA should undergo head, chest, and abdominal imaging.

Presenting signs of GTN include irregular vaginal bleeding, theca lutein cysts, uterine subinvolution, persistently elevated hCG levels, or signs of metastatic disease such as hemoptysis or neurological symptoms. Patients with GTN are categorized into low- and high-risk groups based on the absence or presence of high hCG values, large tumor burden, delay in diagnosis relative to the antecedent pregnancy, and prior failed chemotherapy (Table 4.2). Single-agent chemotherapy with either actinomycin-D or methotrexate is highly effective in the treatment of

Table 4.2 Scoring index for prognosis of gestational trophoblastic tumors

	Risk score			
Prognostic factor	0	1	2	4
Age (years)	<40	≥40		
Antecedent pregnancy	Hydatidiform mole	Abortion	Term pregnancy	
Interval from index pregnancy (months)	<4	4–6	7–12	>12
Pretreatment serum hCG (IU/ml)	<1,000	1,000 to <10,000	10,000 to <100,000	≥100,000
Largest tumor size, including uterus (cm)	<3	3–5	>5	
Site of metastases	Lung	Spleen, kidney	GI tract	Brain, liver
No. of metastases identified		1–4	5–8	>8
Previous failed chemotherapy			Single drug	Two or more drugs

GI gastrointestinal

Caution Box
***

Features of high-risk GTN:
Age ≥40 years
Antecedent term pregnancy
Interval of >12 months from pregnancy
Brain or liver metastases
Tumor size >5 cm
More than eight metastases
β-HCG ≥100,000

nonmetastatic disease and low-risk metastatic disease, with cure rates of 80–100% [7]. High-risk metastatic GTN generally requires combination chemotherapy to obtain remission. Nonmetastatic GTN can cause heavy bleeding and infection and is successfully treated by either chemotherapy or hysterectomy. Historically, hysterectomy has had a secondary role, being particularly reserved for patients with drug-resistant disease or significant hemorrhage.

Hysterectomy and GTN

The role of hysterectomy in GTN has been recently evaluated in several studies. A retrospective study from our institution identified 98 patients who underwent hysterectomy for GTN [36]. These patients were stratified into two groups – those who underwent hysterectomy before 1980 and those who underwent hysterectomy after 1980 – to identify whether the indications for hysterectomy are changing. Hysterectomy was performed for heavy bleeding in the early cohort in 14 (29%) of 49 patients but in only 4 (8%) of 49 patients in the later cohort. This is a statistically significant decline in the number of hysterectomies performed for heavy bleeding ($P=0.02$), likely related to early diagnosis and prompt treatment. In a series from the UK, including 31 patients undergoing hysterectomy as primary treatment for GTN, the indication was major hemorrhage in 18 (58%) patients [37].

In contrast, a series from the Philippines described different indications for hysterectomy performed at their center. Among 134 patients, 31 (24%) underwent hysterectomy for uterine rupture, with only 13 (9%) requiring hysterectomy for control of vaginal bleeding [38]. The authors commented that this may be related to delayed referrals resulting in disease that has perforated the uterus at the time of presentation. We recognize that hysterectomy may remain a mainstay of primary treatment for GTN in parts of the world where access to chemotherapy is limited.

Postterm Choriocarcinoma

Choriocarcinomas may present with irregular vaginal bleeding following an otherwise uncomplicated term pregnancy [39]. Women with persistent vaginal bleeding, lasting more than 6 weeks postpartum, warrant evaluation with a serum hCG test. Positive results should prompt consideration of retained placental tissue or a CCA. Both situations are indications for dilation and curettage, which is diagnostic and potentially therapeutic. If CCA is detected, the patient should undergo prompt evaluation for metastatic disease and begin appropriate chemotherapy.

Bleeding due to Vaginal Metastases

Among potential metastatic sites, GTN involving the vagina is the most likely to present with bleeding. However, vaginal metastases occur in only 4–11% of patients with GTN [40, 41]. Profuse bleeding may result from these vascular and friable lesions, which are most commonly located along the anterior vaginal wall. Significant bleeding necessitating blood transfusion occurred in 13 of the 804 patients in the series by Berry et al. Seven of these patients required one or more procedures for control of bleeding [40]. Yingna et al. [42] noted that 18 of 51 GTN patients (35.3%) with vaginal metastases presented with significant hemorrhage.

Hemorrhage may be controlled with packing, excision, over-sewing, uterine artery ligation (either with our without hysterectomy), or angiographic embolization of the hypogastric arteries.

Bleeding due to AV Malformations

Arteriovenous malformations (AVMs) in the uterine cavity have been described in the setting of molar pregnancy and GTN. Hypervascularity of the uterus may persist after molar pregnancies, even after resolution of hCG levels [43]. Patients with AVMs are at risk of uterine hemorrhage that may be life-threatening. Vascular malformation can cause vaginal or intraperitoneal bleeding in 1–2% of these patients [44, 45]. In addition to hysterectomy and uterine artery ligation, selective arterial embolization has also been described as curative [46]. In the Charing Cross series of 14 patients, 11 experienced successful control of hemorrhage with embolization. This more conservative approach allows preservation of fertility, although repeat embolization may be necessary to entirely control symptoms. Successful pregnancies after arterial embolization of AVMs in the setting of GTN have been described [47].

Placental-Site Trophoblastic Tumors

Placental-site trophoblastic tumors (PSTTs) are uncommon trophoblastic neoplasms characterized by the absence of chorionic villi and proliferation of intermediate cytotrophoblast cells. PSTT is a variant of CCA. Most patients in small case series have presented with irregular vaginal bleeding or amenorrhea [48]. The dimorphic population of syncytiotrophoblast and cytotrophoblast elements that are observed in CCA are lacking in PSTT. The intermediate trophoblastic cells that characterize PSTT secrete low levels of hCG in relation to their volume. PSTT is relatively less sensitive to chemotherapy than CCA. Therefore, it is important to distinguish it from CCA as management is different. Fortunately, PSTT less commonly metastasizes beyond the uterus, although lymphatic involvement has been described when deep myometrial invasion is present. Hysterectomy is the treatment of choice for nonmetastatic PSTT. Combination chemotherapy has been used successfully to treat recurrent or metastatic disease [49].

Summary

Despite the potentially serious outcome, most women with GTN can be successfully diagnosed and treated with preservation of normal reproductive function. Vaginal bleeding during early pregnancy is a common presenting symptom of molar pregnancy and should be evaluated with high-resolution US in combination with a serum hCG level to allow prompt diagnosis and treatment. Postpartum vaginal bleeding is usually related to retained products of conception but on rare occasions is due to GTN.

References

1. Berkowitz RS, Goldstein DP, Bernstein MR. Evolving concepts of molar pregnancy. J Reprod Med. 1991;36(1):40–4.
2. Yamashita K, Wake N, Araki T, Ichinoe K, Makoto K. Human lymphocyte antigen expression in hydatidiform mole: androgenesis following fertilization by a haploid sperm. Am J Obstet Gynecol. 1979;135(5):597–600.
3. Keep D, Zaragoza MV, Hassold T, Redline RW. Very early complete hydatidiform mole. Hum Pathol. 1996;27(7):708–13.
4. Szulman AE, Surti U. The syndromes of hydatidiform mole. II. Morphologic evolution of the complete and partial mole. Am J Obstet Gynecol. 1978;132(1):20–7.
5. Berkowitz RS, Goldstein DP. Management of molar pregnancy and gestational trophoblastic tumors. In: Knapp RC, Berkowitz RS, editors. Gynecologic oncology. New York: McGraw Hill; 1993. p. 328.
6. Benson CB, Genest DR, Bernstein MR, Soto-Wright V, Goldstein DP, Berkowitz RS. Sonographic appearance of first trimester complete hydatidiform moles. Ultrasound Obstet Gynecol. 2000;16(2):188–91.

7. Romero R, Horgan JG, Kohorn EI, Kadar N, Taylor KJ, Hobbins JC. New criteria for the diagnosis of gestational trophoblastic disease. Obstet Gynecol. 1985;66(4):553–8.
8. Genest DR, Laborde O, Berkowitz RS, Goldstein DP, Bernstein MR, Lage J. A clinicopathologic study of 153 cases of complete hydatidiform mole (1980–1990): histologic grade lacks prognostic significance. Obstet Gynecol. 1991;78(3 Pt 1):402–9.
9. Menczer J, Modan M, Serr DM. Prospective follow-up of patients with hydatidiform mole. Obstet Gynecol. 1980;55(3):346–9.
10. Thaker HM, Berlin A, Tycko B, et al. Immunohistochemistry for the imprinted gene product IPL/PHLDA2 for facilitating the differential diagnosis of complete hydatidiform mole. J Reprod Med. 2004;49(8):630–6.
11. Curry SL, Hammond CB, Tyrey L, Creasman WT, Parker RT. Hydatidiform mole: diagnosis, management, and long-term followup of 347 patients. Obstet Gynecol. 1975;45(1):1–8.
12. Kohorn EI. Theca lutein ovarian cyst may be pathognomonic for trophoblastic neoplasia. Obstet Gynecol. 1983;62(3 Suppl):80s–1s.
13. Soto-Wright V, Bernstein M, Goldstein DP, Berkowitz RS. The changing clinical presentation of complete molar pregnancy. Obstet Gynecol. 1995;86(5):775–9.
14. Berkowitz RS, Goldstein DP, Bernstein MR. Natural history of partial molar pregnancy. Obstet Gynecol. 1985;66(5):677–81.
15. Fine C, Bundy AL, Berkowitz RS, Boswell SB, Berezin AF, Doubilet PM. Sonographic diagnosis of partial hydatidiform mole. Obstet Gynecol. 1989;73(3 Pt 1):414–8.
16. Osathanondh R, Berkowitz RS, de Cholnoky C, Smith BS, Goldstein DP, Tyson JE. Hormonal measurements in patients with theca lutein cysts and gestational trophoblastic disease. J Reprod Med. 1986;31(3):179–83.
17. Berkowitz RS, Goldstein DP. Chorionic tumors. N Engl J Med. 1996;335(23):1740–8.
18. Hancock BW, Tidy JA. Current management of molar pregnancy. J Reprod Med. 2002;47(5):347–54.
19. Elias KM, Goldstein DP, Berkowitz RS. Complete hydatidiform mole in women older than age 50. J Reprod Med. 2010;55(5–6):208–12.
20. Orr Jr JW, Austin JM, Hatch KD, Shingleton HM, Younger JB, Boots LR. Acute pulmonary edema associated with molar pregnancies: a high-risk factor for development of persistent trophoblastic disease. Am J Obstet Gynecol. 1980;136(3):412–5.
21. Goldstein DP, Berkowitz RS. Prophylactic chemotherapy of complete molar pregnancy. Semin Oncol. 1995;22(2):157–60.
22. Kim DS, Moon H, Kim KT, Moon YJ, Hwang YY. Effects of prophylactic chemotherapy for persistent trophoblastic disease in patients with complete hydatidiform mole. Obstet Gynecol. 1986;67(5):690–4.
23. Limpongsanurak S. Prophylactic actinomycin D for high-risk complete hydatidiform mole. J Reprod Med. 2001;46(2):110–6.
24. van Trommel NE, Massuger LF, Verheijen RH, Sweep FC, Thomas CM. The curative effect of a second curettage in persistent trophoblastic disease: a retrospective cohort survey. Gynecol Oncol. 2005;99(1):6–13.
25. Pezeshki M, Hancock BW, Silcocks P, et al. The role of repeat uterine evacuation in the management of persistent gestational trophoblastic disease. Gynecol Oncol. 2004;95(3):423–9.
26. Goldstein DP, Garner EI, Feltmate CM, Berkowitz RS. The role of repeat uterine evacuation in the management of persistent gestational trophoblastic disease. Gynecol Oncol. 2004;95(3):421–2.
27. Wolfberg AJ, Growdon WB, Feltmate CM, et al. Low risk of relapse after achieving undetectable HCG levels in women with partial molar pregnancy. Obstet Gynecol. 2006;108(2):393–6.
28. Berkowitz RS, Goldstein DP. Clinical practice. Molar pregnancy. N Engl J Med. 2009;360(16):1639–45.
29. Kohorn EI. Persistent low-level "real" human chorionic gonadotropin: a clinical challenge and a therapeutic dilemma. Gynecol Oncol. 2002;85(2):315–20.
30. Stone M, Bagshawe KD. An analysis of the influences of maternal age, gestational age, contraceptive method, and the mode of primary treatment of patients with hydatidiform moles on the incidence of subsequent chemotherapy. Br J Obstet Gynaecol. 1979;86(10):782–92.

31. Curry SL, Schlaerth JB, Kohorn EI, et al. Hormonal contraception and trophoblastic sequelae after hydatidiform mole (a Gynecologic Oncology Group Study). Am J Obstet Gynecol. 1989;160(4):805–9. discussion 809–11.
32. Berkowitz RS, Goldstein DP, Marean AR, Bernstein M. Oral contraceptives and postmolar trophoblastic disease. Obstet Gynecol. 1981;58(4):474–7.
33. Costa HL, Doyle P. Influence of oral contraceptives in the development of post-molar trophoblastic neoplasia–a systematic review. Gynecol Oncol. 2006;100(3):579–85.
34. Gaffield ME, Kapp N, Curtis KM. Combined oral contraceptive and intrauterine device use among women with gestational trophoblastic disease. Contraception. 2009;80(4):363–71.
35. Garrett LA, Garner EI, Feltmate CM, Goldstein DP, Berkowitz RS. Subsequent pregnancy outcomes in patients with molar pregnancy and persistent gestational trophoblastic neoplasia. J Reprod Med. 2008;53(7):481–6.
36. Clark RM, Nevadunsky NS, Ghosh S, Goldstein DP, Berkowitz RS. The evolving role of hysterectomy in gestational trophoblastic neoplasia at the New England Trophoblastic Disease Center. J Reprod Med. 2010;55(5–6):194–8.
37. Alazzam M, Hancock BW, Tidy J. Role of hysterectomy in managing persistent gestational trophoblastic disease. J Reprod Med. 2008;53(7):519–24.
38. Cagayan MS, Magallanes MS. The role of adjuvant surgery in the management of gestational trophoblastic neoplasia. J Reprod Med. 2008;53(7):513–8.
39. Dobson LS, Gillespie AM, Coleman RE, Hancock BW. The presentation and management of post-partum choriocarcinoma. Br J Cancer. 1999;79(9–10):1531–3.
40. Berry E, Hagopian GS, Lurain JR. Vaginal metastases in gestational trophoblastic neoplasia. J Reprod Med. 2008;53(7):487–92.
41. Cagayan MS. Vaginal metastases complicating gestational trophoblastic neoplasia. J Reprod Med. 2010;55(5–6):229–35.
42. Yingna S, Yang X, Xiuyu Y, Hongzhao S. Clinical characteristics and treatment of gestational trophoblastic tumor with vaginal metastasis. Gynecol Oncol. 2002;84(3):416–9.
43. Cockshott WP, Hendrickse JP. Persistent arteriovenous fistulae following chemotherapy of malignant trophoblastic disease. Radiology. 1967;88(2):329–33.
44. Newlands ES, Bagshawe KD, Begent RH, Rustin GJ, Holden L, Dent J. Developments in chemotherapy for medium- and high-risk patients with gestational trophoblastic tumours (1979–1984). Br J Obstet Gynaecol. 1986;93(1):63–9.
45. McIvor J, Cameron EW. Pregnancy after uterine artery embolization to control haemorrhage from gestational trophoblastic tumour. Br J Radiol. 1996;69(823):624–9.
46. Lim AK, Agarwal R, Seckl MJ, Newlands ES, Barrett NK, Mitchell AW. Embolization of bleeding residual uterine vascular malformations in patients with treated gestational trophoblastic tumors. Radiology. 2002;222(3):640–4.
47. Garner EI, Meyerovitz M, Goldstein DP, Berkowitz RS. Successful term pregnancy after selective arterial embolization of symptomatic arteriovenous malformation in the setting of gestational trophoblastic tumor. Gynecol Oncol. 2003;88(1):69–72.
48. Gillespie AM, Liyim D, Goepel JR, Coleman RE, Hancock BW. Placental site trophoblastic tumour: a rare but potentially curable cancer. Br J Cancer. 2000;82(6):1186–90.
49. Seckl MJ, Sebire NJ, Berkowitz RS. Gestational trophoblastic disease. Lancet. 2010;376(9742): 717–29.

Chapter 5
Gynecological Cancer During Pregnancy

Kristel Van Calsteren and Frédéric Amant

Introduction

Vaginal blood loss during pregnancy can, rarely, be caused by an underlying gynecological malignancy. Cancer is the second leading cause of death in women during the reproductive years and complicates 0.06–0.10% of all pregnancies [1]. In Europe, this number translates into 3,000–5,000 new cases of cancer during pregnancy. As women in developed societies delay childbearing to the third or fourth decade of life, and the incidence of several malignancies rises with increasing age, this coincidence of cancer and pregnancy is likely to become more common in future [2].

The most common malignant tumors associated with pregnancy reflect the most frequently encountered cancer types in women 20–40 years of age. They include breast cancer, hematological malignancies, malignant melanoma, cervical cancer, and thyroid cancer [1, 3].

Gynecological cancers (i.e., cancer of the vulva, vagina, cervix uteri, uterine corpus, ovary, and fallopian tube) typically occur in postmenopausal women, except for cervical cancer. Cervical cancer is the second most common cancer among women worldwide due to the fact that it is the most common gynecological cancer in the developing world [4]. In unscreened populations, the risk of invasive cervical cancer peaks or reaches a plateau from about 35–55 years of age [5]. The increase starts during the second to early third decade of life [5]. This partial overlap with the reproductive era renders pregnant women susceptible to cervical cancer. In contrast, endometrial, vulvar, and ovarian cancer and sarcomas are diagnosed less frequently during the reproductive years. As a result, in the literature data on cancers of the

F. Amant (✉)
Division of Gynecological Oncology, Department of Obstetrics and Gynecology,
University Hospitals of Leuven, Herestraat 49, 3000 Leuven, Belgium
e-mail: Frederic.amant@uzleuven.be

E. Sheiner (ed.), *Bleeding During Pregnancy: A Comprehensive Guide*,
DOI 10.1007/978-1-4419-9810-1_5, © Springer Science+Business Media, LLC 2011

pelvic female reproductive system during pregnancy consist of only case reports or small series.

Cancer affecting the reproductive system during pregnancy is a complex situation that endangers two lives, the pregnant woman and the fetus. Thus, it requires specialized multidisciplinary care [6].

In this chapter, we address the steps in the diagnosis and treatment of gynecological cancers diagnosed during pregnancy. We focus on cervical cancer as it is the most frequently diagnosed tumor in this population.

Cervical Cancer

Epidemiology

The primary risk factor for cervical cancer is a cervical infection with high-risk human papillomavirus (HPV) (subtypes 16, 18, 31, 45), a sexually transmitted disease. After the age of 25 years, the risk of developing cervical cancer begins to increase, although this cancer, or its precancerous changes, can be diagnosed in young women in their early twenties and even their teens. Women who had sexual intercourse at an early age or women who have had many sexual partners are at an increased risk of cervical cancer. Furthermore, women who smoke and women with a weakened immune system are more likely to develop cervical cancer.

The incidence of cervical cancer in pregnancy is estimated to be 1–10 in 10,000 pregnancies, depending on the inclusion of carcinoma in situ and postpartum patients [7]. Approximately 30% of women diagnosed with cervical cancer are in their reproductive years, and 3% of cervical cancers are diagnosed during pregnancy [8].

Diagnosis

Diagnostic evaluation of cervical carcinoma during pregnancy includes a clinical and cytological evaluation, colposcopy, and if indicated directed biopsy, conization, and radiographic imaging examinations. Physiological changes associated with the pregnancy might render the diagnosis more difficult.

Signs and Symptoms

The presenting symptoms and signs of cervical carcinoma during pregnancy are dependent on the clinical stage at diagnosis and the lesion size. Most patients with early stage cervical cancer are asymptomatic at the time of diagnosis. Symptomatic patients may present with abnormal vaginal bleeding, mostly postcoitally, or discharge [8, 9].

Because the symptoms of cervical cancer are also seen in an uncomplicated pregnancy, diagnosis is often delayed to some extent. The average duration of symptoms before diagnosis of cervical cancer during pregnancy is 4.5 months [8].

During *clinical evaluation* complete visualization of the transformation zone is usually possible due to eversion of the squamocolumnar junction that occurs during pregnancy. Early in pregnancy, cervical lesions may be mistaken for an ectropion or a decidualized cervix. Later in pregnancy, the appearance of the lesion and its texture may change with cervical effacement, enlargement, and color changes [8].

Cervical Cytology and Colposcopy During Pregnancy

Abnormal cervical cytology occurs in approximately 5% of pregnancies. Indications for colposcopy are the same as those for nonpregnant patients.

The cervical glands and stroma undergo physiological alterations during pregnancy resulting in an increased cervical volume, stromal edema, glandular hyperplasia, and increased vascularization that alter cytological and colposcopic interpretation [10, 11]. However, if the cytologist and colposcopist are aware of the pregnant state, their reliability is not decreased [7, 11, 12].

Colposcopic arguments for malignancy are based on the same morphological features as in the nonpregnant women: vascular pattern, intercapillary distance, surface pattern, color tone, and clarity of demarcation of the lesion [13].

In case of alterations, a colposcopy-guided biopsy should not be postponed as the colposcopic/cytological concordance can be worse postpartum [14].

Caution Box

The high estrogen levels during pregnancy result in important changes in the glands and stroma of the cervix that can lead to an overestimation of cervical lesions [10, 15]. The cytological differential diagnosis of cellular atypia in pregnant and postpartum women is broad and includes the following.

1. Endocervical gland hyperplasia such as microglandular hyperplasia
2. Pregnancy-related cellular changes such as ectropion, decidual cells, Arias-Stella reaction, and trophoblastic cells
3. Neoplastic and preneoplastic lesions of both squamous and glandular origin

---

Cervical Biopsy and Conization

Colposcopically directed biopsies performed during pregnancy appear to be safe, accurate, and reliable. The concordance between the histological findings of a directed biopsy and the final diagnosis was complete or within one degree of severity in 83.7% and 95.9%, respectively [11, 14]. The risk of bleeding is estimated to be 1–3%, and late in pregnancy it exceptionally induces premature labor [8, 14].

Both the diagnostic importance and technical issues of cervical conization during pregnancy – large loop excision of the transformation zone, loop electrosurgical excision procedure, or traditional cold-knife cone biopsy – deserve special attention. Lesions are usually located on the ectocervix during pregnancy, and a flat cone is appropriate. Its use during pregnancy has been limited by the relatively high complication rate for both mother and fetus. Due to the high rate of positive margins (up to 50%), conization during pregnancy should be seen as a diagnostic, not a therapeutic, procedure [14, 16–18]. The only absolute indication for conization during pregnancy is to confirm or rule out (micro) invasive disease when such a diagnosis would alter the timing or mode of delivery [19]. Therefore, the use of cone biopsy during pregnancy has been reserved for patients with evidence or suspicion of invasive disease on biopsy and/or colposcopy (or in cases of a high grade Papanicolaou smear and no satisfactory colposcopy). Otherwise conization has to be postponed until after delivery [12, 17].

The most frequent complications are hemorrhage (5–15%), spontaneous abortion (25%), premature labor/delivery, and infection [14, 16, 17]. The risk of severe bleeding increases with the duration of pregnancy: insignificant during the first trimester, 5% during the second trimester, and 10% during the third trimester [8, 16, 17]. Abortions during first and second trimester occur in 7–50% [12, 14]. In 12% of the cases there is prematurity, especially among those in which conization is done late in pregnancy [17]. To minimize the risk of spontaneous abortion and blood loss, the optimal time for cervical conization is the second trimester, preferably between 14 and 20 weeks of gestation [8]. Endocervical curettage is discouraged during pregnancy owing to the risk of premature rupture of the membrane.

Caution Box

Indications for conization differ between pregnant and nonpregnant women

Nonpregnant patients	Pregnant patients
Cyto/colpo/histo discrepancy (≥2 grades)	Evaluation of possible microinvasive or invasive cervical carcinoma when such a diagnosis would alter the timing or mode of delivery
Positive endocervical curettage	
Microscopic invasive carcinoma on colposcopy-directed biopsy	
Glandular dysplasia	
Adenocarcinoma in situ	
Inadequate colposcopy	

Management

Preinvasive Cervical Lesions

In cases with well visualized and identified cervical intraepithelial neoplasia (CIN) (on cytology, colposcopy, and biopsy), the lesion can be observed every 6–8 weeks using cytology and colposcopy. Additional directed biopsies are required only if progression to suspected invasive disease is found on colposcopy. At 8–12 weeks postpartum, patients are reevaluated either by cytology, colposcopy, or histology for a final diagnosis and treatment.

The CIN lesions might have been diagnosed and treated with conization performed to exclude (micro)invasive disease. It should be remembered, however, that conization during pregnancy results in high rates of positive section margins and residual disease, and retreatment of premalignant disease during the postpartum period may be required.

Progression of a clearly identified premalignant lesion to (micro)invasive disease is rare during pregnancy [12, 16, 20–22]. Studies report that 10–70% of dysplasia cases diagnosed during pregnancy regress and sometimes even disappear postpartum; persistence in the severity of cervical neoplasia is reported in 25–47% and progression in 3–30% [11, 12, 16, 20–22]. These numbers support a conservative policy during pregnancy with adequate follow-up and definitive management during the postpartum period.

In the presence of preinvasive disease, a vaginal delivery is allowed. Albeit, it does not increase the rate of regression when compared to that seen after cesarean section.

Invasive Cervical Cancer

When cervical cancer complicates pregnancy, both maternal and fetal considerations determine management decisions. The management of cervical cancer during pregnancy depends on the gestational age at diagnosis, the stage of the disease, and the patient's desire to continue the pregnancy and for future fertility.

Staging

To determine the optimal treatment for a patient, exact staging of the disease is required, even during pregnancy.

Ultrasonography (US) and magnetic resonance imaging (MRI) are relative safe and widely used during pregnancy [23, 24]. Radiographic studies expose the fetus to irradiation (Table 5.1). The threshold dose for fetal damage is estimated to be 10–20 cGy. The highest fetal irradiation dosages are generated by computed tomography; therefore, these examination should be replaced by US or MRI in pregnant women. On the other hand, chest radiography with abdominal shielding can be performed safely during pregnancy.

Pregnancy represents an exceptional opportunity for the early diagnosis of cervical cancer as visual inspection, cytological examination, and bimanual palpation are considered part of routine antenatal care [1]. Pregnant women have a two- to threefold higher probability of being diagnosed during an operable stage of disease.

Table 5.1 Approximate fetal absorbed doses during imaging studies

Procedure	Fetal dose (cGy)
Chest radiography (AP, lateral)	0.00006
Abdominal radiography	0.15–0.26
Pelvic radiography	0.2–0.35
Intravenous pyelography	0.4–0.9
Barium enema	0.3–4
Dorsal spine	<0.001
Lumbar spine	0.4–0.6
Lumbosacral spine	0.2–0.6
Mammography	0.1–0.4
Computed tomography	
Thorax	0.1–1.3
Abdomen	0.8–3.0
Pelvis	2.5–8.9
^{99m}Tc bone scan	0.15–0.20

Data are from Toppenberg et al. [25]

A review of the literature on 494 cases of cervical cancer during pregnancy showed that 83.9% of patients were diagnosed in stage I, 11.8% in stage II, 3.1% in stage III, and 1.2% in stage IV [7]. This observation might be explained by the frequent pelvic examinations performed throughout prenatal care, whereas advanced stages would prevent conception. The distribution of histological subtypes was as follows: 82.7% squamous carcinoma, 10.1% adenocarcinoma, and 7.1% adenosquamous carcinoma, which is similar to the distribution in nonpregnant women [7].

FIGO classification of carcinoma of the cervix uteri [26]

Stage I: carcinoma strictly confined to the cervix (extension to the corpus would be disregarded)
  IA: invasive carcinoma; can be diagnosed only by microscopy; deepest invasion ≤5 mm and largest extension ≥7 mm
    IA1: stromal invasion ≤3.0 mm in depth and extension of ≤7.0 mm
    IA2: stromal invasion of >3.0 mm and not >5.0 mm with an extension of not >7.0 mm
  IB: clinically visible lesions limited to the cervix uteri or preclinical cancers greater than stage IA[a]
    IB1: clinically visible lesion ≤4.0 cm in greatest dimension
    IB2: clinically visible lesion >4.0 cm in greatest dimension
Stage II: carcinoma invades beyond the uterus but not to the pelvic wall or to the lower third of the vagina
  IIA: without parametrial invasion
    IIA1: clinically visible lesion ≤4.0 cm in greatest dimension
    IIA2: clinically visible lesion >4 cm in greatest dimension
  IIB: with obvious parametrial invasion
Stage III: tumor extends to the pelvic wall and/or involves lower third of the vagina and/or causes hydronephrosis or a nonfunctioning kidney[b]
  IIIA: tumor involves lower third of the vagina, with no extension to the pelvic wall

(continued)

FIGO classification of carcinoma of the cervix uteri [26]

IIIB: extension to the pelvic wall and/or hydronephrosis or a nonfunctioning kidney
Stage IV: carcinoma extends beyond the true pelvis or involves (biopsy-proven) the mucosa of
       the bladder or rectum; bullous edema, as such, does not permit a case to be allotted to
       stage IV
  IVA: spread of the growth to adjacent organs
  IVB: spread to distant organs

[a]All macroscopically visible lesions – even with superficial invasion – are allotted to stage IB carcinomas. Invasion is limited to a measured stromal invasion with a maximum depth of 5.00 mm and a horizontal extension of not <7.00 mm. Depth of invasion should not be <5.00 mm, measured from the base of the epithelium of the original tissue, superficial or glandular. The depth of invasion should always be reported in millimeters, even in cases of "early (minimal) stromal invasion" (~1 mm). The involvement of vascular/lymphatic spaces should not change the stage allotment.

[b]On rectal examination, there is no cancer-free space between the tumor and the pelvic wall. All cases with hydronephrosis or a nonfunctioning kidney are included unless they are known to be due to another cause.

Treatment

Termination of pregnancy and standard oncological treatment. When the patient, after thorough counseling, decides to end the pregnancy, standard treatment can be executed. Radical hysterectomy of a pregnant uterus is possible. From the second trimester onward, removal of the fetus by hysterotomy improves the accessibility of the pelvis. Dissection of the anatomical structures is not more difficult during pregnancy. Sufficient experience is advised given the increased blood supply. Alternatively, chemoradiotherapy can be used. Irradiation of the pelvis during the first trimester results in spontaneous abortion. During the second trimester, abortion may be protracted and interfere with the radiotherapy. Surgical evacuation (hysterotomy or suction curettage) prior to the start with chemoradiotherapy facilitates subsequent chemoradiotherapy.

Delivery and standard oncological treatment. When fetal maturity is achieved, or if the fetus is mature at the time of diagnosis, immediate delivery – if necessary after steroid therapy to achieve fetal lung maturity – followed by definitive treatment of the mother is preferred. For motivated patients with stage Ia or early stage Ib cervical cancer, a planned treatment delay, with close surveillance, to achieve fetal maturity is a reasonable option [7, 9, 27].

Classic cesarean delivery followed by radical hysterectomy is the recommended treatment. In our experience, a radical hysterectomy is not more hazardous after cesarean section than when done in nonpregnant women. Although a large uterus might render its handling less practical, dissection of the parametria, ureteral mobilization, and blood loss do not seem to differ significantly from that in the nongravid patient. With an advanced-stage lesion, whole-pelvic irradiation may be started immediately postpartum; intracavitary irradiation then follows the external treatment.

Oncological treatment during pregnancy. Limited experience with invasive cervical cancer diagnosed during pregnancy renders every treatment proposal experimental. Therefore, when the patient decides to continue the pregnancy, the experimental nature of the cancer treatment during pregnancy and the potential risks should be discussed with her. The proposed treatment depends on gestational age and the stage of the disease [6].

During the first trimester, a conservative approach is proposed to reach the second trimester. During the second trimester, the stage of the disease determines the treatment strategy. Stage Ia1 disease is treated by a flat cone biopsy [28]. These patients should be closely followed by clinical examination throughout the pregnancy with colposcopy performed every 4 weeks. At 6–8 weeks postpartum, patients should be reevaluated (cytology, colposcopy, and histology) for postpartum diagnostic status. Depending on the postpartum cytology or in case the depth of invasion is in question, repeat conization should be considered [8].

From stage Ia2 on, interventions including lymphadenectomy, neoadjuvant chemotherapy (NACT), and trachelectomy during pregnancy can be considered. Lymphadenectomy is performed during gestation when pregnancy or fertility-saving surgery is possible. Pelvic lymphadenectomy is performed to identify high-risk disease that would exclude a pregnancy-saving policy. A retroperitoneal laparotomy approach or laparoscopy [29–31] could potentially help minimize uterine manipulation and hence contractility. The pathologist should be aware of the pregnant state, as decidual changes in the pelvic lymph nodes may mimic malignant disease [32–36].

Neoadjuvant chemotherapy during pregnancy can be used to stabilize or reduce the size of a cervical cancer [27, 37–43]. Chemotherapy for cervical cancer should be platinum-based, but addition of paclitaxel increases the response rate [44]. During pregnancy, paclitaxel-carboplatin three times a week is proposed, and the number of cycles is guided by the presence of fetal maturity. However, a minimum of two and a maximum of four cycles are advised. When only one cycle of chemotherapy is needed to attain fetal maturity, a waiting policy is preferred.

Trachelectomy has been described as an abdominal [45, 46] or vaginal [47] procedure. Experience during pregnancy is limited, however, and the technique requires sufficient surgical skills. It may be associated with large volumes of blood loss (irrespective of the approach), and the risk of pregnancy loss is considerable [45]. The experimental nature of this approach needs to be addressed.

An algorithm for stage IA2–IB1 <2 cm is presented in Fig. 5.1. In the absence of nodal metastasis, NACT followed by conservative surgery (e.g., trachelectomy) can be considered. However, standard treatment depends on the local policy and is radical hysterectomy or chemoradiotherapy.

An algorithm for stage IB1 2- to 4-cm tumors is presented in Fig. 5.2. Lymphadenectomy is mandatory but can be performed after NACT. The potential to preserve the pregnancy depends mainly on the nodal status and the response to NACT.

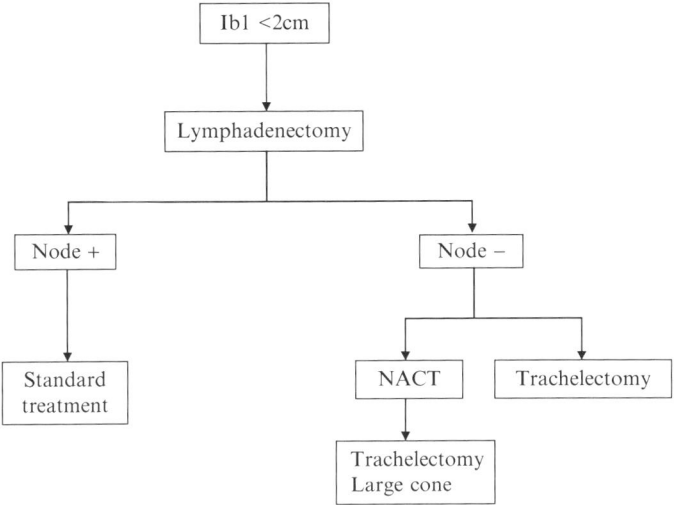

Fig. 5.1 Algorithm for the treatment of cervical cancer stage Ib1, <2 cm treated during the second trimester of pregnancy in patients wishing to preserve the pregnancy and fertility [6]

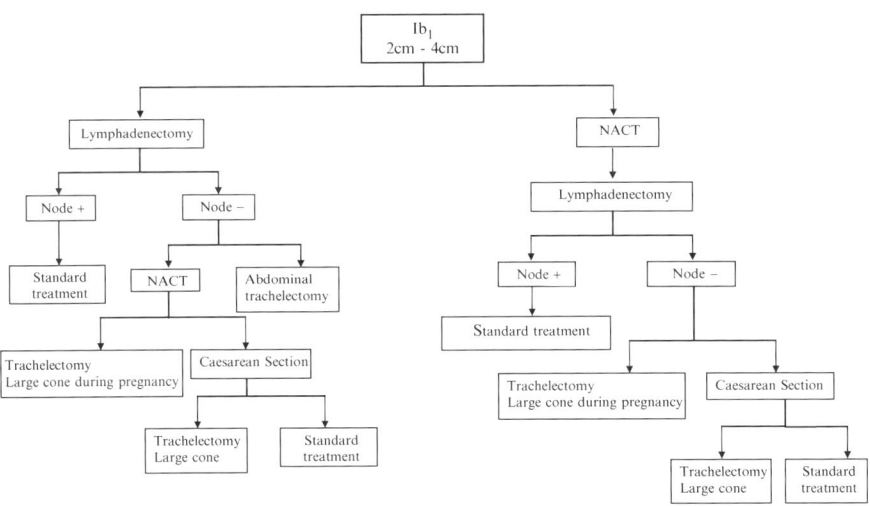

Fig. 5.2 Algorithm for the treatment of cervical cancer stage Ib1, 2–4 cm treated during the second trimester of pregnancy in patients wishing to preserve the pregnancy and fertility [6]

An algorithm for stage IB2–IIB is presented in Fig. 5.3. For these tumors, fertility-sparing surgery has not been sufficiently evaluated. Definitive treatment is performed after delivery. NACT during pregnancy can be applied until fetal maturity, preferably >35 weeks. Cesarean section is followed by the final treatment. In case of a good response (residual tumor <4 cm), fertility-sparing surgery can be performed by an experienced surgeon in an experimental setting, or standard

Fig. 5.3 Algorithm for the treatment of cervical cancer stage Ib2–IIB treated during the second trimester of pregnancy in patients wishing to preserve the pregnancy and fertility [6]

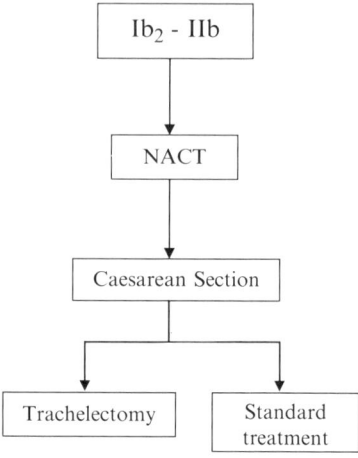

Table 5.2 Recommendations for maternal and fetal surveillance when pregnant women undergo surgery

Anesthesia	Position pregnant patients in left lateral tilt
	Prevent hypoxia, hypotension, and hypoglycemia
	Adequate postoperative analgesia
Fetal monitoring	Screening ultrasonography before surgery
	Assessment fetal well-being immediately before and after surgery
Uterine monitoring	Before and after surgery
Lung maturation	Dexamethasone or betamethasone 24 h before interventions between 24 and 34 weeks
Tocolytic drugs	Case-related: to be discussed with obstetrician
	Consider when uterine manipulation is expected
	Should be started in case of preterm labor
Thrombosis prophylaxis	Low-molecular-weight heparin recommended
Laparoscopy	Open technique
	Limit pressure (maximum 15 mmHg) and time (<90 min) of pneumoperitoneum

These recommendations are based on material in Amant et al. [6]

treatment can be used. Standard treatment is mandatory for nonresponders. Thus, for stage IB2–IIB, lymphadenectomy is postponed until after delivery, when radical trachelectomy or standard treatment is chosen. During the third trimester, fetal maturity is awaited, and a cesarean section followed by standard treatment is proposed.

Surgery during pregnancy. Anesthesia is safe during pregnancy if physiological adaptations for the gestation are considered [48]. The most important recommendations for maternal and fetal surveillance during surgery are summarized in Table 5.2. Adequate maternal monitoring is crucial for preventing hypoxia, hypotension, and hypoglycemia. Pregnant patients should be positioned in the left lateral tilt position to prevent caval compression. Peroperative fetal monitoring is always difficult to interpret and is only useful if clinically relevant. Fetal monitoring during surgery for gynecological cancers is mostly not feasible. Cardiotocography, Doppler scanning (Doptone), or US just before and after the surgery may be useful to exclude direct fetal damage associated with the surgery. With regard to fetal resuscitation, the local policy should be followed.

Surgery might slightly increase preterm delivery, but the numbers are difficult to interpret because there have been no comparisons with a normal pregnant population.

There is no literature to support the prophylactic use of tocolysis in cases of surgery during pregnancy. When signs of preterm labor are present perioperatively, tocolytic agents such as nifedipine, atosiban, or indomethacin (<32 weeks) should be considered [49–52].

Laparoscopic surgery during pregnancy is safe and effective when performed in experienced hands [53].

Chemotherapy and radiotherapy during pregnancy. The potential risk of fetal damage induced by cytotoxic treatment largely depends on the duration of exposure. With regard to this point, a pregnancy can be divided into three stages: fertilization/implantation, organogenesis, and fetal development.

During the first 10 days after conception (fertilization/implantation), cells are omnipotent and can develop in the three embryological layers. Viability depends on the number of cells killed during treatment, which results in an "all-or-nothing" situation. When sufficient cells remain, the embryo develops normally. When too many cells are damaged, a miscarriage occurs. The most vulnerable phase is between 10 days and 8 weeks after conception (organogenesis). Cytotoxic therapy may interfere with organogenesis. The potential for fetal damage varies depending on the agents and dosages used. After single-agent chemotherapy, 7–17% malformations are seen, after combination chemotherapy, the risk increases to 25%. Excluding the folic acid antagonists, a risk of 6% is reported [54]. After radiotherapy, fetal malformations are expected to occur from a threshold dose of 100 mSv [55]. The type of malformation depends on the time of exposure during embryological development. The most frequently described malformations are skeletal problems (face and limbs).

To prevent malformations, administration of chemotherapy and radiotherapy is contraindicated until 10 weeks' gestational age (=duration of amenorrhea). Generally, a "safety period" of 2–4 weeks is added, allowing chemotherapy and radiotherapy to start from a gestational age of 12–14 weeks.

During the second and third trimesters of pregnancy, organogenesis is completed with the exception of the eyes, gonads, and central nervous system. Consequently, no major malformations due to cytotoxic treatment are expected. Nevertheless, growth restriction, prematurity, intrauterine and neonatal death, and hematopoietic suppression have been reported after exposure to chemotherapy or a fetal radiation dose exceeding the threshold of 100 mSv. Moreover, potential problems of neurodevelopmental delay, sterility, carcinogenesis, and genetic defects have to be considered over the long term [56–58].

The most effective cytotoxic drugs for cervical cancer are platinum and paclitaxel. Therapeutic pelvic irradiation induces severe or lethal consequences for the fetus and is not consistent with preserving the pregnancy.

Platinum derivates have a relative low molecular weight (371.3 g/mol for carboplatin) and are known to bind only 24–50% of the plasma proteins [59]. In a recent pharmacokinetic study in baboons, a platinum transfer of around 50% was noted [60]. This relative important transfer fits with the expectations based on the molecular drug characteristics. Review of the literature revealed 37 reported cases of cisplatin exposure during pregnancy and 8 of carboplatin exposure [6]. In the literature, one child was diagnosed with moderate bilateral hearing loss, one child with ventriculomegaly, and one child with microphthalmos after exposure to combination chemotherapy with cisplatin (Dartmouth regimen) during the first trimester [6, 61]. Normal neonatal outcomes have been described in all carboplatin-exposed children. However, either detectable cisplatin levels or platinum DNA adducts were observed in neonates who were exposed to platinum; DNA adducts were observed in neonates who were exposed to platinum derivates during the third trimester, providing evidence for a late-onset transplacental transfer of these drugs. Based on a better toxicity profile, it is recommended that carboplatin is used instead of cisplatin if it has been evaluated regarding the respective tumor entity [6].

A recent pharmacokinetic study in baboons showed a very low concentration of taxanes in fetal plasma. Tissue drug levels revealed a slow and, compared to maternal drug levels, relatively low concentration of taxanes in the fetal compartment [60]. Paclitaxel [molecular weight (MW) 853.9 g/mol] and docetaxel (MW 861.9 g/mol) are highly lipid-soluble, have a wide tissue distribution, are highly protein-bound (>80–90%) and have a long half-life [62]. Furthermore, taxanes are substrates for P-glycoprotein, which is an efflux transporter for various xenobiotics. P-glycoprotein is expressed in bile canaliculi and contributes to their excretion, but it is also postulated as a protective mechanism against toxic xenobiotics in the human placenta [63]. Binding of taxanes to this placental transporter might explain the rather slow increase in fetal (tissue) concentrations. Paclitaxel has been used during pregnancy in 25 cases with a normal neonatal outcome [64, 65].

Chemotherapy should not be administered after 35 weeks because spontaneous labor becomes more likely. This policy minimizes the risk of neutropenia at the time of delivery. Furthermore, neonates, especially preterm babies, have limited capacity to metabolize and eliminate drugs due to liver and renal immaturity. The delay of delivery after chemotherapy allows fetal drug excretion via the placenta [66]. Chemotherapy can be restarted when needed after delivery.

On the other hand, pregnancy is associated with important changes in hemodynamics, renal and hepatic function, and protein binding, among others. Related to these adaptations, pharmacokinetic profiles were altered during pregnancy by various types of drug, among which are some chemotherapeutic agents [48, 63, 67, 68]. In comparison to the nonpregnant state, a decreased maximum plasma concentration (C_{max}), reduced plasma drug exposure (area under the curve, AUC), and increased distribution volume and drug clearance were described in several patients for paclitaxel, carboplatin, doxorubicin, and epirubicin [67, 68].

The pharmacodynamic (antitumor activity and toxicity in relation to the dose administered) consequences of the reduced plasma drug exposure are difficult to predict and require further research. Yet, there are no arguments that pregnant cancer patients have a worse prognosis than nonpregnant patients when the same dosage regimens of chemotherapy are used. Therefore, currently it is recommended to maintain the standard dosage regimens [69].

Obstetrical Management

Prenatal care in women diagnosed with cancer during pregnancy should be performed as in a high-risk obstetrical unit. It is important to estimate correctly the fetal risk caused by the maternal disease and treatment. Therefore, before starting staging examinations and treatment, US of the fetus should be performed to ensure that the fetus has undergone normal development and growth to date [6].

If cytotoxic treatment is administered during pregnancy, the fetal morphology, growth, and well-being must be evaluated by sonographic screening and, if indicated, by Doppler examination including the measurement of peak systolic velocity of the middle cerebral artery, which is a measure of fetal anemia [70]. In the case of abnormal findings, more intense fetal monitoring or even (preterm) delivery may be required. After treatment, it is important to consider fetal well-being and counsel patients to be alert when contractions occur as an increased incidence in preterm contractions was reported after cytotoxic treatment during pregnancy [3].

The timing of delivery should be balanced according to the oncological treatment schedule and the maturation of the fetus. As in noncancer patients, term delivery (≥37 weeks) should be the aim [3]. In the situation that preterm delivery is inevitable, fetal lung maturation should be considered and managed according to local policy.

The mode of delivery is determined by the presence or absence of tumor. When the cervix is cleared of tumor, a vaginal delivery is possible. In the presence of tumor, cesarean section is the preferred route of delivery to prevent (fatal) recurrence in the episiotomy scar [7, 71–78]. Because abdominal wall recurrence has also been described following cesarean section [79, 80] – although fewer have been found – a wound-protective system or a corporeal uterine incision might be useful when the tumor is large.

Although placental metastases from cervical cancer have been described in only one case, histopathological examination of the placenta is advisable [81, 82]. Primary inhibition of milk production is needed because especially lipophilic agents such as taxanes can accumulate in the milk.

Prognosis

It appears that pregnancy-associated cervical carcinoma has an overall better prognosis than that in the nonpregnant population; it is because the relatively high proportion of patients with early stage disease. However, after stratifying for stage, there were no differences between the pregnant and nonpregnant groups with regard to tumor characteristics, the course of the disease, survival analyses, or the rate of complications associated with the treatment [7]. However, larger numbers are required to confirm a lack of impact of pregnancy on the maternal prognosis.

Obstetrical and neonatal outcome is mainly determined by fetal maturity at delivery. Children prenatally exposed to chemotherapy during the second or third trimester of pregnancy have an overall good short-term outcome. However, data on long-term outcomes are lacking [3].

Vulvar Cancer During Pregnancy

Epidemiological evidence to date suggests that vulva carcinogenesis originates from two etiological pathways [83]. The first type, often seen in women over the age of 50 years, is associated with nonneoplastic epithelial disorders. The second type, often seen in women under the age of 50 years, is frequently multifocal and is associated with human papilloma virus infection [83]. Approximately 26% of vulvar intraepithelial neoplasia (VIN) and 19% of invasive vulvar cancers occur in women younger than 40 years [84]. Although single cases of leiomyosarcoma, angiomyxoma, epithelioid sarcoma, and melanoma during pregnancy have been reported [85–88], experience has mainly been with VIN and squamous vulvar cancer.

Diagnosis of VIN is made on a biopsy specimen. VIN can be treated with laser skinning or surgical excision at every stage of pregnancy. Invasive (>1 mm) vulvar cancer with clinically negative nodes during pregnancy should be treated as in nonpregnant women with hemi- or total vulvectomy and uni- or bilateral inguinofemoral lymphadenectomy or the sentinel procedure with technetium-99 m (^{99m}Tc) [6, 89, 90].

Narrow margins should be avoided because recurrence during pregnancy has been described [91]; moreover, since postoperative radiotherapy during pregnancy is contraindicated. From a technical point of view, the increased vascularization of the pelvis during pregnancy increases the perioperative blood loss, and so meticulous hemostasis is the aim. After surgery for vulvar cancer, the route of delivery should be discussed with the gynecological oncologist. Problematic wound healing, important scarring, and a periuretral or perianal scar are considered relative contraindications for a vaginal delivery.

The prognosis is poor if inguinal nodes are involved. Adequate treatment is needed without delay. There is little evidence of a benefit with chemotherapy. Termination of pregnancy with immediate treatment is advocated during the first and second trimesters in patients with metastatic inguinofemoral lymph nodes. During the third trimester, delivery followed by standard treatment is suggested in these patients. Given the potential for spilling into the episiotomy wound and the subsequent risk of an episiotomy scar recurrence, cesarean section is preferred.

Vulvar melanoma deserves the same treatment in pregnant women as in those who are not pregnant. Patients harboring poor-prognosis disease should be informed about the high risk of relapse and death. Metastatic melanoma carries a risk of placental involvement with an approximately 22% risk of fetal metastasis [81, 88].

Endometrial Cancer During Pregnancy

Here, we define endometrial cancer related to pregnancy as any endometrial cancer diagnosed during pregnancy or during the puerperium (defined as the period 6 weeks after delivery). Using our definition, we found 28 published cases [92–97]. Diagnosis was made during curettage ($n=17$, 61%), second–third trimester/at birth ($n=8$, 28%) or during the puerperium ($n=3$, 11%). The distribution of pathological type and grading was as follows: grade I, endometrioid ($n=21$, 75%); grade 2–3, endometrioid ($n=6$, 21%) or serous ($n=1$, 4%). In all but one case, the uterus was empty when the diagnosis was made [98]. In the absence of a fetus, standard treatment for endometrial cancer should be offered.

Genital Sarcoma During Pregnancy

Genital sarcomas are rarely seen during pregnancy. A review on genital sarcomas during pregnancy revealed 40 reported cases between 1955 and 2007 [99]. Most of the cases were uterine sarcoma (37.5%) followed by retroperitoneal sarcoma (27.5%), vulvar sarcoma (22.5%), and vaginal sarcoma (12.5%). The mean age of the patients was 27.8 ± 7.0 years.

Due to a low index of suspicion, there was often a delay in diagnosis. Three major symptoms of genital sarcoma during pregnancy are a growing mass, abdominal pain, and vaginal bleeding, which are similar to the symptoms seen with the nongravid genital sarcoma. However, many cases presented with nonspecific signs and symptoms that are normal during pregnancy.

If a physician encounters a rapidly growing uterine myoma during pregnancy, the tumor is most likely a benign uterine myoma, as sarcomas are rare. Although sarcoma during pregnancy is an extremely unusual clinical entity, any suspicious symptoms should be appropriately investigated. Careful examination is mandatory whenever pelvic examination, US, or surgical intervention is performed. Close observation is needed especially when a definitive tissue diagnosis is not available.

Genital sarcomas, principally leiomyosarcomas, endometrial stromal sarcomas, and adenosarcomas, contain estrogen and progesterone receptors acting as growth factors, which have great potential to induce tumor progression. Estrogen and progesterone receptors are expressed, respectively, in 26–87% and 17–80% of uterine leiomyosarcomas. Pregnancy is characterized by excess placental hormones, which potentially affect these hormone receptors in sarcomas.

Genital sarcomas have affected the pregnancy outcomes in the following aspects compared with a pregnancy without cancer: preterm labor, placenta previa, breech presentation, intrauterine growth restriction (IUGR), and cesarean delivery. The incidence of preterm labor was similar, and the percentage of IUGR infants was higher compared with those from a noncancer pregnancy (13.3–18.2% vs. 10% and 12.5% vs. 4.0%, respectively). The increased incidence of abdominal deliveries (50.0%) and breech fetus positions (7.5%) may be explained by the characteristic location of the tumor in the genital area.

In this review, in more than 80% of cases there was a live birth, and fetal preservation did not alter the prognosis. The 5-year survival rate for women with a genital sarcoma during pregnancy was 17%, which is similar to that of women with stage II–IV sarcoma who were not pregnant (8–12%).

Conclusion

Although rather rare, vaginal bleeding during pregnancy can be caused by gynecological cancer. Of all gynecological cancers, cervical cancer is most frequently seen during pregnancy as a cause of bleeding. The occurrence of vulvar and endometrial cancer and genital sarcomas has been described during pregnancy. However, current knowledge is limited to case reports.

Most important is to consider the option of a malignancy in the differential diagnosis of vaginal bleeding during pregnancy. All abnormal vaginal bleeding or discharge during pregnancy should be carefully evaluated; and in case of a clinically suspicious lesion, additional technical examinations and biopsies should be performed. For cervical cancer, a Papanicolaou smear and colposcopy should be undertaken, as in nonpregnant women. The only absolute indication for conization during pregnancy is to confirm or rule out (micro)invasive disease when such a diagnosis would alter the timing or mode of delivery. Preinvasive disease can be managed conservatively during pregnancy. For invasive disease, a multidisciplinary approach is mandatory because the stage, gestational age, and patient's desire to continue pregnancy will determine the treatment policy. When the cervix is cleared of tumor, a vaginal delivery is possible. In the presence of tumor, cesarean section is the preferred route of delivery to prevent (fatal) recurrence in the episiotomy scar. Stratified for stage, the overall prognosis appears to be similar to that for women who are not pregnant.

References

1. Pavlidis NA. Coexistence of pregnancy and malignancy. Oncologist. 2002;7:279–87.
2. Rendall M, Couet C, Lappegard T, et al. First births by age and education in Britain, France and Norway. *Popul Trends* 2005;Autumn:27–34.
3. Van Calsteren K, Heyns L, De Smet F, et al. Cancer during pregnancy: an analysis of 215 patients emphasizing the obstetrical and the neonatal outcomes. J Clin Oncol. 2010;28:683–9.
4. Sankaranarayanan R, Ferlay J. Worldwide burden of gynaecological cancer: the size of the problem. Best Pract Res Clin Obstet Gynaecol. 2006;20:207–25.
5. Gustafsson L, Ponten J, Zack M, et al. International incidence rates of invasive cervical cancer after introduction of cytological screening. Cancer Causes Control. 1997;8:755–63.
6. Amant F, Van Calsteren K, Halaska MJ, et al. Gynecologic cancers in pregnancy: guidelines of an international consensus meeting. Int J Gynecol Cancer. 2009;19 Suppl 1:S1–12.
7. Van Calsteren K, Vergote I, Amant F. Cervical neoplasia during pregnancy: diagnosis, management and prognosis. Best Pract Res Clin Obstet Gynaecol. 2005;19:611–30.

8. Nguyen C, Montz FJ, Bristow RE. Management of stage I cervical cancer in pregnancy. Obstet Gynecol Surv. 2000;55:633–43.
9. Duggan B, Muderspach LI, Roman LD, et al. Cervical cancer in pregnancy: reporting on planned delay in therapy. Obstet Gynecol. 1993;82:598–602.
10. Michael CW, Esfahani FM. Pregnancy-related changes: a retrospective review of 278 cervical smears. Diagn Cytopathol. 1997;17:99–107.
11. Baldauf JJ, Dreyfus M, Ritter J, et al. Colposcopy and directed biopsy reliability during pregnancy: a cohort study. Eur J Obstet Gynecol Reprod Biol. 1995;62:31–6.
12. Douvier S, Filipuzzi L, Sagot P. Management of cervical intra-epithelial neoplasm during pregnancy. Gynécol Obstét Fertil. 2003;31:851–5.
13. Stafl A, Wilbanks GD. An international terminology of colposcopy: report of the Nomenclature Committee of the International Federation of Cervical Pathology and Colposcopy. Obstet Gynecol. 1991;77:313–4.
14. Economos K, Perez VN, Delke I, et al. Abnormal cervical cytology in pregnancy: a 17-year experience. Obstet Gynecol. 1993;81:915–8.
15. Chhieng DC, Elgert P, Cangiarella JF, et al. Significance of AGUS Pap smears in pregnant and postpartum women. Acta Cytol. 2001;45:294–9.
16. Palle C, Bangsboll S, Andreasson B. Cervical intraepithelial neoplasia in pregnancy. Acta Obstet Gynecol Scand. 2000;79:306–10.
17. Robinson WR, Webb S, Tirpack J, et al. Management of cervical intraepithelial neoplasia during pregnancy with LOOP excision. Gynecol Oncol. 1997;64:153–5.
18. Hannigan EV, Whitehouse III HH, Atkinson WD, et al. Cone biopsy during pregnancy. Obstet Gynecol. 1982;60:450–5.
19. Fader AN, Alward EK, Niederhauser A, et al. Cervical dysplasia in pregnancy: a multi-institutional evaluation. Am J Obstet Gynecol. 2010;203:113–6.
20. Yost NP, Santoso JT, McIntire DD, et al. Postpartum regression rates of antepartum cervical intraepithelial neoplasia II and III lesions. Obstet Gynecol. 1999;93:359–62.
21. Vlahos G, Rodolakis A, Diakomanolis E, et al. Conservative management of cervical intraepithelial neoplasia (CIN(2–3)) in pregnant women. Gynecol Obstet Invest. 2002;54:78–81.
22. Robova H, Rob L, Pluta M, et al. Squamous intraepithelial lesion-microinvasive carcinoma of the cervix during pregnancy. Eur J Gynaecol Oncol. 2005;26:611–4.
23. Nagayama M, Watanabe Y, Okumura A, et al. Fast MR imaging in obstetrics. Radiographics. 2002;22:563–80.
24. Reddy UM, Filly RA, Copel JA. Prenatal imaging: ultrasonography and magnetic resonance imaging. Obstet Gynecol. 2008;112:145–57.
25. Toppenberg KS, Hill DA, Miller DP. Safety of radiographic imaging during pregnancy. Am Fam Physician. 1999;59:1813–8.
26. Pecorelli S. Revised FIGO staging for carcinoma of the vulva, cervix, and endometrium. Int J Gynaecol Obstet. 2009;105:103–4.
27. Tewari K, Cappuccini F, Gambino A, et al. Neoadjuvant chemotherapy in the treatment of locally advanced cervical carcinoma in pregnancy: a report of two cases and review of issues specific to the management of cervical carcinoma in pregnancy including planned delay of therapy. Cancer. 1998;82:1529–34.
28. Yahata T, Numata M, Kashima K, et al. Conservative treatment of stage IA1 adenocarcinoma of the cervix during pregnancy. Gynecol Oncol. 2008;109:49–52.
29. Hertel H, Possover M, Kuhne-Heid R, et al. Laparoscopic lymph node staging of cervical cancer in the 19th week of pregnancy. A case report. Surg Endosc. 2001;15:324.
30. Alouini S, Rida K, Mathevet P. Cervical cancer complicating pregnancy: implications of laparoscopic lymphadenectomy. Gynecol Oncol. 2008;108:472–7.
31. Favero G, Chiantera V, Oleszczuk A, et al. Invasive cervical cancer during pregnancy: laparoscopic nodal evaluation before oncologic treatment delay. Gynecol Oncol. 2010;118:123–7.
32. Covell LM, Disciullo AJ, Knapp RC. Decidual change in pelvic lymph nodes in the presence of cervical squamous cell carcinoma during pregnancy. Am J Obstet Gynecol. 1977;127:674–6.

33. Ashraf M, Boyd CB, Beresford WA. Ectopic decidual cell reaction in para-aortic and pelvic lymph nodes in the presence of cervical squamous cell carcinoma during pregnancy. J Surg Oncol. 1984;26:6–8.
34. Burnett RA, Millan D. Decidual change in pelvic lymph nodes: a source of possible diagnostic error. Histopathology. 1986;10:1089–92.
35. Cobb CJ. Ectopic decidua and metastatic squamous carcinoma: presentation in a single pelvic lymph node. J Surg Oncol. 1988;38:126–9.
36. Hogg R, Ungar L, Hazslinszky P. Radical hysterectomy for cervical carcinoma in pregnant women – a case of decidua mimicking metastatic carcinoma in pelvic lymph nodes. Eur J Gynaecol Oncol. 2005;26:499–500.
37. Giacalone PL, Laffargue F, Benos P, et al. Cis-platinum neoadjuvant chemotherapy in a pregnant woman with invasive carcinoma of the uterine cervix. Br J Obstet Gynaecol. 1996;103:932–4.
38. Marana HR, De Andrade JM, Silva Mathes AC, et al. Chemotherapy in the treatment of locally advanced cervical cancer and pregnancy. Gynecol Oncol. 2001;80:272–4.
39. Caluwaerts S, Van Calsteren K, Mertens L, et al. Neoadjuvant chemotherapy followed by radical hysterectomy for invasive cervical cancer diagnosed during pregnancy: report of a case and review of the literature. Int J Gynecol Cancer. 2006;16:905–8.
40. Bader AA, Petru E, Winter R. Long-term follow-up after neoadjuvant chemotherapy for high-risk cervical cancer during pregnancy. Gynecol Oncol. 2007;105:269–72.
41. Karam A, Feldman N, Holschneider CH. Neoadjuvant cisplatin and radical cesarean hysterectomy for cervical cancer in pregnancy. Nat Clin Pract Oncol. 2007;4:375–80.
42. Palaia I, Pernice M, Graziano M, et al. Neoadjuvant chemotherapy plus radical surgery in locally advanced cervical cancer during pregnancy: a case report. Am J Obstet Gynecol. 2007;197:e5–6.
43. Robova H, Pluta M, Hrehorcak M, et al. High-dose density chemotherapy followed by simple trachelectomy: full-term pregnancy. Int J Gynecol Cancer. 2008;18:1367–71.
44. Benedetti PP, Bellati F, Pastore M, et al. An update in neoadjuvant chemotherapy in cervical cancer. Gynecol Oncol. 2007;107:S20–2.
45. Ungar L, Smith JR, Palfalvi L, et al. Abdominal radical trachelectomy during pregnancy to preserve pregnancy and fertility. Obstet Gynecol. 2006;108:811–4.
46. Mandic A, Novakovic P, Nincic D, et al. Radical abdominal trachelectomy in the 19th gestation week in patients with early invasive cervical carcinoma: case study and overview of literature. Am J Obstet Gynecol. 2009;201:e6–8.
47. van de Nieuwenhof HP, van Ham MA, Lotgering FK, et al. First case of vaginal radical trachelectomy in a pregnant patient. Int J Gynecol Cancer. 2008;18:1381–5.
48. Ni Mhuireachtaigh R, O'Gorman DA. Anesthesia in pregnant patients for nonobstetric surgery. J Clin Anesth. 2006;18:60–6.
49. Giles W, Bisits A. Preterm labour. The present and future of tocolysis. Best Pract Res Clin Obstet Gynaecol. 2007;21:857–68.
50. Rizzo AG. Laparoscopic surgery in pregnancy: long-term follow-up. J Laparoendosc Adv Surg Tech A. 2003;13:11–5.
51. Mathevet P, Nessah K, Dargent D, et al. Laparoscopic management of adnexal masses in pregnancy: a case series. Eur J Obstet Gynecol Reprod Biol. 2003;108:217–22.
52. Yuen PM, Ng PS, Leung PL, et al. Outcome in laparoscopic management of persistent adnexal mass during the second trimester of pregnancy. Surg Endosc. 2004;18:1354–7.
53. Jackson H, Granger S, Price R, et al. Diagnosis and laparoscopic treatment of surgical diseases during pregnancy: an evidence-based review. Surg Endosc. 2008;22:1917–27.
54. Ebert U, Loffler H, Kirch W. Cytotoxic therapy and pregnancy. Pharmacol Ther. 1997;74:207–20.
55. Mazonakis M, Damilakis J, Theoharopoulos N, et al. Brain radiotherapy during pregnancy: an analysis of conceptus dose using anthropomorphic phantoms. Br J Radiol. 1999;72:274–8.
56. Kal HB, Struikmans H. Radiotherapy during pregnancy: fact and fiction. Lancet Oncol. 2005;6:328–33.

57. De Santis M, Di Gianantonio E, Straface G, et al. Ionizing radiations in pregnancy and terato-genesis: a review of literature. Reprod Toxicol. 2005;20:323–9.
58. Cardonick E, Iacobucci A. Use of chemotherapy during human pregnancy. Lancet Oncol. 2004;5:283–91.
59. De Vita VJ, Hellman S, Rosenberg S. Cancer principles & practice of oncology. 6th ed. Philadelphia: Lippincott Williams & Wilkins; 2001.
60. Van Calsteren K, Verbesselt R, Devlieger R, et al. Transplacental transfer of paclitaxel, docetaxel, carboplatin and trastuzumab in a baboon model. Int J Gynecol Cancer. 2010;20(9):456–64.
61. Mir O, Berveiller P, Ropert S, et al. Use of platinum derivatives during pregnancy. Cancer. 2008;113:3069–74.
62. Gligorov J, Lotz JP. Preclinical pharmacology of the taxanes: implications of the differences. Oncologist. 2004;9 Suppl 2:3–8.
63. Syme MR, Paxton JW, Keelan JA. Drug transfer and metabolism by the human placenta. Clin Pharmacokinet. 2004;43:487–514.
64. Mir O, Berveiller P, Goffinet F, et al. Taxanes for breast cancer during pregnancy: a systematic review. Ann Oncol. 2010;21:425–6.
65. Chun KC, Kim DY, Kim JH, et al. Neoadjuvant chemotherapy with paclitaxel plus platinum followed by radical surgery in early cervical cancer during pregnancy: three case reports. Jpn J Clin Oncol. 2010;40(7):694–8.
66. Sorosky JI, Sood AK, Buekers TE. The use of chemotherapeutic agents during pregnancy. Obstet Gynecol Clin North Am. 1997;24:591–9.
67. Lycette JL, Dul CL, Munar M, et al. Effect of pregnancy on the pharmacokinetics of paclitaxel: a case report. Clin Breast Cancer. 2006;7:342–4.
68. Van Calsteren K, Verbesselt R, Ottevanger P, et al. Pharmacokinetics of chemotherapeutic agents in pregnancy: a preclinical and clinical study. Acta Obstet Gynecol Scand. 2010;89:1338–45.
69. Loibl S, von Minckwitz G, Gwyn K, et al. Breast carcinoma during pregnancy. International recommendations from an expert meeting. Cancer. 2006;106:237–46.
70. Delle CL, Buck G, Grab D, et al. Prediction of fetal anemia with Doppler measurement of the middle cerebral artery peak systolic velocity in pregnancies complicated by maternal blood group alloimmunization or parvovirus B19 infection. Ultrasound Obstet Gynecol. 2001;18: 232–6.
71. Gordon AN, Jensen R, Jones III HW. Squamous carcinoma of the cervix complicating preg-nancy: recurrence in episiotomy after vaginal delivery. Obstet Gynecol. 1989;73:850–2.
72. Khalil AM, Khatib RA, Mufarrij AA, et al. Squamous cell carcinoma of the cervix implanting in the episiotomy site. Gynecol Oncol. 1993;51:408–10.
73. Cliby WA, Dodson MK, Podratz KC. Cervical cancer complicated by pregnancy: episiotomy site recurrences following vaginal delivery. Obstet Gynecol. 1994;84:179–82.
74. Van den Broek NR, Lopes AD, Ansink A, et al. "Microinvasive" adenocarcinoma of the cervix implanting in an episiotomy scar. Gynecol Oncol. 1995;59:297–9.
75. Goldman NA, Goldberg GL. Late recurrence of squamous cell cervical cancer in an episiotomy site after vaginal delivery. Obstet Gynecol. 2003;101:1127–9.
76. Heron DE, Axtel A, Gerszten K, et al. Villoglandular adenocarcinoma of the cervix recurrent in an episiotomy scar: a case report in a 32-year-old female. Int J Gynecol Cancer. 2005;15: 366–71.
77. Baloglu A, Uysal D, Aslan N, et al. Advanced stage of cervical carcinoma undiagnosed during antenatal period in term pregnancy and concomitant metastasis on episiotomy scar during delivery: a case report and review of the literature. Int J Gynecol Cancer. 2007;17:1155–9.
78. Neumann G, Rasmussen KL, Petersen LK. Cervical adenosquamous carcinoma: tumor implantation in an episiotomy scar. Obstet Gynecol. 2007;110:467–9.
79. Sivanesaratnam V, Jayalakshmi P, Loo C. Surgical management of early invasive cancer of the cervix associated with pregnancy. Gynecol Oncol. 1993;48:68–75.
80. Method MW, Brost BC. Management of cervical cancer in pregnancy. Semin Surg Oncol. 1999;16:251–60.

81. Alexander A, Samlowski WE, Grossman D, et al. Metastatic melanoma in pregnancy: risk of transplacental metastases in the infant. J Clin Oncol. 2003;21:2179–86.
82. Dildy III GA, Moise Jr KJ, Carpenter Jr RJ, et al. Maternal malignancy metastatic to the products of conception: a review. Obstet Gynecol Surv. 1989;44:535–40.
83. Madeleine MM, Daling JR, Carter JJ, et al. Cofactors with human papillomavirus in a population-based study of vulvar cancer. J Natl Cancer Inst. 1997;89:1516–23.
84. Stroup AM, Harlan LC, Trimble EL. Demographic, clinical, and treatment trends among women diagnosed with vulvar cancer in the United States. Gynecol Oncol. 2008;108:577–83.
85. Moore RG, Steinhoff MM, Granai CO, et al. Vulvar epithelioid sarcoma in pregnancy. Gynecol Oncol. 2002;85:218–22.
86. Bagga R, Keepanasseril A, Suri V, et al. Aggressive angiomyxoma of the vulva in pregnancy: a case report and review of management options. Med Gen Med. 2007;9:16.
87. Di Gilio AR, Cormio G, Resta L, et al. Rapid growth of myxoid leiomyosarcoma of the vulva during pregnancy: a case report. Int J Gynecol Cancer. 2004;14:172–5.
88. Alexander A, Harris RM, Grossman D, et al. Vulvar melanoma: diffuse melanosis and metastasis to the placenta. J Am Acad Dermatol. 2004;50:293–8.
89. Gitsch G, van Eijkeren M, Hacker NF. Surgical therapy of vulvar cancer in pregnancy. Gynecol Oncol. 1995;56:312–5.
90. Couvreux-Dif D, Lhomme C, Querleu D, et al. Cancer of the vulva and pregnancy: two cases and review of the literature. J Gynécol Obstét Biol Reprod. 2003;32:46–50.
91. Ogunleye D, Lewin SN, Huettner P, et al. Recurrent vulvar carcinoma in pregnancy. Gynecol Oncol. 2004;95:400–1.
92. Vaccarello L, Apte SM, Copeland LJ, et al. Endometrial carcinoma associated with pregnancy: a report of three cases and review of the literature. Gynecol Oncol. 1999;74:118–22.
93. Schammel DP, Mittal KR, Kaplan K, et al. Endometrial adenocarcinoma associated with intrauterine pregnancy. A report of five cases and a review of the literature. Int J Gynecol Pathol. 1998;17:327–35.
94. Ayhan A, Gunalp S, Karaer C, et al. Endometrial adenocarcinoma in pregnancy. Gynecol Oncol. 1999;75:298–9.
95. Foersterling DL, Blythe JG. Ovarian carcinoma, endometrial carcinoma, and pregnancy. Gynecol Oncol. 1999;72:425–6.
96. Ichikawa Y, Takano K, Higa S, et al. Endometrial carcinoma coexisting with pregnancy, presumed to derive from adenomyosis: a case report. Int J Gynecol Cancer. 2001;11:488–90.
97. Itoh K, Shiozawa T, Shiohara S, et al. Endometrial carcinoma in septate uterus detected 6 months after full-term delivery: case report and review of the literature. Gynecol Oncol. 2004;93:242–7.
98. Wall JA, Lucci Jr JA. Adenocarcinoma of the corpus uteri and pelvic tuberculosis complicating pregnancy; report of case with delivery of live infant and successful recovery. Obstet Gynecol. 1953;2:629–35.
99. Matsuo K, Eno ML, Im DD, et al. Pregnancy and genital sarcoma: a systematic review of the literature. Am J Perinatol. 2009;26:507–18.

Part III
Bleeding During the Second Half of Pregnancy

Chapter 6
Vaginal Bleeding and Preterm Delivery

**Offer Erez, Idit Erez-Weiss, Ruth Beer-Weisel, Vered Kleitman-Meir,
and Moshe Mazor**

Introduction

Vaginal bleeding during gestation is an ominous sign indicating an adverse pregnancy outcome. Bleeding can occur during all stages of gestation. It complicates up
to 20% of pregnancies during the first trimester and is regarded as a sign of threatened abortion. During the second and third trimesters, vaginal bleeding was found
to be a risk factor for adverse maternal and neonatal outcomes including preterm
labor (PTL), preterm prelabor rupture of membranes (PROM), placental abruption,
placenta previa, and stillbirth.

The hemochorial maternofetal interface of the human villous placenta puts the
mother at risk for bleeding that in some of the cases (i.e., abruption) can be life-
threatening. To address this risk especially during implantation [1] and after delivery [2] adequate hemostasis in the maternal circulation and the placental bed is
sustained by the physiological changes of the coagulation system in both compart-
ments. Indeed, pregnancy is regarded as a hypercoagulable state, with pregnant
women have an increased plasma concentration of fibrinogen and clotting factors
(VII, VIII, IX, X, and XII) [3–8], a low plasma concentration of anticoagulation
proteins (i.e., protein S [9–13]), and decreased activated protein C sensitivity [13–15].
Moreover, during gestation, there is reduced fibrinolysis [3, 16–20] due to low
activation of plasminogen activator inhibitors I and II [21–23]. In addition to the
systemic changes in the maternal circulation, local changes are observed in the
decidua and the maternofetal interface, including an abundance of tissue factor,
the most potent initiator of the coagulation cascade in the uterine decidua [24, 25],
fetal membranes, and amniotic fluid [26–28].

O. Erez (✉)
Department of Obstetrics and Gynecology "B", Soroka University Medical Center,
School of Medicine, Faculty of Health Sciences, Ben Gurion University of the Negev,
Beer-Sheva, Israel
e-mail: erezof@bgu.ac.il

E. Sheiner (ed.), *Bleeding During Pregnancy: A Comprehensive Guide*,
DOI 10.1007/978-1-4419-9810-1_6, © Springer Science+Business Media, LLC 2011

When these mechanisms fail and bleeding occurs owing to vascular pathology, infection/inflammation, or trauma, activation of the coagulation cascade and increased thrombin generation comprise a pathophysiological process that can lead to preterm birth. This chapter discusses the epidemiology, underlying mechanisms linking clinically evident vaginal bleeding and occult subchorionic bleeding/hematoma to spontaneous preterm birth, and the diagnostic and treatment framework of preterm parturition.

Epidemiology of Vaginal Bleeding During Pregnancy

Preterm birth is the leading cause of perinatal morbidity and mortality worldwide [29]. The annual societal economic burden associated with preterm birth in the USA exceeded $26.2 billion in 2005 [29]. Preterm birth is associated with short- and long-term maternal and fetal sequelae. The mothers are at risk for recurrent preterm birth and cardiovascular disease later in life [30, 31]. The premature newborn is at risk for acute respiratory distress syndrome (RDS), necrotizing enterocolitis (NEC), and intraventricular hemorrhage (IVH). Chronic illness [i.e., retinopathy of prematurity (ROP), cerebral palsy (CP), and bronchopulmonary dysplasia (BPD)] are also risks for the newborn; and social and behavioral maladjustment may occur later in life [32], as in the Barker hypothesis.

Vaginal Bleeding

The overall prevalence of vaginal bleeding during pregnancy is about 12.2%, and it is associated with an increased risk for pregnancy loss and preterm birth [odds ratio (OR) 2.3, 95% confidence interval (CI) 2.1–2.5] [33]. Bleeding is a common feature of early gestation, affecting about 15–25% of pregnant women during the first trimester, about half of whom have a fetal loss [34, 35]. Hasan et al. reported that the risk of miscarriage in women with vaginal bleeding during the first trimester was higher among patients with heavy bleeding accompanied by abdominal pain (OR 3.0, 95% CI 1.9–4.6) [35].

The typical patient with vaginal bleeding who delivers preterm is a privately insured, white, older, parous, college-educated woman [36]. Indeed, Caucasian women with an episode of first trimester bleeding had an increased risk for: (1) preterm delivery that correlated with the severity of prematurity (delivery at 20–27 weeks: OR 3.3, 95% CI 2.6–4.2; at 28–31 weeks: OR 3.0, 95% CI 2.5–3.5; and at 32–36 weeks: OR 1.6, 95% CI 1.5–1.8); (2) PROM (OR 1.2, 95% CI 1.1–1.3); and (3) placental abruption (OR 1.5, 95% CI 1.3–1.7) [37].

The association of vaginal bleeding with preterm PROM was further established by the following: (1) Vaginal bleeding during at least one trimester occurred in 41.4% (141/341) of patients with preterm PROM and in 17.3% (44/253) of patients without this complication ($P=0.001$) [38]. (2) The risk for preterm PROM was increased twofold in the presence of first trimester bleeding and four- or sixfold when occurring during the second or third trimester, respectively. (3) If vaginal bleeding is present during more than one trimester, the odds ratio for preterm PROM is 7.4 (95% CI 2.2–25.6) [38]. In addition, among patients with a singleton gestation who conceived by assisted reproductive technologies (ART), first trimester vaginal bleeding was associated with an increased risk for second trimester bleeding (OR 4.6, 95% CI 2.8–7.6) and third-trimester bleeding (OR 2.9, 95% CI 1.4–5.7), preterm PROM (OR 2.4, 95% CI 1.4–4.3), preterm contractions (OR 2.3, 95% CI 1.5–3.5), increased risk of preterm birth (OR 1.6, 95% CI 1.1–2.6) and extreme preterm birth (OR 3.1, 95% CI 1.1–8.3) and neonatal intensive care unit (NICU) admission (OR 1.8, 95% CI 1.2–2.5), [39].

Subchorionic Hematoma

Decidual or placental bleeding is not always clinically evident in the outward appearance of vaginal bleeding. In some cases, the bleeding is confined to the uterine cavity and therefore can be detected only by ultrasonography (US) examination. The incidence of intrauterine hematoma in the general obstetrical population is 1.3–3.1% [40–42]. Subchorionic hematoma, which is a form of intrauterine bleeding, correlates with an increased risk for adverse maternal and neonatal outcome.

Evidence in support of this is as follows: (1) Ball et al. [40] reported that the incidence of subchorionic hemorrhage was 1.3%. In comparison to women without subchorionic hemorrhage or bleeding, the presence of hematoma was associated with an increased risk of miscarriage (OR 2.8, 95% CI 1.7–7.4), stillbirth (OR 4.5, 95% CI 1.5–13.2), placental abruption (OR 11.2, 95% CI 2.7–46.4), PTL (OR 2.6, 95% CI 1.5–4.6), and lower mean birth weight. (2) Nagy et al. [41] reported that the rates of gestational hypertension [relative risk (RR) 2.1, 95% CI 1.5–2.9], preeclampsia (RR 4.0, 95% CI 2.4–6.7), placental abruption (RR 5.6, 95% CI 2.8–11.1), operative vaginal delivery (RR 1.9, 95% CI 1.1–3.2), placental separation abnormalities (RR 3.2, 95% CI 2.2–4.7), and cesarean delivery (RR 1.4, 95% CI 1.1–1.8), were significantly greater in the hematoma group. Perinatal complications, including the rate of preterm delivery (RR 2.3, 95% CI 1.6–3.2), fetal growth restriction (RR 2.4, 95% CI 1.4–4.1), fetal distress (RR 2.6, 95% CI 1.9–3.5), meconium-stained amniotic fluid (RR 2.2, 1.7–2.9), and NICU admission (RR 5.6, 95% CI 4.1–7.6), were also significantly increased in this group. The presence or absence of symptoms of threatened abortion did not affect these outcomes. (3) Norman et al. [42] reported that among 63,966 women the incidence of subchorionic hemorrhage was 1.7% (1,081/63,966). Patients with a subchorionic hemorrhage were at increased risk of abruption (OR 2.6, 95% CI 1.8–3.7) and preterm delivery (OR 1.3, 95% CI 1.1–1.5), even after adjusting for bleeding during pregnancy, chronic hypertension, body mass index, race, diabetes mellitus, tobacco use, and previous preterm birth.

The magnitude of the risk for preterm birth attributable to bleeding may be related not only to the amount of bleeding and the gestational age at which bleeding occurs during pregnancy but also to the cause(s) of the bleeding.

Underlying Mechanisms Leading to Preterm Birth in Patients with Vaginal Bleeding

Vaginal bleeding may be the clinical presentation of several pathological processes leading to preterm parturition. The most prominent are placental abruption and placenta previa (discussed in other chapters), vascular pathology of the placenta and/or the decidua, and intrauterine infection and/or inflammation (IAI), which will be discussed in this chapter.

Vascular Pathology

The origin of vaginal bleeding associated with preterm birth can be decidual or placental. Evidence of decidual bleeding, including hemosiderin depositions and retrochorionic hematoma formation, are present in 37.5% of patients with preterm PROM at 22–32 weeks of gestation and in 36.0% of patients with PTL and intact membranes who delivered before term. In contrast, these lesions are found only in 0.8% of placentas of those who deliver at term [43]. Vascular pathology is one of the mechanisms leading to decidual hemorrhage and subsequent preterm birth. Arias et al. [44] reported that the rate of vascular lesions in placentas of patients with PTL was 34%, and it was 35% in those with preterm PROM, in comparison to only in 12% among women who delivered at term [44]. The rate of failure of transformation of spiral arteries, a vascular lesion usually associated with preeclampsia, is higher among patients with PTL with intact membranes and those with preterm PROM than in patients who delivered at term [45, 46].

Role of Thrombin in Preterm Birth

The effect of decidual bleeding on the activation of premature uterine contractions and/or rupture of membranes is thought to be mediated by thrombin, the last enzyme generated by the coagulation cascade. Thrombin cleaves fibrinogen into fibrin but also has a role in the activation of inflammatory and angiogenic processes. Decidual bleeding, even minor, leads to generation of thrombin owing to the abundance of tissue factor, the most potent activator of the coagulation process. PTL and preterm PROM are both associated with increased activation of the coagulation cascade and thrombin generation. Evidence in support of this view include the following: (1) Patients with PTL or preterm PROM have a higher median concentration of maternal plasma thrombin–antithrombin III complexes than that of women with a normal pregnancy [47]. (2) Among patients with a history of spontaneous preterm birth, the maternal concentration of plasma thrombin–antithrombin III complexes concentration during the midtrimester were lower in patients who subsequently delivered preterm than in those who delivered at term [48]. (3) Regardless to the presence of intraamniotic IAI, women with PTL and intact membranes have higher median tissue factor activity and lower median tissue factor pathway inhibitor (TFPI) than those with a normal pregnancy [49]. (4) Patients with preterm PROM have a higher median maternal plasma tissue factor concentration and a lower median TFPI concentrations than normal pregnant women [50]. (5) Women with spontaneous PTL without intraamniotic IAI and women with vaginal bleeding who delivered preterm have a lower median plasma protein Z (a cofactor of protein Z-dependent protease inhibitor that inhibits the activity of factor X) than that of normal pregnant women [51]. Moreover, increased thrombin generation was detected not only in the maternal circulation but also in the amniotic fluid. Women with PTL who delivered preterm had a higher median concentration of thrombin–antithrombin III complexes than those who delivered at term. This was particularly evident among those without intraamniotic IAI, in whom elevated concentrations of amniotic fluid thrombin–antithrombin III complex were associated with a shorter amniocentesis-to-delivery interval and a lower gestational age at delivery than those with normal or low concentrations of this complex [52]. Collectively, these reports support the hypothesis that PTL and preterm PROM are associated with increased thrombin generation. Yet, it is not clear whether it is due to increased activation of the coagulation cascade or inadequate activity of anticoagulation proteins.

Caution Box

Vaginal bleeding at any stage of pregnancy is a risk factor for induced and spontaneous preterm birth. These patients should be treated as high risk pregnancies especially if they had preterm birth in previous pregnancies.

Thrombin can activate preterm parturition through several mechanisms: (1) It has uterotonic activity. Indeed, administration of whole blood into a nonpregnant uterus generated uterine contractions, which were not evident when saline or heparinized blood was introduced into the uterine cavity [53–55]. (2) Thrombin and activated coagulation factor X can induce proinflammatory cytokine production [56–63], which may lead to prostaglandin generation, premature myometrial activation, and contractions. (3) Thrombin activates matrix-degrading enzymes such as matrix metalloproteinases (MMPs) 1, 3, and 9 which can degrade the chorioamniotic membranes, leading to rupture of membranes [64–66] (Fig. 6.1).

Fig. 6.1 Underlying
mechanisms by which
increased thrombin generation
may lead to preterm birth

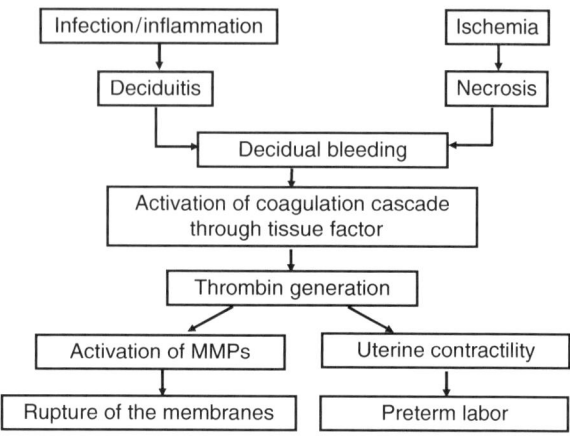

Intraamniotic Infection and Inflammation

Vaginal bleeding may be the only presenting symptom of intraamniotic infection that leads to PTL, preterm PROM, and eventually preterm birth. Indeed, microbial invasion of the amniotic cavity (MIAC) was detected in 14% of patients with idiopathic vaginal bleeding and was associated with subsequent preterm PROM and early preterm delivery [67]. Thus, vaginal bleeding may be the only clinical manifestation of MIAC, and it predisposes to an adverse outcome. Additional support to this observation were the findings that the median total hemoglobin concentration in amniotic fluid, a marker for intraamniotic bleeding, was higher among patients with PTL or preterm PROM who had intraamniotic IAI than in those with PTL or preterm PROM without intraamniotic IAI [68]. Of interest, the proportion of fetal hemoglobin in the total amniotic fluid hemoglobin was lower in patients with intraamniotic IAI than in those without it [69]. This point suggests that bleeding from the maternal compartment, such as decidual bleeding, contributes to the higher total hemoglobin detected in the amniotic fluid of patients with PTL or preterm PROM who had IAI.

Caution Box

Vaginal bleeding in the midtrimester can be the only manifestation of intraamniotic infection.

Intrauterine infection and/or inflammation is one of the leading underlying mechanisms contributing to preterm parturition. Indeed, Goncalves et al. [70] reviewed the results of amniotic fluid cultures from 33 studies regarding the rate of positive amniotic fluid cultures for microorganisms in women with PTL and intact membranes and found that the prevalence of microbial invasion of amniotic fluid among patients with PTL was 12.8% [70, 71], and about 30% of them were polymicrobial. The MIAC rate in patients with preterm PROM was higher and reached 32.4% [70, 71]. However, when amniocenteses were performed in patients with preterm PROM at the time of the onset of labor, 75% of patients had MIAC [72], suggesting that some patients were infected prior to the clinical rupture of membranes, while others were infected after they had ruptured. In addition, the MIAC rate among patients with cervical insufficiency in the midtrimester is around 33% (range 13–52%) [73, 74] and 45–51% during the early third trimester [74]. The most common microbial organisms isolated from the amniotic fluid of women with PTL and intact membranes, preterm PROM, or cervical insufficiency were *Ureaplasma urealyticum*, *Mycoplasma hominis*, and *Fusobacterium* species and other anaerobic bacteria [72, 73, 75–81]. The MIAC rate in patients with PTL and intact membranes is gestational age-dependent. It is as high as 45% at 23–26 weeks of gestation and decreases to 11.5% at 31–34 weeks [82]. Thus, the earlier the gestational age at preterm birth, the more likely it is that MIAC is present [82].

Diagnosis of PTL/Preterm PROM

The diagnosis of PTL or preterm PROM is based on the clinical assessment of all the components of the common pathway of parturition, meaning signs of uterine contraction, cervical ripening and/or dilatation, and rupture of the chorioamniotic membranes. The presence of six or more uterine contractions per hour during fetal monitoring and a cervical dilatation of >3 cm with >80% effacement ascertains the diagnosis of PTL. This is already a late stage in the progress of the disease, but lowering these cutoffs ended in a higher rate of false-positive diagnosis of PTL. Additional factors that contribute to the diagnosis of preterm parturition are the presence of vaginal bleeding and rupture of the chorioamniotic membranes.

The initial assessment of patients with symptoms suggestive of PTL is presented in Fig. 6.2. Maternal examination includes (1) fetal monitoring, performed for the presence of contraction and fetal assessment; (2) sterile speculum examination for evidence of PROM, vaginal bleeding or bulging membranes; (3) digital examination for cervical dilatation can be performed only after placenta previa and rupture of membranes (PROM) have been rulled out; (4) abdominal US for locating the placenta, estimating fetal weight and well-being and the amniotic fluid volume. Transvaginal US is an important tool in the assessment of patients presenting with PTL, especially those with vaginal bleeding. This sonographic examination is needed to determination placental location, rule out placenta previa, and measure the cervical length as part of the assessment of the risk of impending preterm birth.

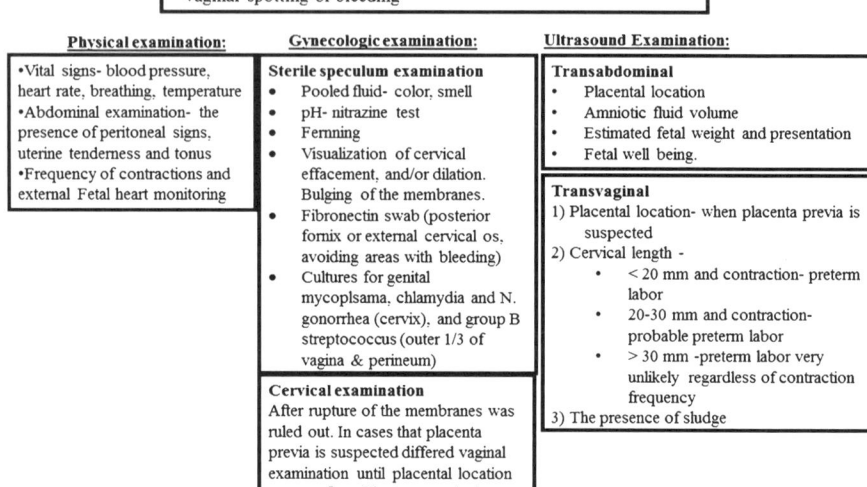

	Patient presents with signs / symptoms of preterm labor: • Uterine contractions (painful or painless)- at least 6/hour • Intermittent abdominal cramping, pelvic pressure, or backache • Vaginal spotting or bleeding	
Physical examination:	**Gynecologic examination:**	**Ultrasound Examination:**
•Vital signs- blood pressure, heart rate, breathing, temperature •Abdominal examination- the presence of peritoneal signs, uterine tenderness and tonus •Frequency of contractions and external Fetal heart monitoring	**Sterile speculum examination** • Pooled fluid- color, smell • pH- nitrazine test • Fernning • Visualization of cervical effacement, and/or dilation. Bulging of the membranes. • Fibronectin swab (posterior fornix or external cervical os, avoiding areas with bleeding) • Cultures for genital mycoplsama, chlamydia and N. gonorrhea (cervix), and group B streptococcus (outer 1/3 of vagina & perineum)	**Transabdominal** • Placental location • Amniotic fluid volume • Estimated fetal weight and presentation • Fetal well being. **Transvaginal** 1) Placental location- when placenta previa is suspected 2) Cervical length - • < 20 mm and contraction- preterm labor • 20-30 mm and contraction- probable preterm labor • > 30 mm -preterm labor very unlikely regardless of contraction frequency 3) The presence of sludge
	Cervical examination After rupture of the membranes was ruled out. In cases that placenta previa is suspected differed vaginal examination until placental location was confirmed by trans vaginal ultrasound	

Fig. 6.2 Initial clinical assessment of patients with preterm labor

Management of a PTL Episode

After establishing a diagnosis of PTL, the underlying cause leading to this clinical presentation has to be identified (Fig. 6.3).

When vaginal bleeding is part of the presenting symptoms of a patient with PTL, the clinician assessment of the patients should include the following: (1) a diagnosis of placental abruption – the presence of hypertonic uterine contraction, uterine tenderness, and in some of the cases sonographic evidence of intrauterine bleeding or blood clots; (2) the presence of placenta previa – in most cases the patient reports vaginal bleeding with mild abdominal cramping. In both cases the clinician must (1) estimate whether the bleeding is compromising the mother or the fetus in a way that necessitates prompt delivery, preventing the administration of tocolysis and corticosteroids; (2) treat possible maternal coagulopathy with blood products; and (3) in cases of mild vaginal bleeding or spotting during the course of progression of preterm delivery, administer tocolysis and corticosteroids.

Intraamniotic infection can be clinically evident as maternal chorioamnionitis, presenting with a fever of >37.8°C with no other evident source (i.e., pneumonia, pyelonephritis), fetal tachycardia, uterine tenderness, high leukocyte counts, and foul-smelling amniotic fluid in the case of preterm PROM. The treatment of these patients includes the administration of intravenous antibiotics, preferably penicillin and aminoglycoside, and delivery of the fetus. However, in most cases, intraamniotic infection is subclinical, and the only clinical manifestation is premature contractions and/or vaginal bleeding. Amniocentesis is an important diagnostic tool for

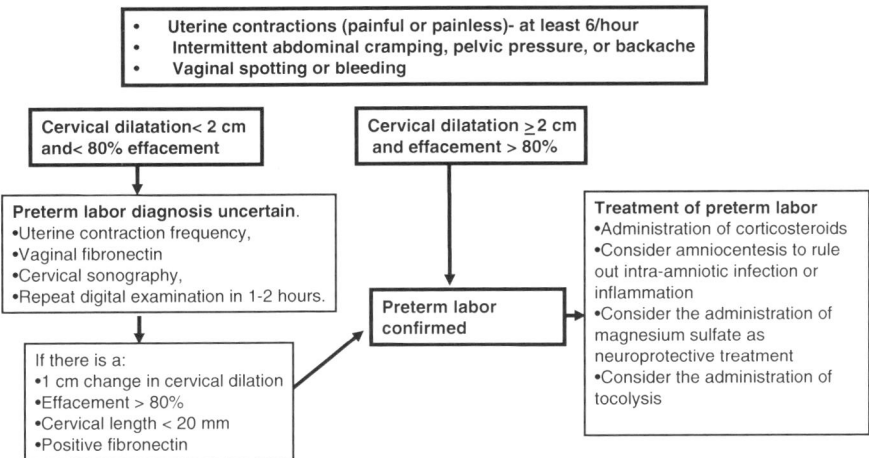

Fig. 6.3 Management of episode of preterm labor <34 weeks of gestation

detecting intraamniotic IAI. It can also be used to determine fetal lung maturity and the fetal karyotype when needed.

The three interventions that were shown to reduce neonatal morbidity and mortality include administration of corticosteroids, antibiotic treatment to prevent group B streptococcal (GBS) infection during active labor, and transferring the patient to a hospital capable of treating premature neonates.

Corticosteroids

The administration of corticosteroids, usually two doses of intramuscular betamethasone 12 mg 24 h apart, is associated with a significant reduction in neonatal RDS, IVH, NEC, patent ductus arteriosus (PDA), and neonatal mortality in preterm neonates. Glucocorticoids promote maturation overgrowth and accelerate the maturation process of fetal organs including the lungs, brain, kidneys, and gut. This process is especially prominent in the fetal lungs as corticosteroids increase lung compliance, reduce vascular permeability, and promote surfactant synthesis in utero; they also generate an enhanced response to postnatal surfactant treatment [83, 84]. A single course of corticosteroids increases the maternal white blood cells and the platelet count and challenges her glucose tolerance during the 48 h following the treatment. In addition, reduced fetal movements and reduce fetal heart rate variability are observed up to 48 h after administration of antenatal corticosteroids. The duration of the beneficial effect of a single course of corticosteroids is 1 week, and repeated courses of corticosteroids were found to have maternal and fetal side effects without a beneficial effect. However, there is accumulating evidence that when the interval from the initial dose of corticosteroids to the recurrent PTL episode is more than 2 weeks the administration of a rescue dose may be beneficial.

Antibiotics

During active PTL, prophylactic antibiotic treatment against GBS infection is indicated because premature neonates are at higher risk for neonatal GBS infection than those born at term [85]. However, the administration of prophylactic antibiotic to prolong the latency period from the PTL event until delivery yielded disappointing results in randomized controlled trials. Moreover, a follow-up study after 7 years found that the risk of cerebral palsy was increased in children of mothers treated by antibiotics, and there was increased functional impairment among the children at 7 years of age born to women who received erythromycin. Therefore, antibiotics should not be administered routinely to women with PTL because it is not effective and may even be harmful to the fetus/neonate.

Tocolysis

Tocolysis refers to the treatment for the uterine component of the common pathway of parturition by drugs aimed to stop the contractions. However, the available data today suggest that the beneficial effect of these drugs is to delay delivery by 48 h, which is the time needed for the beneficial effect of corticosteroids to take effect. The various groups of tocolytic agents along with their potency and side effects are presented in Table 6.1. Recent Cochrane's meta-analyses of tocolytic agents indicate that (1) calcium channel blockers [86] and oxytocin antagonists [87] may delay delivery by 2–7 days with the most favorable benefit-to-risk ratio, (2) β-mimetic drugs delay delivery by 48 h but are associated with greater side effects [88], (3) there is insufficient evidence regarding cyclooxygenase inhibitors [89], and (4) magnesium sulfate is ineffective [90]. None of these agents reduced the rate of preterm births in patients admitted with PTL.

Neuroprotection

Cerebral palsy (CP) is one of the long-term complications of preterm birth. The incidence of CP is negatively proportional to the gestational age at delivery, ranging from 14.6% among newborns that were born at 22–27 weeks of gestation to 0.7% among children born at 32–36 weeks. IAI was associated with increased risk for the subsequent development of CP. Some reports suggest that intrapartum administration of magnesium sulfate ($MgSO_4$) has a role in reducing the overall incidence of CP and of that of severe cerebral palsy. Indeed, a large, double-masked, placebo-controlled trial conducted by the Maternal Fetal Medicine network of the National Institute of Child Health and Human Development (NICHHD) in 2,241 women with imminent preterm birth (91% with PPROM) before 32 weeks' gestation found a 55% reduction (RR 0.45, CI 0.23–0.87) in the rate of CP at age 2 years among survivors who received antenatal magnesium just before delivery [91]. In addition,

Table 6.1 Tocolytic agents currently in use for the treatment of an episode of preterm labor with intact membranes

Parameter	β-Adrenergic agonist	Magnesium sulfate	Prostaglandin synthesis inhibitors	Calcium channel blockers	Oxytocin receptor antagonist
Mechanism	Stimulates receptors to relax smooth muscle	Competes for calcium ions during depolarization	Inhibits prostaglandin synthesis and release	Decreases intracellular calcium ions	Blocks oxytocin bindings to its receptor
Agent	Ritrodine, terbutaline	Magnesium sulfate	Indomethacin	Nifedipine	Atociban
Side effects	Cardiovascular, pulmonary, hypokalemia, hyperglycemia	Muscle weakness, respiratory depression, pulmonary edema	PDA closure in utero, oligohydramnios, increases NEC, GI irritation, IVH	Tachycardia, hypotension, myocardial depression	Nausea and vomiting, headache, dizziness, flushes, tachycardia, hypotension, hyperglycemia

PDA patent ductus arteriosus, *NEC* necrotizing enterocolitis, *GI* gastrointestinal, *IVH* intraventricular hemorrhage a Cochrane Systematic Review [92] that reviewed findings regarding the effect of antenatal $MgSO_4$ administration on the CP rate found that it was associated with a significant reduction in the incidence of CP (RR 0.68, 95% CI 0.54–0.87) but had no effect on fetal/infant mortality (RR 1.04, 95% CI 0.92–1.17) [92]. However, when only studies indicating that neuroprotection was their specific intent were included in the analysis, antenatal $MgSO_4$ was associated with a reduction in the CP rate and in the combined outcome of CP and fetal/infant death (RR 0.85, 95% CI 0.74–0.98) [92]. These data suggest that there may be a role for prenatally administered $MgSO_4$ as a neuroprotectant for infants born before 32 weeks' gestation.

In cases where the acute episode of PTL is arrested, management of the patient is aimed at maintaining uterine quiescence and a prolonged gestation. However, prolonged uterine contraction suppression was not associated with a reduction in the incidence of preterm birth. The gestational age and the cervical length, dilatation, and effacement, the frequency of uterine contractions, and the maternal obstetrical history should be taken into account when deciding whether to follow the patient in an outpatient clinic or as an inpatient. Of note, outpatient follow-up was not associated with a better outcome in relation to the rate of preterm birth and birth weight.

Diagnosis and Management of Preterm PROM

Women with vaginal bleeding are at increased risk for preterm PROM, and this diagnosis should be ruled out in these patients. The diagnosis of preterm PROM is based on visualization of a vaginal pool or obvious leakage of fluid from the cervix into the posterior fornix. Additional tests include that for the presence of ferning, or changes in vaginal pH, which is determined by a nitrazine test. The latter may be difficult in patients with vaginal bleeding as the presence of blood in the vagina changes its pH and leads to a false-positive result. Additional biochemical tests include diamine oxidase (DAO) activity [93], prolactin levels [94–96], α-fetoprotein (AFP) [94, 97], insulin-like growth factor-binding protein-1 (IGFB-1) [98], and placental $α_1$-microglobulin. However, these markers are not yet in routine clinical use. In cases in which there is inconsistency in the diagnosis of preterm PROM, transabdominal injection of dye into the amniotic sac along with placement of a vaginal tampon can be used for ascertaining the diagnosis. Indigo carmine, Evans blue, and fluorescein are commonly used [99–102]. Of note, methylene blue should not be used as it can cause fetal methemoglobinemia [103–105] (Fig. 6.4).

After the diagnosis of preterm PROM is established and occult cord prolapse is excluded, the initial evaluation of a patient with preterm PROM includes (1) accurate assessment of gestational age as the management of these patients is dependent on the gestational age at which the membrane rupture has occurred (Fig. 6.5) – precise dating of the pregnancy is crucial for tailoring the appropriate treatment; (2) estimation of fetal weight and presentation; (3) assessment of fetal well-being; (4) evaluation for the presence of intrauterine infection; and (5) determination of lung maturity.

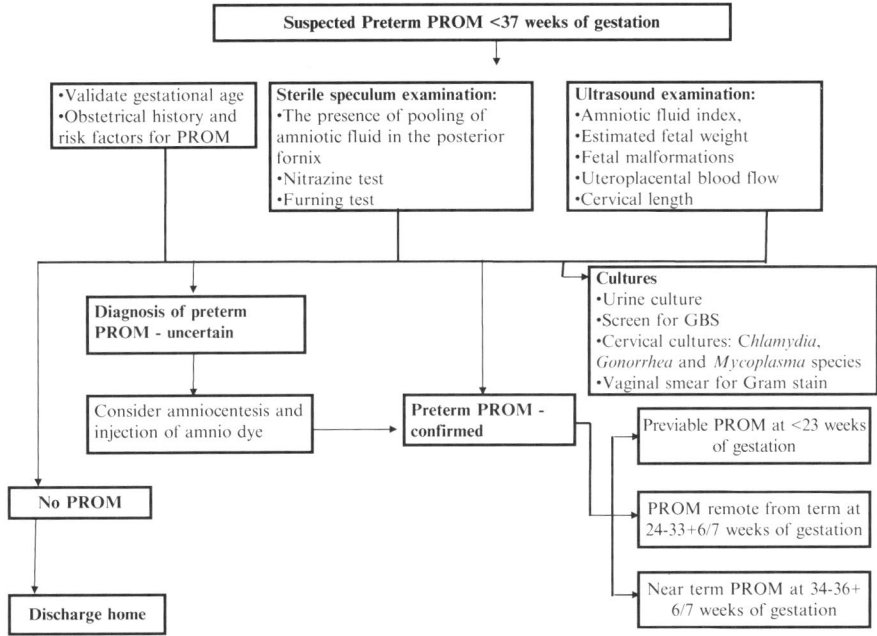

Fig. 6.4 Initial clinical assessment of patients with preterm premature rupture of the membrane (PROM)

The management of preterm PROM before the threshold of viability (<24 weeks' gestation) include (1) assessment for the presence of clinical chorioamnionitis; (2) consideration of amniocentesis for fetal karyotype and diagnosis of intraamniotic IAI; (3) consult the patient regarding the possible neonatal outcome when PROM occurs at this stage of pregnancy, including the risk for lung hypoplasia (Fig. 6.5) and fetal contractures. In case the patient decides to continue the pregnancy, recommend bed rest and constantly assess her for signs of chorioamnionitis or abruption, in which case terminating the pregnancy is warranted.

The management of preterm PROM remote from term (24–34 weeks of gestation) is aimed at postponing the preterm birth as much as possible to reduce the sequelae associated with early prematurity. After the initial assessment for the presence of clinical chorioamnionitis of abruption that would necessitate prompt delivery, expectant management can be established. In contrast to PTL with intact membranes, the administration of prophylactic antibiotic treatment prolongs the latency period from membrane rupture to delivery and reduces neonatal morbidity. Indeed, Mercer et al. [106] in a randomized trial allocating patients with preterm PROM at 24–32 weeks' gestation to receive intravenous ampicillin (2 g every 6 h) and erythromycin (250 mg every 6 h) for 48 h followed by 5 days of oral amoxicillin and erythromycin base (every 8 h) vs. placebos. Antibiotic administration was associated with prolongation of pregnancy and a significant reduction in the incidence of RDS [RR 0.83, 95% CI 0.69–0.99], NEC [RR 0.4, 95% CI 0.17–0.95], clinical

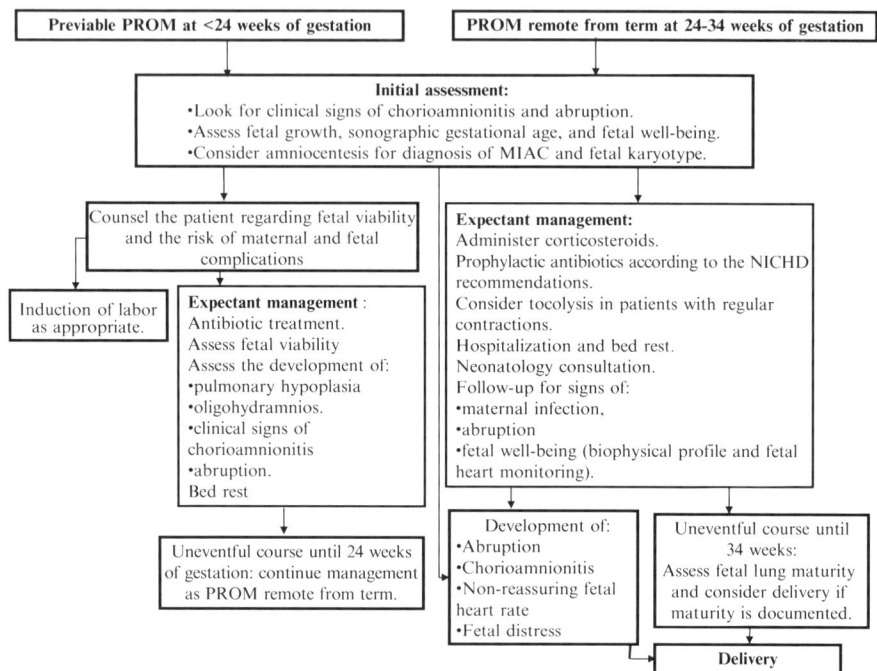

Fig. 6.5 Management of preterm PROM before the threshold of viability and between 24 and 34 weeks of gestation. *MIAC* microbial invasion of the amniotic cavity, *GBS* group B streptococci. Modified from Mercer et al. (Clinics in Perinatology 2004;31:765–82, with permission)

chorioamnionitis, and the composite neonatal outcome (fetal or infant death, RDS, severe IVH, stage II or III of NEC, or sepsis within 72 h of birth [106]) (RR 0.84, 95% CI 0.71–0.99). Although the beneficial effect of corticosteroids in reducing neonatal morbidity is under debate, the current recommendation is to treat all patients with preterm PROM between 24 and 32 weeks of gestation.

There in no evidence to support the use of tocolytic agents to prolong the latency period from membrane rupture to delivery. However, a survey among Maternal Fetal Medicine specialists in the USA reported that 56% of them are giving tocolysis for patients with preterm RPOM who have contractions, and 32% also treat patients with tocolysis who have preterm PROM without contractions [107] (Fig. 6.5). There is a debate regarding the timing of delivery of a patient with preterm PROM remote from term. While the general approach is to deliver at or after 34 weeks of gestation, there is evidence that delivering at 32–34 weeks is not associated with a higher rate of neonatal morbidity [108]. During the expectant management of preterm PROM, the main maternal complications are chorioamnionitis (39%), endometritis (14%), placental abruption (3%), and postpartum hemorrhage due to retained placenta that requires curettage (12%) [109]. No relation between the duration of membrane rupture and chorioamnionitis has been noted. However, patients with septicemia requiring a hysterectomy, septic shock, or maternal death were reported [110–113]. The current approach is that patients with preterm PROM after 34 weeks of gestation should undergo delivery.

Summary

Vaginal bleeding during gestation is an ominous sign that presents an increased risk for spontaneous preterm delivery (PTL with intact membranes, preterm PROM) or indicated preterm delivery (abruption and placenta previa). Vascular disease and infection are the main mechanisms leading to preterm parturition in patients with an episode of vaginal bleeding. The current treatment modalities for patients with vaginal bleeding do not suggest any effective intervention for the prevention of preterm birth. Nevertheless, women presenting with vaginal bleeding during pregnancy should be defined as being at high risk for preterm birth and should be followed accordingly. In cases in which bleeding is jeopardizing the mother or the fetus, prompt intervention is warranted.

References

1. Lockwood CJ, Schatz F. A biological model for the regulation of peri-implantational hemostasis and menstruation. J Soc Gynecol Investig. 1996;3:159–65.
2. Hahn L. On fibrinolysis and coagulation during parturition and menstruation. Acta Obstet Gynecol Scand Suppl. 1974;28:7–40.
3. Hellgren M, Blomback M. Studies on blood coagulation and fibrinolysis in pregnancy, during delivery and in the puerperium. I. Normal condition. Gynecol Obstet Invest. 1981;12:141–54.
4. Stirling Y, Woolf L, North WR, Seghatchian MJ, Meade TW. Haemostasis in normal pregnancy. Thromb Haemost. 1984;52:176–82.
5. Beller FK, Ebert C. The coagulation and fibrinolytic enzyme system in pregnancy and in the puerperium. Eur J Obstet Gynecol Reprod Biol. 1982;13:177–97.
6. Donohoe S, Quenby S, Mackie I, Panal G, Farquharson R, Malia R, et al. Fluctuations in levels of antiphospholipid antibodies and increased coagulation activation markers in normal and heparin-treated antiphospholipid syndrome pregnancies. Lupus. 2002;11:11–20.
7. Bremme KA. Haemostatic changes in pregnancy. Best Pract Res Clin Haematol. 2003;16:153–68.
8. Brenner B. Haemostatic changes in pregnancy. Thromb Res. 2004;114:409–14.
9. Clark P, Brennand J, Conkie JA, McCall F, Greer IA, Walker ID. Activated protein C sensitivity, protein C, protein S and coagulation in normal pregnancy. Thromb Haemost. 1998;79:1166–70.
10. Faught W, Garner P, Jones G, Ivey B. Changes in protein C and protein S levels in normal pregnancy. Am J Obstet Gynecol. 1995;172:147–50.
11. Oruc S, Saruc M, Koyuncu FM, Ozdemir E. Changes in the plasma activities of protein C and protein S during pregnancy. Aust N Z J Obstet Gynaecol. 2000;40:448–50.
12. Lefkowitz JB, Clarke SH, Barbour LA. Comparison of protein S functional and antigenic assays in normal pregnancy. Am J Obstet Gynecol. 1996;175:657–60.

13. Mahieu B, Jacobs N, Mahieu S, Naelaerts K, Vertessen F, Weyler J, et al. Haemostatic changes and acquired activated protein C resistance in normal pregnancy. Blood Coagul Fibrinolysis. 2007;18:685–8.

14. Mimuro S, Lahoud R, Beutler L, Trudinger B. Changes of resistance to activated protein C in the course of pregnancy and prevalence of factor V mutation. Aust N Z J Obstet Gynaecol. 1998;38:200–4.

15. Cumming AM, Tait RC, Fildes S, Yoong A, Keeney S, Hay CR. Development of resistance to activated protein C during pregnancy. BrJ Haematol. 1995;90:725–7.

16. Biezenski JJ, Moore HC. Fibrinolysis in normal pregnancy. J Clin Pathol. 1958;11:306–10.

17. Naidoo SS, Hathorn M, Gillman T. Fibrinolytic and antifibrinolytic activity in pregnancy. J Clin Pathol. 1960;13:224–5.

18. Thorsen S. The inhibition of tissue plasminogen activator and urokinase-induced fibrinolysis by some natural proteinase inhibitors and by plasma and serum from normal and pregnant subjects. Scand J Clin Lab Invest. 1973;31:51–9.

19. Kleiner GJ, Greston WM. Current concepts of defibrination in the pregnant woman. J Reprod Med. 1976;17:309–17.

20. Arias F, Andrinopoulos G, Zamora J. Whole-blood fibrinolytic activity in normal and hypertensive pregnancies and its relation to the placental concentration of urokinase inhibitor. Am J Obstet Gynecol. 1979;133:624–9.

21. Ishii A, Yamada S, Yamada R, Hamada H. t-PA activity in peripheral blood obtained from pregnant women. J Perinat Med. 1994;22:113–7.

22. Kruithof EK, Tran-Thang C, Gudinchet A, Hauert J, Nicoloso G, Genton C, et al. Fibrinolysis in pregnancy: a study of plasminogen activator inhibitors. Blood. 1987;69:460–6.

23. Wright JG, Cooper P, Astedt B, Lecander I, Wilde JT, Preston FE, et al. Fibrinolysis during normal human pregnancy: complex inter-relationships between plasma levels of tissue plasminogen activator and inhibitors and the euglobulin clot lysis time. BrJ Haematol. 1988;69: 253–8.

24. Lockwood CJ, Krikun G, Schatz F. The decidua regulates hemostasis in human endometrium. Semin Reprod Endocrinol. 1999;17:45–51.

25. Lockwood CJ, Krikun G, Schatz F. Decidual cell-expressed tissue factor maintains hemostasis in human endometrium. Ann NY Acad Sci. 2001;943:77–88.

26. Erez O, Gotsch F, Mazaki-Tovi S, Vaisbuch E, Kusanovic JP, Kim CJ, et al. Evidence of maternal platelet activation, excessive thrombin generation, and high amniotic fluid tissue factor immunoreactivity and functional activity in patients with fetal death. J Matern Fetal Neonatal Med. 2009;22:672–87.

27. Lockwood CJ, Bach R, Guha A, Zhou XD, Miller WA, Nemerson Y. Amniotic fluid contains tissue factor, a potent initiator of coagulation. Am J Obstet Gynecol. 1991;165:1335–41.

28. Uszynski M, Zekanowska E, Uszynski W, Kuczynski J. Tissue factor (TF) and tissue factor pathway inhibitor (TFPI) in amniotic fluid and blood plasma: implications for the mechanism of amniotic fluid embolism. Eur J Obstet Gynecol Reprod Biol. 2001;95:163–6.

29. Goldenberg RL, Culhane JF, Iams JD, Romero R. Epidemiology and causes of preterm birth. Lancet. 2008;371:75–84.

30. Nardi O, Zureik M, Courbon D, Ducimetiere P, Clavel-Chapelon F. Preterm delivery of a first child and subsequent mothers' risk of ischaemic heart disease: a nested case-control study. Eur J Cardiovasc Prev Rehabil. 2006;13:281–3.

31. Smith GC, Pell JP, Walsh D. Pregnancy complications and maternal risk of ischaemic heart disease: a retrospective cohort study of 129,290 births. Lancet. 2001;357:2002–6.

32. Moster D, Lie RT, Markestad T. Long-term medical and social consequences of preterm birth. N Engl J Med. 2008;359:262–73.

33. Ananth CV, Savitz DA. Vaginal bleeding and adverse reproductive outcomes: a meta-analysis. Paediatr Perinat Epidemiol. 1994;8:62–78.

34. Hasan R, Baird DD, Herring AH, Olshan AF, Jonsson Funk ML, Hartmann KE. Patterns and predictors of vaginal bleeding in the first trimester of pregnancy. Ann Epidemiol. 2010;20: 524–31.

35. Hasan R, Baird DD, Herring AH, Olshan AF, Jonsson Funk ML, Hartmann KE. Association between first-trimester vaginal bleeding and miscarriage. Obstet Gynecol. 2009;114:860–7.
36. Strobino B, Pantel-Silverman J. Gestational vaginal bleeding and pregnancy outcome. Am J Epidemiol. 1989;129:806–15.
37. Lykke JA, Dideriksen KL, Lidegaard O, Langhoff-Roos J. First-trimester vaginal bleeding and complications later in pregnancy. Obstet Gynecol. 2010;115:935–44.
38. Harger JH, Hsing AW, Tuomala RE, Gibbs RS, Mead PB, Eschenbach DA, et al. Risk factors for preterm premature rupture of fetal membranes: a multicenter case-control study. Am J Obstet Gynecol. 1990;163:130–7.
39. De Sutter P, Bontinck J, Schutysers V, Van der EJ, Gerris J, Dhont M. First-trimester bleeding and pregnancy outcome in singletons after assisted reproduction. Hum Reprod. 2006;21:1907–11.
40. Ball RH, Ade CM, Schoenborn JA, Crane JP. The clinical significance of ultrasonographically detected subchorionic hemorrhages. Am J Obstet Gynecol. 1996;174:996–1002.
41. Nagy S, Bush M, Stone J, Lapinski RH, Gardo S. Clinical significance of subchorionic and retroplacental hematomas detected in the first trimester of pregnancy. Obstet Gynecol. 2003;102:94–100.
42. Norman SM, Odibo AO, Macones GA, Dicke JM, Crane JP, Cahill AG. Ultrasound-detected subchorionic hemorrhage and the obstetric implications. Obstet Gynecol. 2010;116:311–5.
43. Arias F, Rodriquez L, Rayne SC, Kraus FT. Maternal placental vasculopathy and infection: two distinct subgroups among patients with preterm labor and preterm ruptured membranes. Am J Obstet Gynecol. 1993;168:585–91.
44. Kim YM, Chaiworapongsa T, Gomez R, Bujold E, Yoon BH, Rotmensch S, et al. Failure of physiologic transformation of the spiral arteries in the placental bed in preterm premature rupture of membranes. Am J Obstet Gynecol. 2002;187:1137–42.
45. Kim YM, Bujold E, Chaiworapongsa T, Gomez R, Yoon BH, Thaler HT, et al. Failure of physiologic transformation of the spiral arteries in patients with preterm labor and intact membranes. Am J Obstet Gynecol. 2003;189:1063–9.
46. Salafia CM, Lopez-Zeno JA, Sherer DM, Whittington SS, Minior VK, Vintzileos AM. Histologic evidence of old intrauterine bleeding is more frequent in prematurity. Am J Obstet Gynecol. 1995;173:1065–70.
47. Chaiworapongsa T, Espinoza J, Yoshimatsu J, Kim YM, Bujold E, Edwin S, et al. Activation of coagulation system in preterm labor and preterm premature rupture of membranes. J Matern Fetal Neonatal Med. 2002;11:368–73.
48. Hackney DN, Catov JM, Simhan HN. Low concentrations of thrombin-inhibitor complexes and the risk of preterm delivery. Am J Obstet Gynecol. 2010;203:184–6.
49. Erez O, Romero R, Vaisbuch E, Kusanovic JP, Mazaki-Tovi S, Chaiworapongsa T, et al. High tissue factor activity and low tissue factor pathway inhibitor concentrations in patients with preterm labor. J Matern Fetal Neonatal Med. 2010;23:23–33.
50. Erez O, Espinoza J, Chaiworapongsa T, Gotsch F, Kusanovic JP, Than NG, et al. A link between a hemostatic disorder and preterm PROM: a role for tissue factor and tissue factor pathway inhibitor. J Matern Fetal Neonatal Med. 2008;21:732–44.
51. Kusanovic JP, Espinoza J, Romero R, Hoppensteadt D, Nien JK, Kim CJ, et al. Plasma protein Z concentrations in pregnant women with idiopathic intrauterine bleeding and in women with spontaneous preterm labor. J Matern Fetal Neonatal Med. 2007;20:453–63.
52. Erez O, Romer R, Vaisbuch E, Chaiworapongsa T, Kusanovic JP, Mazaki-Tovi S, et al. Changes in amniotic fluid concentration of thrombin-antithrombin III complexes in patients with preterm labor: evidence of an increased thrombin generation. J Matern Fetal Neonatal Med. 2009;22:971–82.
53. Elovitz MA, Saunders T, Ascher-Landsberg J, Phillippe M. Effects of thrombin on myometrial contractions in vitro and in vivo. Am J Obstet Gynecol. 2000;183:799–804.
54. Elovitz MA, Ascher-Landsberg J, Saunders T, Phillippe M. The mechanisms underlying the stimulatory effects of thrombin on myometrial smooth muscle. Am J Obstet Gynecol. 2000;183:674–81.

55. Elovitz MA, Baron J, Phillippe M. The role of thrombin in preterm parturition. Am J Obstet Gynecol. 2001;185:1059–63.
56. Daubie V, Cauwenberghs S, Senden NH, Pochet R, Lindhout T, Buurman WA, et al. Factor Xa and thrombin evoke additive calcium and proinflammatory responses in endothelial cells subjected to coagulation. Biochim Biophys Acta. 2006;1763:860–9.
57. Borensztajn K, Stiekema J, Nijmeijer S, Reitsma PH, Peppelenbosch MP, Spek CA. Factor Xa stimulates proinflammatory and profibrotic responses in fibroblasts via protease-activated receptor-2 activation. Am J Pathol. 2008;172:309–20.
58. Johnson K, Aarden L, Choi Y, De GE, Creasey A. The proinflammatory cytokine response to coagulation and endotoxin in whole blood. Blood. 1996;87:5051–60.
59. Kranzhofer R, Clinton SK, Ishii K, Coughlin SR, Fenton JW, Libby P. Thrombin potently stimulates cytokine production in human vascular smooth muscle cells but not in mononuclear phagocytes. Circ Res. 1996;79:286–94.
60. Senden NH, Jeunhomme TM, Heemskerk JW, Wagenvoord R, van't VC, Hemker HC, et al. Factor Xa induces cytokine production and expression of adhesion molecules by human umbilical vein endothelial cells. J Immunol. 1998;161:4318–24.
61. Naldini A, Pucci A, Carney DH, Fanetti G, Carraro F. Thrombin enhancement of interleukin-1 expression in mononuclear cells: involvement of proteinase-activated receptor-1. Cytokine. 2002;20:191–9.
62. Fan Y, Zhang W, Mulholland M. Thrombin and PAR-1-AP increase proinflammatory cytokine expression in C6 cells. J Surg Res. 2005;129:196–201.
63. Li T, Wang H, He S. Induction of interleukin-6 release from monocytes by serine proteinases and its potential mechanisms. Scand J Immunol. 2006;64:10–6.
64. Lockwood CJ, Krikun G, Papp C, Toth-Pal E, Markiewicz L, Wang EY, et al. The role of progestationally regulated stromal cell tissue factor and type-1 plasminogen activator inhibitor (PAI-1) in endometrial hemostasis and menstruation. Ann NY Acad Sci. 1994;734:57–79.
65. Lockwood CJ, Krikun G, Aigner S, Schatz F. Effects of thrombin on steroid-modulated cultured endometrial stromal cell fibrinolytic potential. J Clin Endocrinol Metab. 1996;81:107–12.
66. Rosen T, Schatz F, Kuczynski E, Lam H, Koo AB, Lockwood CJ. Thrombin-enhanced matrix metalloproteinase-1 expression: a mechanism linking placental abruption with premature rupture of the membranes. J Matern Fetal Neonatal Med. 2002;11:11–7.
67. Gomez R, Romero R, Nien JK, Medina L, Carstens M, Kim YM, et al. Idiopathic vaginal bleeding during pregnancy as the only clinical manifestation of intrauterine infection. J Matern Fetal Neonatal Med. 2005;18:31–7.
68. Vaisbuch E, Romero R, Erez O, Kusanovic JP, Gotsch F, Than NG, et al. Total hemoglobin concentration in amniotic fluid is increased in intraamniotic infection/inflammation. Am J Obstet Gynecol. 2008;199:426–7.
69. Vaisbuch E, Kusanovic JP, Erez O, Mazaki-Tovi S, Gotsch F, Kim CJ, et al. Amniotic fluid fetal hemoglobin in normal pregnancies and pregnancies complicated with preterm labor or prelabor rupture of membranes. J Matern Fetal Neonatal Med. 2009;22:388–97.
70. Goncalves LF, Chaiworapongsa T, Romero R. Intrauterine infection and prematurity. Ment Retard Dev Disabil Res Rev. 2002;8:3–13.
71. Romero R, Espinoza J, Chaiworapongsa T, Kalache K. Infection and prematurity and the role of preventive strategies. Semin Neonatol. 2002;7:259–74.
72. Romero R, Quintero R, Oyarzun E, Wu YK, Sabo V, Mazor M, et al. Intraamniotic infection and the onset of labor in preterm premature rupture of the membranes. Am J Obstet Gynecol. 1988;159:661–6.
73. Romero R, Gonzalez R, Sepulveda W, Brandt F, Ramirez M, Sorokin Y, et al. Infection and labor. VIII. Microbial invasion of the amniotic cavity in patients with suspected cervical incompetence: prevalence and clinical significance. Am J Obstet Gynecol. 1992;167:1086–91.
74. Bujold E, Morency AM, Rallu F, Ferland S, Tetu A, Duperron L, et al. Bacteriology of amniotic fluid in women with suspected cervical insufficiency. J Obstet Gynaecol Can. 2008;30:882–7.
75. Romero R, Mazor M. Infection and preterm labor. Clin Obstet Gynecol. 1988;31:553–84.

76. Averbuch B, Mazor M, Shoham-Vardi I, Chaim W, Vardi H, Horowitz S, et al. Intra-uterine infection in women with preterm premature rupture of membranes: maternal and neonatal characteristics. Eur.J Obstet Gynecol. Reprod Biol. 1995;62:25–9.
77. Carroll SG, Papaioannou S, Ntumazah IL, Philpott-Howard J, Nicolaides KH. Lower genital tract swabs in the prediction of intrauterine infection in preterm prelabour rupture of the membranes. Br J Obstet Gynaecol. 1996;103:54–9.
78. Cotton DB, Hill LM, Strassner HT, Platt LD, Ledger WJ. Use of amniocentesis in preterm gestation with ruptured membranes. Obstet Gynecol. 1984;63:38–43.
79. Coultrip LL, Grossman JH. Evaluation of rapid diagnostic tests in the detection of microbial invasion of the amniotic cavity. Am J Obstet Gynecol. 1992;167:1231–42.
80. Garite TJ, Freeman RK, Linzey EM, Braly P. The use of amniocentesis in patients with premature rupture of membranes. Obstet Gynecol. 1979;54:226–30.
81. Zlatnik FJ, Cruikshank DP, Petzold CR, Galask RP. Amniocentesis in the identification of inapparent infection in preterm patients with premature rupture of the membranes. J Reprod Med. 1984;29:656–60.
82. Watts DH, Krohn MA, Hillier SL, Eschenbach DA. The association of occult amniotic fluid infection with gestational age and neonatal outcome among women in preterm labor. Obstet Gynecol. 1992;79:351–7.
83. Ballard PL, Ballard RA. Scientific basis and therapeutic regimens for use of antenatal glucocorticoids. Am J Obstet Gynecol. 1995;173:254–62.
84. Crowley P. Prophylactic corticosteroids for preterm birth. Cochrane Database Syst Rev. 1996; Issue 1, Wiley, Chichester, UK. DOI: 10.1002./14651858.CD000065.
85. Schrag S, Gorwitz R, Fultz-Butts K, Schuchat A. Prevention of perinatal group B streptococcal disease. Revised guidelines from CDC. MMWR Recomm Rep. 2002;51:1–22.
86. King JF, Flenady VJ, Papatsonis DN, Dekker GA, Carbonne B. Calcium channel blockers for inhibiting preterm labour. Cochrane Database Syst Rev. 2003;CD002255.
87. Papatsonis D, Flenady V, Cole S, Liley H. Oxytocin receptor antagonists for inhibiting preterm labour. Cochrane Database Syst Rev. 2005;CD004452.
88. Anotayanonth S, Subhedar NV, Garner P, Neilson JP, Harigopal S. Betamimetics for inhibiting preterm labour. Cochrane Database Syst Rev. 2004;CD004352.
89. King J, Flenady V, Cole S, Thornton S. Cyclo-oxygenase (COX) inhibitors for treating preterm labour. Cochrane Database Syst Rev. 2005;CD001992.
90. Crowther CA, Hiller JE, Doyle LW. Magnesium sulphate for preventing preterm birth in threatened preterm labour. Cochrane Database Syst Rev. 2002;CD001060.
91. Rouse DJ, Hirtz DG, Thom E, Varner MW, Spong CY, Mercer BM, et al. A randomized, controlled trial of magnesium sulfate for the prevention of cerebral palsy. N Engl J Med. 2008;359:895–905.
92. Doyle LW, Crowther CA, Middleton P, Marret S, Rouse D. Magnesium sulphate for women at risk of preterm birth for neuroprotection of the fetus. Cochrane Database Syst Rev. 2009; CD004661.
93. Gahl W, Kazina TR, Furmann D, et al. Diamine oxidase in the diagnosis of ruptured fetal membranes. Am J Obstet Gynecol. 1969;104:544.
94. Huber JF, Bischof P, Extermann P, Beguin F, Herrmann WL. Are vaginal fluid concentrations of prolactin, alpha-fetoprotein and human placental lactogen useful for diagnosing ruptured membranes? Br J Obstet Gynaecol. 1983;90:1183–5.
95. Koninckx PR, Trappeniers H, Van Assche FA. Prolactin concentration in vaginal fluid: a new method for diagnosing ruptured membranes. Br J Obstet Gynaecol. 1981;88:607–10.
96. Phocas I, Sarandakou A, Kontoravdis A, Chryssicopoulos A, Zourlas PA. Vaginal fluid prolactin: a reliable marker for the diagnosis of prematurely ruptured membranes. Comparison with vaginal fluid alpha-fetoprotein and placental lactogen. Eur J Obstet Gynecol Reprod Biol. 1989;31: 133–41.
97. Gaucherand P, Guibaud S, Rudigoz RC, Wong A. Diagnosis of premature rupture of the membranes by the identification of alpha-feto-protein in vaginal secretions. Acta Obstet Gynecol Scand. 1994;73:456–9.

98. Kishida T, Hirao A, Matsuura T, Katamine T, Yamada H, Sagawa T, et al. Diagnosis of premature rupture of membranes with an improved alpha-fetoprotein monoclonal antibody kit. Clin Chem. 1995;41:1500–3.

99. Atlay RD, Sutherst JR. Premature rupture of the fetal membranes confirmed by intra-amniotic injection of dye (Evans blue T-1824). Am J Obstet Gynecol. 1970;108:993–4.

100. Diaz-Garzon J. Indigocarmine test of preterm rupture of membranes. Rev Columb Obstet Gynecol. 1969;20:373.

101. Fujimoto S, Kishida T, Sagawa T, Negishi H, Okuyama K, Hareyama H, et al. Clinical usefulness of the dye-injection method for diagnosing premature rupture of the membranes in equivocal cases. J Obstet Gynaecol. 1995;21:215–20.

102. Meyer BA, Gonik B, Creasy RK. Evaluation of phenazopyridine hydrochloride as a tool in the diagnosis of premature rupture of the membranes. Am J Perinatol. 1991;8:297–9.

103. Cowett RM, Hakanson DO, Kocon RW, Oh W. Untoward neonatal effect of intraamniotic administration of methylene blue. Obstet Gynecol. 1976;48:74S–5.

104. Mc Enerney J, Mc Enerney L. Unfavourable neotal outcomes after intraamniotic injection of methylene blue. Obstet Gynecol. 1983;61:35S–7S.

105. Troche BI. Methylene blue baby. N Engl J Med. 1989;320:1756–7.

106. Mercer BM, Miodovnik M, Thurnau GR, Goldenberg RL, Das AF, Ramsey RD, et al. Antibiotic therapy for reduction of infant morbidity after preterm premature rupture of the membranes. A randomized controlled trial. National Institute of Child Health and Human Development Maternal-Fetal Medicine Units Network. JAMA. 1997;278:989–95.

107. Fox NS, Gelber SE, Kalish RB, Chasen ST. Contemporary practice patterns and beliefs regarding tocolysis among u.s. Maternal-fetal medicine specialists. Obstet Gynecol. 2008; 112:42–7.

108. Cox SM, Leveno KJ. Intentional delivery versus expectant management with preterm ruptured membranes at 30–34 weeks' gestation. Obstet Gynecol. 1995;86:875–9.

109. Beydoun SN, Yasin SY. Premature rupture of the membranes before 28 weeks: conservative management. Am J Obstet Gynecol. 1986;155:471–9.

110. Taylor J, Garite TJ. Premature rupture of membranes before fetal viability. Obstet Gynecol. 1984;64:615–20.

111. Moretti M, Sibai BM. Maternal and perinatal outcome of expectant management of premature rupture of membranes in the midtrimester. Am J Obstet Gynecol. 1988;159:390–6.

112. Major CA, Kitzmiller JL. Perinatal survival with expectant management of midtrimester rupture of membranes. Am J Obstet Gynecol. 1990;163:838–44.

113. Bengtson JM, VanMarter LJ, Barss VA, Greene MF, Tuomala RE, Epstein MF. Pregnancy outcome after premature rupture of the membranes at or before 26 weeks' gestation. Obstet Gynecol. 1989;73:921–7.

Chapter 7
Placental Abruption

Cande V. Ananth and Wendy L. Kinzler

Introduction

In normal pregnancies placental separation occurs immediately following birth, but in cases of abruption the placental detachment occurs prematurely [1]. There are no standard criteria for diagnosing placental abruption, but the clinical hallmarks of the condition are vaginal bleeding and abdominal pain accompanied by uterine hypertonicity, tachysystole, and a nonreassuring fetal heart rate pattern. Abruption is strongly associated with disproportionately increased risks of stillbirth and neonatal and infant mortality, as well as preterm delivery and intrauterine growth restriction.

In this chapter, we review the literature on placental abruption, focusing on the epidemiology and risk factors, and clinical diagnosis. We provide directions for effective and optimal obstetrical management of patients diagnosed with placental abruption.

Epidemiology

Placental abruption complicates roughly 0.6–1.2% of all pregnancies [2–7], with higher risks seen with increasing plurality. A retrospective cohort study [8] based on 15,051,872 singletons, 413,619 twins, and 22,585 triplets delivered in the USA

C.V. Ananth (✉)
Department of Obstetrics and Gynecology, College of Physicians and Surgeons,
Columbia University, New York, NY, USA
e-mail: cva2111@columbia.edu

E. Sheiner (ed.), *Bleeding During Pregnancy: A Comprehensive Guide*,
DOI 10.1007/978-1-4419-9810-1_7, © Springer Science+Business Media, LLC 2011

Table 7.1 Risk factors for placental abruption

Advanced maternal age
Advanced parity
African American race
Smoking before/during pregnancy
Cocaine and drug use
Single marital status
Underweight maternal BMI
Chronic hypertension
Preeclampsia/eclampsia
Oligohydramnios/polyhydramnios
Preterm PROM
Multiple pregnancy
Folate deficiency
Assisted reproduction
Intrapartum fever
Maternal anemia
Diabetes
Prior cesarean delivery
Maternal vascular disease
Abdominal trauma during pregnancy
Fibroids/uterine malformations
History of ischemic placental disease[a]
History of stillbirth
Short umbilical cord

BMI body mass index, *PROM* premature rupture of membranes
[a]Includes preeclampsia, intrauterine growth restriction, and placental abruption

during the years 1995–1998 reported risks of 0.6% in singletons, 1.2% among twins, and 1.6% among triplet births ($P_{trend} < 0.0001$).

Several studies have identified a number of predisposing risk factors for abruption (Table 7.1). Risk factors that are associated with abruptions of acute onset include abdominal trauma, short umbilical cord, and sudden uterine decompression [9–13]. Women of advanced maternal age, multiparity, folate deficiency, tobacco and cocaine use, chronic hypertension, preeclampsia, intraamniotic infection, and prolonged rupture of membranes are also at an increased risk for abruption [2–4, 6, 7, 9, 14–26]. Studies suggest that surgical disruption of the uterine cavity (e.g., prior cesarean delivery) and a short interpregnancy interval are risk factors for abruption [27, 28]. Studies have also suggested that maternal uterine fibroids predispose women to increased susceptibility to abruption [29], although this finding remains uncorroborated. Other putative risk factors for abruption include maternal iron deficiency anemia [30], hyperhomocysteinemia [31], and maternal infection and inflammation [15, 18]. The strongest predictor of placental abruption, however, is abruption during a previous pregnancy [24, 32–40].

Familial Predisposition

Studies have recently shown that placental abruption tends to aggregate more in families of women who have experienced an abruption. This was first demonstrated by Toivonen et al. [41] in a Finnish study. They compared rates of abruption in first-degree female relatives (mothers and sisters) to that of 29,605 women in a general obstetrical population. The risk of abruption in first-degree relatives of abruption probands (0.4%) was similar to that in the general population (0.6%). However, when these data were restricted to probands with recurrent placental abruption, the odds ratio for familial aggregation of abruption in mothers and sisters combined was 5.6 [95% confidence interval (CI) 1.4–23.2].

A population-based study of Missouri residents [42] reported that the sibling–sibling odds ratio for placental abruption was 3.8 (95% CI 2.6–5.5). In a large, population-based Norwegian cohort study, Rasmussen and Irgens [43] reported that following a severe abruption (defined as placental abruption resulting in preterm delivery), odds ratios for abruption in the proband's sisters were 1.7–2.1, whereas mild abruption (i.e., those delivered at term gestations) was not associated with any increased risk in sisters. The estimated heritability of placental abruption between sisters of abruption was 11% (95% CI 5–17), whereas the heritability coefficient for severe abruption between sisters was 16%. However, these authors found no excess risk of abruption between sisters and brothers' partners or from brothers' partners to sisters.

Placental Abruption and Adverse Perinatal Outcomes

Placental abruption is implicated in disproportionately high rates of an array of adverse perinatal outcomes, including preterm delivery, IUGR, stillbirth, and perinatal mortality [6, 16, 23, 24, 39, 44–47]. Placental abruption is the strongest known "trigger" of spontaneous preterm labor and preterm premature rupture of membranes (PROM) [44, 48] – both leading to excessively high rates of preterm birth [24, 49, 50]. Women with abruption tend to deliver 3–4 weeks earlier than nonabruption births, and newborns weigh, on average, 300–700 g less [44]. Placental abruption is associated with a four- to sixfold higher risk of preterm birth and with a two- to fourfold higher risk of IUGR. Risks of stillbirth and neonatal mortality in the USA in relation to abruption are 22-fold higher (95% CI 21.1–22.9) and 13-fold higher (95% CI 12.2–13.9), respectively [45]. The high incidence of mortality with abruption was due, in part, to its strong association with preterm delivery. In all, 55% of the excess deaths associated with placental abruption were due to early delivery (<37 weeks) and an additional 9% to IUGR [45].

Pathophysiology

The immediate cause of the premature placental separation is often the rupture of maternal vessels in the decidua basalis, where it interfaces with the anchoring villi in the placenta. Rarely, the bleeding can originate from the fetoplacental vessels. The accumulating blood splits the decidua and its placental attachment from the uterus. The resultant hematoma may be small and self-limited, or it may continue to dissect through the placenta–decidua interface, leading to complete or near-complete placental separation. Because the detached portion of the placenta is unable to exchange gases and nutrients, fetal growth and development remain compromised.

Placental abruption can be "revealed" when the blood tracks between the membranes and the decidua and escapes through the cervix into the vagina. In other instances, although relatively less common, the blood accumulates and is entrapped behind the placenta with no obvious external evidence of bleeding. This type of abruption is called "concealed" abruption [51].

Signs and Symptoms

The clinical manifestations of placental abruption can be quite variable, depending on the severity and the chronicity of the hemorrhage. Classically, an acute clinical abruption presents with vaginal bleeding, abdominal and/or back pain, and uterine contractions. The bleeding may be scant or severe and its color may vary between bright red and maroon ("port wine"). Unfortunately, the amount of vaginal bleeding correlates poorly with the severity of placental separation and potential fetal risk [1]. The contractions are often of high frequency and low amplitude, but a mild to moderate contraction pattern is also possible. There may be an elevated resting tone of the uterus, resulting in a firm, tender fundus on palpation. In up to 20% of abruption cases the hemorrhage is concealed within the uterus, and the presentation includes preterm labor without vaginal bleeding [1, 51]. Fetal heart rate abnormalities or fetal death may also be present. Owing to the wide range of presentations, any woman with preterm labor, with or without vaginal bleeding, should be suspected as having a placental abruption.

Caution Box
_____

Classically, an acute clinical abruption presents with vaginal bleeding, abdominal and/or back pain, and uterine contractions. Nevertheless, the amount of vaginal bleeding correlates poorly with the severity of placental separation and potential fetal risk as a large amount of blood can remain concealed within the uterine cavity.

With more than 50% of the placenta separated from the maternal surface, both fetal and maternal compromise is likely [44, 51]. There are large releases of tissue factor into the maternal circulation within a short time, acutely triggering the coagulation cascade and massive generation of thrombin, resulting in disseminated intravascular coagulation (DIC). The coagulation mechanisms subsequently become overwhelmed, and the clinical consequence is significant, with profound systemic bleeding and tissue ischemia. Hypovolemic shock and multiorgan system failure can result, with kidney, liver, lung, cardiac, and central nervous system injury. As a result, abruption is associated with an increased incidence of blood transfusions and hysterectomy [18, 51], DIC, hemorrhagic shock, uterine rupture, and acute renal failure [52, 53].

Placental abruption can also be a chronic process and a manifestation of ischemic placental disease [54, 55]. Affected patients experience mild to moderate intermittent bleeding throughout the second and third trimesters. Associated findings may include oligohydramnios, fetal growth restriction, and preterm PROM. These women are also at increased risk of developing preeclampsia, a maternal manifestation of ischemic placental disease [23].

Caution Box

With more than 50% of the placenta separated from the maternal surface, both fetal and maternal compromise is likely. With large releases of tissue factor into the maternal circulation in a short time, there is acute triggering of the coagulation cascade and massive generation of thrombin, resulting in DIC.

Clinical Diagnosis

Placental abruption can be one of the most devastating complications in all of obstetrics. In the presence of vaginal bleeding or hemorrhage, it is often a diagnosis of exclusion. Roughly, one-third of all bleeding episodes are attributable to placental abruption, about one-fifth to placenta previa, and the remainder of undetermined etiology [56–58]. The diagnosis of placental abruption is based on clinical hallmarks, including vaginal bleeding (in the absence of placenta previa) at presentation accompanied by at least one of the following conditions: fetal distress, uterine tenderness, or hypertonic uterus (without other causes, such as those due to hyperstimulation from pitocin augmentation). In addition, if the delivered placenta shows any evidence of a tightly adherent clot consistent with retroplacental bleeding or if sonographic signs of abruption are present, the diagnosis of abruption is recorded [59].

Ultrasonography (US), laboratory, and placental pathological findings often support the clinical diagnosis. Because of the potential variability in presentations, a high index of suspicion is important, particularly for women with underlying risk factors. These factors include a prior pregnancy complicated by ischemic placental disease, recent trauma, smoking and/or cocaine use, preterm PROM, hypertension, and other co-morbid vascular disease.

History

Obstetrical History

Uteroplacental underperfusion, chronic hypoxia, and uteroplacental ischemia can result in placental abruption, IUGR, or preeclampsia, otherwise known as ischemic placental disease. When any one of these manifestations has complicated a prior pregnancy, subsequent pregnancies are at increased risk for abruption, preeclampsia, or small for gestational age (SGA) infants. If abruption complicated a prior pregnancy, there is a threefold increased risk of recurrent abruption [33].

Trauma

Maternal trauma during pregnancy may cause external compression–decompression stress at the placenta–decidua interface or rapid acceleration–deceleration injury. Uterine stretch without concomitant placental stretch can lead to a shearing force between the placenta and attached decidua basalis and the uterine wall, resulting in placental abruption. Other causes of rapid uterine decompression, such as after rupture of membranes in the setting of polyhydramnios or after delivery of a first twin, can also trigger placental abruption [60].

Social Exposures

Smoking is associated with a 60% increased risk of placental ischemia in a dose–response relation [61]. Smoking is also associated with a 2.5-fold increased risk of abruption severe enough to result in fetal death in a dose-dependent fashion, with the risk increasing by 40% for each pack per day smoked [49].

As many as 10% of women using cocaine during the third trimester suffer placental abruption [62, 63]. It has been hypothesized that this increased risk is associated with cocaine-induced acute vasoconstriction, ischemia, and reflex vasodilation. Women who consume alcohol during pregnancy may have an up to 33% greater likelihood of placental abruption [64].

Preterm Premature Rupture of Membranes

Placental abruption occurs in 2–5% of pregnancies complicated by preterm PROM [7, 15, 65]. The risk is increased seven- to ninefold in those in whom there is an intrauterine infection or oligohydramnios associated with the preterm PROM [15, 65].

The risk of placental abruption increases with increasing pregnancy latency following preterm PROM, suggesting that inflammation prior to membrane rupture may induce placental separation [15]. In addition, decidual hemorrhage and thrombin release results in degradation of the extracellular matrix and decidual inflammation, which may lead to subsequent preterm PROM [66].

Maternal Medical Conditions

Hypertensive disorders of pregnancy, including chronic hypertension, preeclampsia, and preeclampsia superimposed on chronic hypertension, are strong risk factors for placental abruption [2, 6, 7, 23, 26, 32, 49, 67]. Unfortunately, antihypertensive therapy does not appear to reduce the risk of placental abruption [68]. Underweight women also have an increased risk of placental abruption in both singletons and twins [69, 70]. Although much attention has been given to the association of maternal thrombophilia and an increased risk of placental disorders and adverse pregnancy outcomes, they have not been consistently linked to increased risks of abruption [71–75]. Caution should always be taken when evaluating women with other conditions associated with vascular disease, including long-standing diabetes, systemic lupus erythematosus, renal disease, and anti-phospholipid antibody syndrome.

Obstetrical Factors

Early markers of placental abruption can be detected during routine prenatal care and should increase the index of suspicion for abruption when a woman presents with vaginal bleeding and/or preterm labor. The presence of a subchorionic hemorrhage and/or first trimester bleeding increases the risk of placental abruption later in the pregnancy [76, 77]. Obtaining this history from a patient may be helpful in determining her risk status. First and second trimester maternal serum screening for aneuploidy can also provide insight as to the possibility of underlying placental dysfunction. Low pregnancy-associated plasma protein-A (PAPP-A) levels are possibly linked to inadequate trophoblast invasion. First trimester values of PAPP-A < 0.4 multiples of the median (MoM) have been associated with increased risks of preeclampsia, fetal loss, preterm delivery and fetal growth restriction [78]. Likewise, these same adverse outcomes, in addition to placental abruption, are increased with elevations of second trimester α-fetoprotein (AFP>2.0 MoM) [79–81]. These high values are thought to be the result of disruptions of the maternal-fetal-placental barrier with vascular damage and uteroplacental ischemia [82–85]. Elevations in AFP that are not explained by fetal abnormalities carry up to a tenfold risk of subsequent abruption [86, 87]. Similar risks have been noted with elevated second trimester human chorionic gonadotropin (hCG) (>3.0 MoM) [79, 80] and inhibin A (>2.0 MoM) [78].

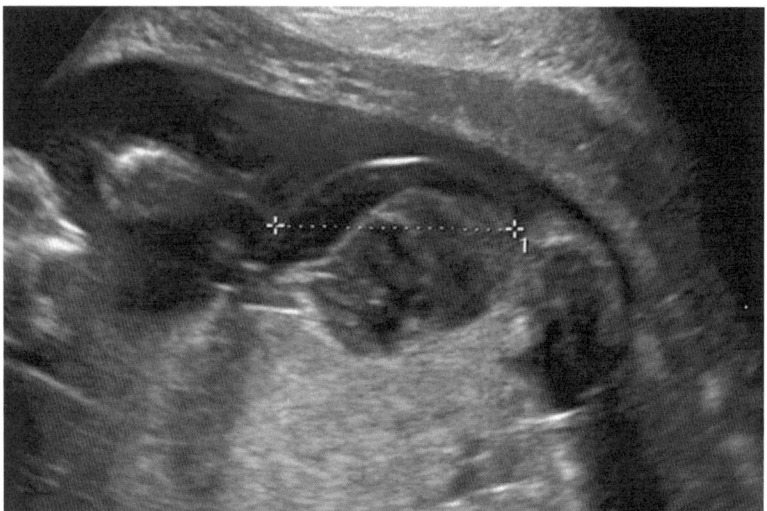

Fig. 7.1 Preplacental subchorionic hematoma

Sonographic Findings

Several sonographic features can increase the diagnostic certainty of an abruption. A retroplacental clot (Fig. 7.1) is the classic US finding, but identification of a clot depends on the extent of the hemorrhage, the chronicity of the bleeding, and whether there has been escape of blood through the cervix. Other sonographic findings include subchorionic collections of fluid, which can be located at the margins of the placenta, along the chorionic surface of the placenta, or even remote from the placental attachment site. Echogenic debris (free-floating blood) in the amniotic fluid can be seen; it swirls with movement but settles at dependent portions of the uterus (posterior wall and lower uterine segment at the level of the cervix). This picture is sometimes confused with a placenta previa in a woman presenting with vaginal bleeding. A thickened placenta (Fig. 7.2), especially if it shimmers with maternal movement ("jello"-like sign), can indicate parenchymal or retroplacental bleeding [88]. In the setting of trauma, placental abruption may be identified during the maternal evaluation by computed tomography [89, 90].

Laboratory Findings

Laboratory testing is not useful in making the diagnosis of placental abruption, but coagulopathy, particularly hypofibrinogenemia, supports the diagnosis of severe abruption. It is important to remember that placental abruption is a clinical diagnosis. Histologic and gross pathology findings may be supportive, but also have limitations.

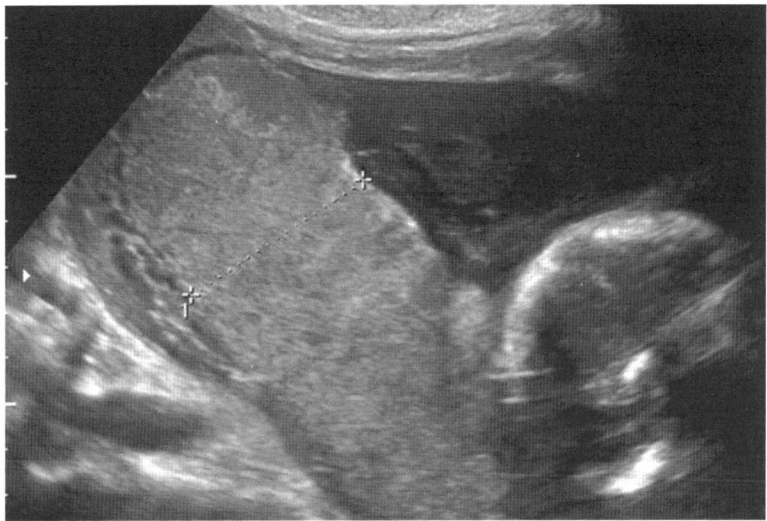

Fig. 7.2 Increased placental thickness associated with intraparenchymal placental bleeding

The presence of a retroplacental clot, especially when associated with a compression defect, is the most common finding, along with microscopic evidence of hemorrhage, particularly at preterm gestations [91]. Other less specific lesions such as acute chorioamnionitis and placental infarcts have also been associated with clinical abruption, such that the overall concordance between clinical abruption and histologic findings is low [59].

Obstetrical Management of Pregnancies Diagnosed with Placental Abruption

Management of placental abruption depends on several factors, including the severity of the abruption, the gestational age, the immediate maternal and fetal risks, and the anticipated subsequent maternal and neonatal risks.

In cases of suspected abruption, the initial evaluation consists of continuous fetal monitoring and assessment of the maternal hemodynamic status. Adequate maternal intravenous access and close monitoring of vital signs and urine output is essential. Laboratory evaluation includes a complete blood count, blood type and Rh status, and coagulation studies. A low fibrinogen level is the most sensitive indicator of coagulopathy related to abruption. The blood bank should be notified if blood product replacement is anticipated. Anti-D immunoglobulin in a dose determined by Kleihauer-Betke testing is also necessary for women who are Rh-negative. It is important to remember that the extent of blood loss is not accurately determined by the amount of vaginal bleeding as a large amount of blood can remain concealed in the uterine cavity.

In stable patients, bedside US is suggested to evaluate for sonographic signs of abruption, assess fetal presentation and estimated fetal weight, and assess amniotic fluid volume.

Delivery at Term and Late Preterm Gestations

Delivery is recommended at term gestational ages ($\geq$37 weeks). At gestational ages 34–36$^{6/7}$ weeks, if there is a high index of suspicion for abruption, especially in the setting of underlying risk factors, the maternal and fetal benefits of delivery likely outweigh the risks of preterm delivery. Inpatient monitoring and delivery should be considered. Tocolysis is not recommended in these circumstances. Vaginal delivery is reasonable if the maternal status is stable and the fetal heart tracing is reassuring. Prompt cesarean delivery is indicated if the fetal heart tracing is nonreassuring, if there is ongoing major blood loss or other serious maternal complications, or if vaginal delivery is otherwise contraindicated. If maternal coagulopathy is present, rapid replacement of blood products is necessary to limit maternal surgical morbidity. Extravasation of blood into the myometrium due to a placental abruption is called a Couvelaire uterus and can be identified at the time of cesarean delivery. It is associated with an increased risk of postpartum atony and hemorrhage. Close monitoring of the maternal hemodynamic status and fluid balance is essential, even during the postpartum period.

Delivery at Preterm Gestational Ages

At preterm gestational ages <34 weeks, there may be benefit in delaying delivery when fetal status is reassuring and there is no evidence of ongoing major blood loss or maternal hemodynamic instability. Antenatal glucocorticoids should be administered to promote fetal lung maturity and to reduce the risk of neonatal death. Many experts believe that tocolysis is contraindicated in the presence of placental abruption. Results from a few small studies have suggested that women with clinically stable suspected abruptions may benefit by administration of tocolytics to prolong gestation [92, 93]. These data should be interpreted with caution, however, as the studies were neither randomized nor controlled. Nevertheless, no adverse complications of tocolytic administration were reported. If tocolytics are considered, they should be utilized only for short courses to achieve the maximal corticosteroid effect and only when the maternal and fetal status is stable. It is prudent to avoid β-sympathomimetics because of potentially adverse cardiovascular effects in bleeding patients. The risk of maternal hypotension with the use of calcium-channel blockers should also be taken into consideration.

There are no compelling data to guide the length of hospital stay for women with acute or chronic abruptions that are stable. Because of the unpredictable nature of recurrent episodes, close surveillance in the hospital is reasonable until bleeding has stopped for several days. Outpatient management should be considered only for patients who are able to return to the hospital quickly and reliably if bleeding recurs. They should have normal hematological parameters, reassuring fetal testing, and no active bleeding. Outpatient maternal and fetal assessments should occur at least weekly and include nonstress tests and biophysical profiles. Serial sonographic estimated fetal weights every 3–4 weeks are suggested because of the increased risk of fetal growth restriction.

Fetal Demise

Management of pregnancies complicated by placental abruption and fetal demise should focus on minimizing maternal morbidity and mortality while expediting delivery. Vaginal delivery is preferred unless there are maternal contraindications to a vaginal birth or there is severe maternal hemorrhage remote from delivery. As the frequency of coagulopathy is higher in abruptions associated with fetal demise, close monitoring of maternal vital signs, urine output, and fluid and blood/blood product resuscitation is paramount.

Significance and Importance of Studying Placental Abruption

Despite the increased recurrence and the importance of abruption as a determinant of adverse pregnancy outcomes, there are no reliable methods for risk assessment or biological markers for predicting risk [94]. This leaves the undesired consequence of uncertain obstetrical management of patients with abruption in a previous pregnancy or those at impending risk. With an estimated 1.34 million births complicated by abruption annual worldwide (and more than 40,000 in the USA alone), statistics on maternal/infant consequences of placental abruption and its impact on societal economic implications are insurmountable. Efforts to predict and subsequently prevent women from having to endure this devastating obstetrical complication should focus on understanding abruption as a chronic process with origins early in pregnancy and perhaps even extending back to the stage of placental implantation [45].

References

1. Clark SL. Placenta previa and abruptio placentae. In: Creasy RK, Resnik R, editors. Maternal fetal medicine. Philadelphia, PA: WB Saunders Company; 2004. p. 715–7.
2. Ananth CV, Smulian JC, Vintzileos AM. Incidence of placental abruption in relation to cigarette smoking and hypertensive disorders during pregnancy: a meta-analysis of observational studies. Obstet Gynecol. 1999;93:622–8.

3. Ananth CV, Oyelese Y, Yeo L, et al. Placental abruption in the United States, 1979 through 2001: temporal trends and potential determinants. Am J Obstet Gynecol. 2005;192:191–8.
4. Cnattingius S. Maternal age modifies the effect of maternal smoking on intrauterine growth retardation but not on late fetal death and placental abruption. Am J Epidemiol. 1997;145:319–23.
5. Rasmussen S, Irgens LM, Bergsjo P, et al. The occurrence of placental abruption in Norway 1967–1991. Acta Obstet Gynecol Scand. 1996;75:222–8.
6. Raymond EG, Mills JL. Placental abruption. Maternal risk factors and associated fetal conditions. Acta Obstet Gynecol Scand. 1993;72:633–9.
7. Williams MA, Lieberman E, Mittendorf R, et al. Risk factors for abruptio placentae. Am J Epidemiol. 1991;134:965–72.
8. Salihu HM, Bekan B, Aliyu MH, et al. Perinatal mortality associated with abruptio placenta in singletons and multiples. Am J Obstet Gynecol. 2005;193:198–203.
9. Brink AL, Odendaal HJ. Risk factors for abruptio placentae. S Afr Med J. 1987;72:250–2.
10. Cook KE, Jenkins SM. Pathologic uterine torsion associated with placental abruption, maternal shock, and intrauterine fetal demise. Am J Obstet Gynecol. 2005;192:2082–3.
11. Kettel LM, Branch DW, Scott JR. Occult placental abruption after maternal trauma. Obstet Gynecol. 1988;71:449–53.
12. Lavin Jr JP, Miodovnik M. Delayed abruption after maternal trauma as a result of an automobile accident. J Reprod Med. 1981;26:621–4.
13. Munro KI, Horne AW, Martin CW, et al. Uterine torsion with placental abruption. J Obstet Gynaecol. 2006;26:167–9.
14. Ananth CV, Smulian JC, Demissie K, et al. Placental abruption among singleton and twin births in the United States: risk factor profiles. Am J Epidemiol. 2001;153:771–8.
15. Ananth CV, Oyelese Y, Srinivas N, et al. Preterm premature rupture of membranes, intrauterine infection, and oligohydramnios: risk factors for placental abruption. Obstet Gynecol. 2004;104:71–7.
16. Ananth CV, Smulian JC, Srinivas N, et al. Risk of infant mortality among twins in relation to placental abruption: contributions of preterm birth and restricted fetal growth. Twin Res Hum Genet. 2005;8:524–31.
17. Ananth CV, Oyelese Y, Prasad V, et al. Evidence of placental abruption as a chronic process: Associations with vaginal bleeding early in pregnancy and placental lesions. Eur J Obstet Gynecol Reprod Biol. 2006;128:15–21.
18. Ananth CV, Getahun D, Peltier MR, et al. Placental abruption in term and preterm gestations: evidence for heterogeneity in clinical pathways. Obstet Gynecol. 2006;107:785–92.
19. Cnattingius S, Granath F, Petersson G, et al. The influence of gestational age and smoking habits on the risk of subsequent preterm deliveries. N Engl J Med. 1999;341:943–8.
20. Dafallah SE, Babikir HE. Risk factors predisposing to abruptio placentae. Maternal and fetal outcome. Saudi Med J. 2004;25:1237–40.
21. Eriksen G, Wohlert M, Ersbak V, et al. Placental abruption. A case-control investigation. Br J Obstet Gynaecol. 1991;98:448–52.
22. Faiz AS, Demissie K, Ananth CV, et al. Risk of abruptio placentae by region of birth and residence among African-American women in the USA. Ethn Health. 2001;6:247–53.
23. Rasmussen S, Irgens LM, Dalaker K. A history of placental dysfunction and risk of placental abruption. Paediatr Perinat Epidemiol. 1999;13:9–21.
24. Rasmussen S, Irgens LM, Dalaker K. Outcome of pregnancies subsequent to placental abruption: a risk assessment. Acta Obstet Gynecol Scand. 2000;79:496–501.
25. Sanchez SE, Pacora PN, Farfan JH, et al. Risk factors of abruptio placentae among Peruvian women. Am J Obstet Gynecol. 2006;194:225–30.
26. Williams MA, Mittendorf R, Monson RR. Chronic hypertension, cigarette smoking, and abruptio placentae. Epidemiology. 1991;2:450–3.
27. Getahun D, Oyelese Y, Salihu HM, et al. Previous cesarean delivery and risks of placenta previa and placental abruption. Obstet Gynecol. 2006;107:771–8.

28. Lydon-Rochelle M, Holt VL, Easterling TR, et al. First-birth cesarean and placental abruption or previa at second birth. Obstet Gynecol. 2001;97:765–9.

29. Rice JP, Kay HH, Mahony BS. The clinical significance of uterine leiomyomas in pregnancy. Am J Obstet Gynecol. 1989;160:1212–6.

30. Duthie SJ, King PA, To WK, et al. A case controlled study of pregnancy complicated by severe maternal anaemia. Aust N Z J Obstet Gynaecol. 1991;31:125–7.

31. Ray JG, Laskin CA. Folic acid and homocyst(e)ine metabolic defects and the risk of placental abruption, pre-eclampsia and spontaneous pregnancy loss: a systematic review. Placenta. 1999;20:519–29.

32. Ananth CV, Savitz DA, Williams MA. Placental abruption and its association with hypertension and prolonged rupture of membranes: a methodologic review and meta-analysis. Obstet Gynecol. 1996;88:309–18.

33. Ananth CV, Cnattingius S. Influence of maternal smoking on placental abruption in successive pregnancies: a population-based prospective cohort study in Sweden. Am J Epidemiol. 2007;166:289–95.

34. Ananth CV, Peltier MR, Chavez MR, et al. Recurrence of ischemic placental disease. Obstet Gynecol. 2007;110:128–33.

35. Furuhashi M, Kurauchi O, Suganuma N. Pregnancy following placental abruption. Arch Gynecol Obstet. 2002;267:11–3.

36. Karegard M, Gennser G. Incidence and recurrence rate of abruptio placentae in Sweden. Obstet Gynecol. 1986;67:523–8.

37. Karri K, Dwarakanath L. Recurrent preterm abruption – case report. Med Gen Med. 2005;7:63.

38. Misra DP, Ananth CV. Risk factor profiles of placental abruption in first and second pregnancies: heterogeneous etiologies. J Clin Epidemiol. 1999;52:453–61.

39. Rasmussen S, Irgens LM, Dalaker K. The effect on the likelihood of further pregnancy of placental abruption and the rate of its recurrence. Br J Obstet Gynaecol. 1997;104:1292–5.

40. Tikkanen M, Nuutila M, Hiilesmaa V, et al. Prepregnancy risk factors for placental abruption. Acta Obstet Gynecol Scand. 2006;85:40–4.

41. Toivonen S, Keski-Nisula L, Saarikoski S, et al. Risk of placental abruption in first-degree relatives of index patients. Clin Genet. 2004;66:244–6.

42. Plunkett J, Borecki I, Morgan T, et al. Population-based estimate of sibling risk for preterm birth, preterm premature rupture of membranes, placental abruption and pre-eclampsia. BMC Genet. 2008;9:44.

43. Rasmussen S, Irgens LM. Occurrence of placental abruption in relatives. BJOG. 2009;116: 693–9.

44. Ananth CV, Berkowitz GS, Savitz DA, et al. Placental abruption and adverse perinatal outcomes. JAMA. 1999;282:1646–51.

45. Ananth CV, Wilcox AJ. Placental abruption and perinatal mortality in the United States. Am J Epidemiol. 2001;153:332–7.

46. Kayani SI, Walkinshaw SA, Preston C. Pregnancy outcome in severe placental abruption. BJOG. 2003;110:679–83.

47. Kyrklund-Blomberg NB, Gennser G, Cnattingius S. Placental abruption and perinatal death. Paediatr Perinat Epidemiol. 2001;15:290–7.

48. Ananth CV, Demissie K, Hanley ML. Birth weight discordancy and adverse perinatal outcomes among twin gestations in the United States: the effect of placental abruption. Am J Obstet Gynecol. 2003;188:954–60.

49. Kramer MS, Usher RH, Pollack R, et al. Etiologic determinants of abruptio placentae. Obstet Gynecol. 1997;89:221–6.

50. Rasmussen S, Irgens LM, Bergsjo P, et al. Perinatal mortality and case fatality after placental abruption in Norway 1967–1991. Acta Obstet Gynecol Scand. 1996;75:229–34.

51. Oyelese Y, Ananth CV. Placental abruption. Obstet Gynecol. 2006;108:1005–16.

52. Brame RG, Harbert Jr GM, McGaughey Jr HS, et al. Maternal risk in abruption. Obstet Gynecol. 1968;31:224–7.

53. Leunen K, Hall DR, Odendaal HJ, et al. The profile and complications of women with placental abruption and intrauterine death. J Trop Pediatr. 2003;49:231–4.
54. Ananth CV, Vintzileos AM. Maternal-fetal conditions necessitating a medical intervention resulting in preterm birth. Am J Obstet Gynecol. 2006;195:1557–63.
55. Ananth CV, Peltier MR, Kinzler WL, et al. Chronic hypertension and risk of placental abruption: is the association modified by ischemic placental disease? Am J Obstet Gynecol. 2007;197:273.e1–7.
56. Hibbard BM, Jeffcoate TN. Abruptio placentae. Obstet Gynecol. 1966;27:155–67.
57. Lowe TW, Cunningham FG. Placental abruption. Clin Obstet Gynecol. 1990;33:406–13.
58. Nielson EC, Varner MW, Scott JR. The outcome of pregnancies complicated by bleeding during the second trimester. Surg Gynecol Obstet. 1991;173:371–4.
59. Elsasser DA, Ananth CV, Prasad V, et al. Diagnosis of placental abruption: relationship between clinical and histopathological findings. Eur J Obstet Gynecol Reprod Biol. 2010;148:125–30.
60. Benedetti TJ. Obstetrical hemorrhage. In: Gabbe SG, Niebyl JR, Simpson JL, editors. Obstetrics: normal and problem pregnancies. New York, NY: Churchill Livingston Inc.; 1996.
61. Dafopoulos A, Dafopoulos K, Georgoulias P, et al. Smoking and AMH levels in women with normal reproductive history. Arch Gynecol Obstet. 2010;282:215–9.
62. Bauer CR, Shankaran S, Bada HS, et al. The Maternal Lifestyle Study: drug exposure during pregnancy and short-term maternal outcomes. Am J Obstet Gynecol. 2002;186:487–95.
63. Hoskins IA, Friedman DM, Frieden FJ, et al. Relationship between antepartum cocaine abuse, abnormal umbilical artery Doppler velocimetry, and placental abruption. Obstet Gynecol. 1991;78:279–82.
64. Aliyu MH, Lynch O, Nana PN, et al. Alcohol consumption during pregnancy and risk of placental abruption and placenta previa. Matern Child Health J. 2010; May 1. [Epub ahead of print].
65. Vintzileos AM, Campbell WA, Nochimson DJ, et al. Preterm premature rupture of the membranes: a risk factor for the development of abruptio placentae. Am J Obstet Gynecol. 1987;156:1235–8.
66. Lockwood CJ, Paidas M, Murk WK, et al. Involvement of human decidual cell-expressed tissue factor in uterine hemostasis and abruption. Thromb Res. 2009;124:516–20.
67. Ananth CV, Savitz DA, Bowes Jr WA, et al. Influence of hypertensive disorders and cigarette smoking on placental abruption and uterine bleeding during pregnancy. Br J Obstet Gynaecol. 1997;104:572–8.
68. Sibai BM, Mabie WC, Shamsa F, et al. A comparison of no medication versus methyldopa or labetalol in chronic hypertension during pregnancy. Am J Obstet Gynecol. 1990;162:960–6. discussion 6–7.
69. Aliyu MH, Alio AP, Lynch O, et al. Maternal pre-gravid body weight and risk for placental abruption among twin pregnancies. J Matern Fetal Neonatal Med. 2009;22:745–50.
70. Deutsch AB, Lynch O, Alio AP, et al. Increased risk of placental abruption in underweight women. Am J Perinatol. 2010;27:235–40.
71. Alfirevic Z, Roberts D, Martlew V. How strong is the association between maternal thrombophilia and adverse pregnancy outcome? A systematic review. Eur J Obstet Gynecol Reprod Biol. 2002;101:6–14.
72. Dizon-Townson D, Miller C, Sibai B, et al. The relationship of the factor V Leiden mutation and pregnancy outcomes for mother and fetus. Obstet Gynecol. 2005;106:517–24.
73. Silver RM, Zhao Y, Spong CY, et al. Prothrombin gene G20210A mutation and obstetric complications. Obstet Gynecol. 2010;115:14–20.
74. Gargano JW, Holzman CB, Senagore PK, et al. Polymorphisms in thrombophilia and renin-angiotensin system pathways, preterm delivery, and evidence of placental hemorrhage. Am J Obstet Gynecol. 2009;201:317.e1–9.
75. Said JM, Higgins JR, Moses EK, et al. Inherited thrombophilia polymorphisms and pregnancy outcomes in nulliparous women. Obstet Gynecol. 2010;115:5–13.
76. Norman SM, Odibo AO, Macones GA, et al. Ultrasound-detected subchorionic hemorrhage and the obstetric implications. Obstet Gynecol. 2010;116:311–5.

77. Lykke JA, Dideriksen KL, Lidegaard O, et al. First-trimester vaginal bleeding and complications later in pregnancy. Obstet Gynecol. 2010;115:935–44.
78. Dugoff L. First- and second-trimester maternal serum markers for aneuploidy and adverse obstetric outcomes. Obstet Gynecol. 2010;115:1052–61.
79. Chandra S, Scott H, Dodds L, et al. Unexplained elevated maternal serum alpha-fetoprotein and/or human chorionic gonadotropin and the risk of adverse outcomes. Am J Obstet Gynecol. 2003;189:775–81.
80. Spencer K. Second-trimester prenatal screening for Down syndrome and the relationship of maternal serum biochemical markers to pregnancy complications with adverse outcome. Prenat Diagn. 2000;20:652–6.
81. Krause TG, Christens P, Wohlfahrt J, et al. Second-trimester maternal serum alpha-fetoprotein and risk of adverse pregnancy outcome(1). Obstet Gynecol. 2001;97:277–82.
82. Berkeley AS, Killackey MA, Cederqvist LL. Elevated maternal serum alpha-fetoprotein levels associated with breakdown in fetal-maternal-placental barrier. Am J Obstet Gynecol. 1983; 146:859–61.
83. Yaron Y, Cherry M, Kramer RL, et al. Second-trimester maternal serum marker screening: maternal serum alpha-fetoprotein, beta-human chorionic gonadotropin, estriol, and their various combinations as predictors of pregnancy outcome. Am J Obstet Gynecol. 1999;181: 968–74.
84. Perkes EA, Baim RS, Goodman KJ, et al. Second-trimester placental changes associated with elevated maternal serum alpha-fetoprotein. Am J Obstet Gynecol. 1982;144:935–8.
85. Spong CY, Ghidini A, Walker CN, et al. Elevated maternal serum midtrimester alpha-fetoprotein levels are associated with fetoplacental ischemia. Am J Obstet Gynecol. 1997; 177:1085–7.
86. Katz VL, Chescheir NC, Cefalo RC. Unexplained elevations of maternal serum alpha-fetoprotein. Obstet Gynecol Surv. 1990;45:719–26.
87. Tikkanen M, Hamalainen E, Nuutila M, et al. Elevated maternal second-trimester serum alpha-fetoprotein as a risk factor for placental abruption. Prenat Diagn. 2007;27:240–3.
88. Yeo L, Ananth CV, Vintzileos AM. Placental abruption. In: Sciarra J, editor. Gynecology and obstetrics. Hagerstown, MD: Lippincott Williams & Wilkins; 2003.
89. Wei SH, Helmy M, Cohen AJ. CT evaluation of placental abruption in pregnant trauma patients. Emerg Radiol. 2009;16:365–73.
90. Manriquez M, Srinivas G, Bollepalli S, et al. Is computed tomography a reliable diagnostic modality in detecting placental injuries in the setting of acute trauma? Am J Obstet Gynecol. 2010;202:611.e1–5.
91. Gargano JW, Holzman CB, Senagore PK, et al. Evidence of placental haemorrhage and pre-term delivery. BJOG. 2010;117:445–55.
92. Saller Jr DN, Nagey DA, Pupkin MJ, et al. Tocolysis in the management of third trimester bleeding. J Perinatol. 1990;10:125–8.
93. Towers CV, Pircon RA, Heppard M. Is tocolysis safe in the management of third-trimester bleeding? Am J Obstet Gynecol. 1999;180:1572–8.
94. Neilson JP. Interventions for treating placental abruption. Cochrane Database Syst Rev, 2003;CD003247.

Chapter 8
Placenta Previa and Placenta Accreta

Yinka Oyelese and Joseph C. Canterino

Placenta Previa

The term placenta previa refers to a placenta that is abnormally located in the lower part of the uterus, often covering the cervix. The words are derived from the Latin pre, meaning before, and via, which comes from the same derivation as "viaduct" and "avenue," meaning passageway. Thus, placenta previa means that the placenta lies before the baby in the birth canal. The placenta normally implants in the upper uterus, but in fewer than 1% of pregnancies it implants in the lower uterine segment. It was probably the French man-midwife Portal in 1683 who first described a placenta previa [1]. Placenta previa is one of the leading causes of bleeding during the third trimester. The condition is associated with significantly increased perinatal and maternal mortality and morbidity [2]. Perhaps the most important fetal consequence is prematurity with its associated sequelae, such as respiratory distress syndrome, high perinatal mortality, and long-term neurodevelopmental handicap. Placenta previa is also associated with significant maternal hemorrhage, a need for surgical delivery, placenta accreta, and cesarean hysterectomy [2].

With placenta previa, because the placenta covers the cervix, as the cervix dilates during labor or in late pregnancy the placenta separates from the uterine wall and bleeding ensues. During labor, this bleeding becomes severe and life-threatening. Therefore, these women need a cesarean delivery.

Y. Oyelese (✉)
Division of Maternal Fetal Medicine, Department of Obstetrics and Gynecology,
Jersey Shore University Medical Center,
Neptune, NJ, USA

UMDNJ-Robert Wood Johnson Medical School,
New Brunswick, NJ, USA
e-mail: Yinkamd@aol.com

E. Sheiner (ed.), *Bleeding During Pregnancy: A Comprehensive Guide*,
DOI 10.1007/978-1-4419-9810-1_8, © Springer Science+Business Media, LLC 2011

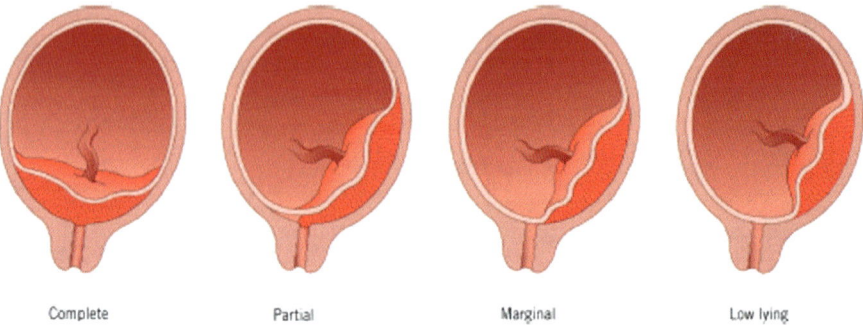

Complete   Partial   Marginal   Low lying

Fig. 8.1 Traditional classification of placenta previa. Complete type totally overlies the internal os. Partial type only partially overlies a dilated cervix but does not overlie the cervix with increasing dilation. Marginal type just reaches the internal os. Low-lying type is in the lower segment but does not reach the internal os (generally considered to be within 5 cm of the internal os). From Oyelese and Smulian. Placenta previa, placenta accreta, and vasa previa. Obstet Gynecol. 2006;107:771–8. With permission from the American Congress of Obstetricians and Gynecologists

Classification

Traditionally, placenta previa has been classified into four types: complete, partial, marginal, and low-lying (Fig. 8.1). This classification was based on digital vaginal examination during an era prior to the availability of ultrasonography (US). The patient who was bleeding was examined in the operating room, often under anesthesia, with the ability to perform a cesarean if heavy bleeding occurred. If the placenta was palpated through the cervix and the finger could not reach the placental edge, it was called a complete placenta previa. The term partial placenta previa was used when the placenta covered the closed cervical os but not the dilated cervix. When the lower placental edge did not cover the cervix, but the edge could easily be felt, it was called a marginal placenta previa. A low-lying placenta was one that did not implant over the cervix and whose lower edge could only be felt with difficulty [3].

Ultrasonography has revolutionized the management of patients with placenta previa, and a newer classification using sonographic findings has been advocated [3–5]. It has been noted that the classification should be clinically relevant and should answer two critical questions: What is the risk of significant antepartum hemorrhage? What is the likelihood of requiring a cesarean delivery?

Incidence

Placenta previa complicates approximately 0.4% of deliveries [6, 7]. In a study from the Duke University Medical Center covering a 20-year period, Crenshaw and coworkers found that 1 in 271 pregnancies (0.37%) were affected by placenta previa [8]. Hibbard reviewed 102,670 deliveries at the University of Southern California Medical Center in Los Angeles over the years 1948–1953 and found a 0.46% rate of placenta previa [9]. Iyasu et al., in a population-based study using data from the U.S. National Hospital Discharge Survey, found an average incidence of placenta previa of 0.48% [10]. Similarly, rates of placenta previa of 0.4% have been reported in Croatia and Israel [6, 11].

However, the reported incidence depends on the gestational age at diagnosis, how placenta previa is defined, and the accuracy of the diagnosis [12]. For instance, some studies include cases of low-lying placenta, whereas others exclude them. The use of transvaginal US (TVUS) is resulting in a much lower incidence of placenta previa because transabdominal US is associated with a high false-positive rate [13]. The incidence is higher in the mid-trimester. Approximately 90% of cases of placenta previa at 20 weeks resolve by term. Thus, the earlier patients are delivered, the higher is the rate of placenta previa. If the earlier pregnancies were allowed to continue to term, more cases of placenta previa would have resolved, resulting in a lower incidence.

Risk Factors

Probably the most important risk factor for developing placenta previa is a prior cesarean delivery [7, 14]. Bender was one of the earliest to suggest this relation [15]. This increased risk has subsequently been confirmed in several studies [14, 16]. In a meta-analysis by Faiz and Ananth, the odds ratio (OR) of developing a placenta previa among women who had a prior cesarean was 2.6 [95% confidence interval (CI) 2.3–3.0] [7]. These authors also found a dose–response pattern for developing a placenta previa with increasing numbers of prior cesareans.

Prior intrauterine surgery, including termination of pregnancy, is considered a risk factor for placenta previa [6, 17]. However, a small case–control study by Grimes and Techman did not find that prior legal abortion was associated with increased risk for placenta previa [18]. Other risk factors include a history of uterine surgery, smoking, multiparity [19], and increasing maternal age [6].

Zhang and Savitz, in a population-based study from North Carolina, found that women who were aged ≥ 34 years had a two- to threefold higher rate of placenta previa than women aged <20 [20]. Sheiner and coworkers found in a case–control study that women aged >40 years had an odds ratio of 3.1 for placenta previa (95% CI 2.0–4.9) [6]. Although increasing age is associated with greater parity, this association remains when parity is taken into account.

Smoking has been associated with an increased risk for placenta previa, with the risk increasing with the number of years the woman has smoked, rather than with the amount [21, 22]. In a population-based study from Washington State, Kramer and coworkers found that, after adjusting for confounders, smoking doubled the risk for placenta previa (OR 2.1, 95% CI 1.7–2.5) [23]. Also, some data suggest that cocaine use during pregnancy is associated with an increased risk for placenta previa [24].

Clinical Presentation

In the past, most cases of placenta previa presented with painless bleeding during the early third trimester. It was the absence of pain that was used to differentiate placenta previa from placental abruption, the other major cause of third trimester bleeding, which is often associated with pain. Placenta previa may also present with fetal malpresentation. The placenta in the lower segment frequently prevents engagement of the fetal head. Consequently, placenta previa is associated with an unstable lie. However, more recently, with the advent of US, almost all cases are diagnosed at the time of the mid-trimester anatomy scan in asymptomatic women.

In 1966, Gottesfeld et al. first described the use of US for placental location [25]. Prior to that, such techniques as X-ray placentography had been used [4], which involved radiation and the intravenous injection of such radioactive substances as technetium. The advent of widespread use of US made the diagnosis of placenta previa much easier.

In 1988, Farine and coworkers described the use of TVUS for the diagnosis of placenta previa [26]. In that initial study of 35 patients, they found that TVUS could accurately identify the cervical internal os and its relation to the placenta in all patients, whereas this was possible in only 24 patients (69%) using transabdominal US. Furthermore, they found that TVUS ruled out placenta previa in 13 cases thought to have it based on transabdominal US. At the time, the use of TVUS was contrary to the teaching in most obstetrics textbooks in that it was contraindicated to put anything in the vagina of patients with placenta previa. However, shortly afterward, the authors and others demonstrated that not only was TVUS more accurate than transabdominal US but it was safe and did not lead to increased bleeding [26, 27]. Transabdominal US for placenta previa may be associated with false-positive and false-negative rates as high as 12% [27, 28]. There are several reasons that TVUS is more accurate than transabdominal sonography for evaluating placenta previa [4].

1. In some cases, the exact location of the cervix and the internal os cannot be accurately demonstrated using transabdominal US.
2. For examining the cervix, transabdominal sonography often requires a full bladder. This apposes the anterior and posterior walls of the lower uterine segment and may give a false-positive diagnosis of placenta previa.
3. The fetal head may obscure the actual location of the placenta and the cervix.
4. A posterior placenta may be difficult to visualize using transabdominal US.
5. TVUS uses higher-frequency transducers, allowing improved resolution. In addition, the probe is closer to the region of interest (the internal os and the lower placental edge), allowing better visualization than that achieved with transabdominal US.

Several studies have found that TVUS used to evaluate placenta previa during the second trimester has some advantages [4, 27]. First, when TVUS is used, it is more accurate, and so there are fewer false-positive diagnoses [29] (Figures 8.2 and 8.3). Furthermore, the degree to which the placenta overlies the internal os at 20 weeks is predictive of persistence to term. Lauria et al. found 100% sensitivity and 85% specificity of persistence to term when the placental edge overlay the cervix by >1 cm at 16–24 weeks using TVS [29]. A study by Becker et al. using TVUS suggested that the degree of overlap at 20–23 weeks predicted persistence to term. These investigators found that an overlap of ≥2.5 cm seemed incompatible with future vaginal delivery [30]. Placenta previa found during the mid-trimester is more likely to resolve by term if the placenta is anterior, rather than posterior [31]. In a study of 131 women who were thought to have a placenta within 2 cm of the internal os on transabdominal US, Smith et al. found that in 50% of cases landmarks were poorly seen [28]. In 26% of cases, the diagnosis was changed after TVUS was performed [28] (Figs. 8.2–8.4).

Most cases of placenta previa found during the second trimester resolve by term [32]. However, a second-trimester placenta previa that resolves is still a risk factor for vasa previa, especially when the placenta covers the cervix during the second trimester [33]. In a large study, we found that approximately two-thirds of patients with vasa previa had second-trimester placenta previa. By the time of delivery, however, two-thirds of the placenta previas had resolved, although the patients had vasa previas [33]. Thus, in women who have complete placenta previas during the second trimester, TVUS with color Doppler should be performed during the third trimester to rule out vasa previa (see Chap. 9).

Management

Patients with placenta previa fall into two main groups: asymptomatic patients in whom a placenta previa is identified on routine US and those who have been

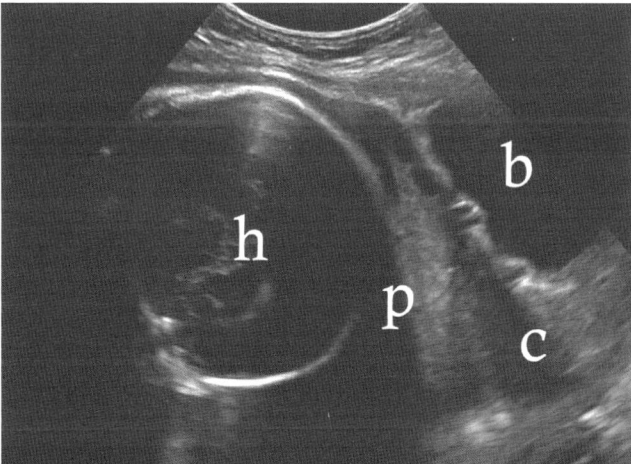

Fig. 8.2 Transabdominal ultrasonography of a complete posterior placenta previa. It is difficult to locate the cervical internal os accurately in this image h=fetal head, p=placenta, c=cervix, b=bladder, a=anterior lip of cervix, p=posterior lip of cervix

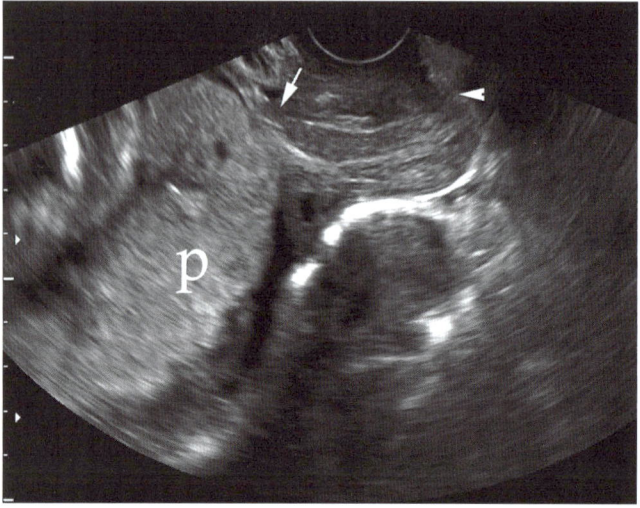

Fig. 8.3 Transvaginal sonogram of the same patient as depicted in Fig. 8.2. Note that the internal os is clearly seen, as is its relation with the lower placental edge (p). It is clear that this is a posterior complete placenta previa that just overlies the internal os. (Long arrow=internal cervical os, Arrow head=external os)

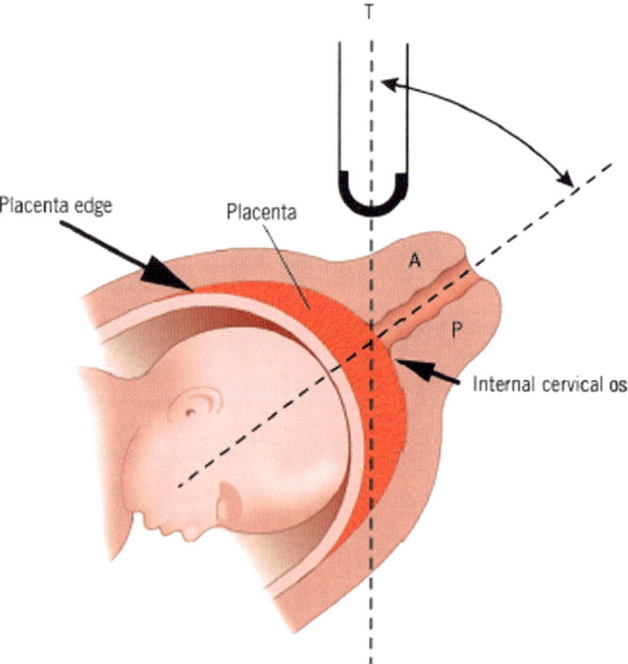

Fig. 8.4 Drawing showing why transvaginal sonography is safe. The transducer does not enter the internal os. Rather, it is directed to the anterior lip of the cervix. Thus, it does not cause increased bleeding. From Oyelese and Smulian. Placenta previa, placenta accreta, and vasa previa. Obstet Gynecol. 2006;107:771–8. With permission from the American Congress of Obstetricians and Gynecologists

diagnosed as a result of their symptoms, such as bleeding. In asymptomatic women, no change in obstetrical management is necessary prior to 36 weeks. Women who have bleeding, on the other hand, should be admitted for evaluation [12]. Typically, the first bleed occurs at about 26–30 weeks and is usually painless. In the past, these patients were often delivered immediately. However, in 1945, MacAfee and Phillips demonstrated that these babies who were delivered early had an extremely high perinatal mortality rate and that perinatal outcomes could be improved drastically [34]. They proposed that rather than deliver these pregnancies the first time bleeding was experienced conservative expectant management with the aim of prolonging gestation and delivering the babies at a more advanced gestational age would lead to improved perinatal outcomes without worsening outcomes for the mother. This study has formed the framework for the modern management of placenta previa.

A few small studies have evaluated inpatient vs. outpatient management of placenta previa. An initial small study by D'Angelo and Irwin of 38 patients with placenta previa found that those managed as outpatients had worse perinatal outcomes [35]. A subsequent retrospective study by Rosen and Peek found that patients with placenta previa who had no bleeding could be managed safely as outpatients, without an increase in adverse outcomes [36]. Mouer reviewed the records of 104 women with placenta previa [37]. He compared outcomes in the 49 patients who were managed as outpatients with the 55 managed as inpatients. He found no difference in gestational age or birth weight at delivery, postpartum hemoglobin levels, or neonatal outcomes. Of course, several of these retrospective studies are biased by patient selection. In a randomized trial, Wing et al. found that women with placenta previa managed as outpatients had outcomes similar to those of patients managed in hospital [38].

Bleeding with placenta previa is often associated with uterine contractions. These contractions cause further cervical effacement, which in turn leads to more bleeding – a vicious cycle. The use of tocolytics in patients with bleeding has long been a subject of great controversy in obstetrics. However, several small studies have demonstrated that cautious use of tocolytics in patients with placenta previa who are contracting is safe and may lead to prolongation of gestation [39].

At least two small studies have evaluated prophylactic cervical cerclage in treating placenta previa [40, 41]. One suggested some benefit of cerclage with regard to prolongation of gestation and perinatal outcomes [41], whereas the other found no such a benefit [40]. Cerclage is invasive and carries risks, and routine cerclage placement for placenta previa is not justified.

Delivery

There is consensus that women with a placenta that overlies the internal os at term should be delivered by cesarean. What is more controversial is the appropriate route of delivery for women who have a placenta that is close to the internal os but does not cover it. In an initial study of 24 women, Oppenheimer et al. assessed the delivery route in women based on distance between the lower placental edge and the internal cervical os using TVUS [42]. These authors found that women could safely have a vaginal delivery if the placenta–os distance was >2 cm. In a larger study, Bhide and coworkers in a retrospective study of 64 women with placenta previa who were allowed to go into labor found that the risk of cesarean increased with decreasing placental edge–os distance [43]. Women who had a lower placental edge >2 cm from the internal os safely had a vaginal delivery in 63% of cases, whereas only 10% successfully delivered vaginally when the placental edge was <2 cm from the internal os; these women generally required a cesarean. A major flaw of both these studies was that the physicians were not blinded to the sonographic findings. Thus, they may have been biased in determining who would have a cesarean and who would have a vaginal delivery. Two more studies have evaluated the relation between placenta–os distance and mode of delivery. In a retrospective study of 45 women with a placenta–os distance of <2 cm who were allowed to go into labor, Bronsteen et al. found that 29 (64.4%) successfully delivered vaginally [44]. When this distance was <1 cm, the vaginal delivery rate was only 27.3%, whereas it was 76.5% when the placenta–os distance was 1–2 cm. Vergani and coworkers similarly found a high rate of successful vaginal delivery (69%) when the placental edge was 11–20 mm from the internal os, whereas the cesarean delivery rate was high: 75% among women who had a placental edge–os distance of 1–10 mm [45].

Summary

When the placenta does not overlie the internal os and there are no contraindications to vaginal delivery, it appears that women may safely attempt a vaginal delivery if the placental edge–internal os distance in >1 cm. It must be emphasized that this assessment of placental edge–os distance can only be made accurately using TVUS. Based on the fact that the placental edge–os distance is probably the most important

---

Caution Box

Placenta previa tips

1. Most cases of placenta previa found in the second trimester will resolve prior to full term. Thus patients can be reassured in most cases.
2. Transvaginal sonography is the ideal method for diagnosing a placenta previa. Transabdominal sonography is not sufficiently accurate, and will overdiagnose placenta previa. Transvaginal sonography is safe and accurate.
3. Women with a complete placenta previa will need a cesarean delivery. Women in whom the placental edge is greater than 1 cm from the internal os may attempt for vaginal delivery, in the absence of other contraindications.

determinant of the ability to undergo a vaginal delivery successfully, Oppenheimer and Farine have proposed that the old classification of types of placenta previa be abandoned and a more contemporary classification be adopted based on the placenta–os relation as demonstrated on TVUS [3].

It is preferable that the women who require cesarean delivery be delivered under controlled circumstances rather than as an emergency when the patient is acutely or massively bleeding. Hence, cesarean delivery at 37–38 weeks is advisable, even without demonstrating fetal lung maturity.

Placenta Accreta

The term placenta accreta is used to describe collectively various degrees of abnormal adherence of the placenta to the myometrium. It is used when the placenta is abnormally adherent to the myometrium. Placenta increta describes a placenta that invades the myometrium. The term placenta percreta is used when the placenta invades through the myometrium into the uterine serosa and into adjacent structures, such as the bladder, ureters, bowel, and omentum.

Placenta accreta is important because it is a cause of massive hemorrhage, with a significant risk of serious maternal morbidity and, in some cases, death [46]. In a study of 76 cases of placenta accreta from two tertiary care hospitals in Utah (USA), Silver and colleagues found that the mean estimated blood loss was in excess of 2.5 L and that more than one-fourth of women with accreta were admitted to the intensive care unit [47].

Incidence

Estimates of the incidence of placenta accreta vary, which may be due to the different criteria used for the diagnosis. However, it is clear that the incidence of placenta accreta is rising [48], primarily the consequence of the rising cesarean delivery rate. In several centers, placenta accreta is now the leading reason for peripartum hysterectomy [49]. In a hospital-based study, Miller et al. found that histologically confirmed placenta accreta complicated 62 of 155,670 deliveries (1:2,510) [50]. Estimates of the incidence of placenta accreta range between 1:1,000 and 1:2,500 pregnancies.

Risk Factors

Risk factors include prior cesarean delivery. The risk for placenta accreta increases with the number of prior cesarean deliveries. A study by Clark et al. found that placenta accreta complicated only 0.26% of deliveries with an unscarred uterus [51].

However, in patients with four or more prior cesarean deliveries, the risk was 10% [51]. In the presence of a single prior cesarean and a placenta previa, the risk of placenta accreta was 24% [51]. This risk rose with the number of prior cesareans to 67% in women with four or more prior cesareans and a placenta previa in the current pregnancy. Importantly, a woman with a placenta previa and no prior cesarean had a 5% risk for placenta accreta [51]. Prior uterine artery embolization may also be associated with an increased risk for placenta accreta.

Pathophysiology

In the normal pregnancy, the placenta is separated from the uterus by Nitabuch's layer, and the placenta usually separates from the uterine wall without difficulty. With placenta accreta, however, this layer is deficient, and the placenta is abnormally adherent to the uterine wall. Recent US studies suggest that placenta accreta starts off as an abnormal implantation into the myometrium rather than the decidua [52]. Reviews of first trimester sonograms on patients who had placenta accreta found that most had gestational sacs that were located abnormally low in the uterine cavity and that they were located in close proximity to the anterior wall [52].

Diagnosis

Placenta accreta may be diagnosed prenatally [53]. Generally, the diagnosis is based on the use of US [46, 54–57] or magnetic resonance imaging (MRI) [54, 58, 59]. Perhaps the most important aid to prenatal diagnosis is a high index of suspicion, paying attention to the aforementioned risk factors.

A sonographic finding suggestive of placenta accreta is echolucent spaces (lacunae) in the placenta, giving it a moth-eaten appearance [56]. Obliteration of the placental–myometrial interface is not a very reliable sign, as it is present in women who have had prior cesareans without an accreta [56]. There may also be abnormal turbulent Doppler flow through these spaces. The protrusion of placenta into the bladder is pathognomonic of placenta percreta. US has good sensitivity (90%) and a reasonable positive predictive value for placenta accreta (about 68%) [57]. Some have suggested that MRI be used in the diagnosis of placenta accreta. The modality used, however, depends on availability and expertise.

Placenta accreta may be associated with elevated levels of α-fetoprotein (AFP) [60, 61]. A small study by Zelop et al. found that 5 of 11 women with placenta accreta requiring hysterectomy had elevated second-trimester maternal serum AFP levels [61]. None of the 14 controls who had placenta previa but not accreta had elevated AFP levels.

Occasionally, placenta accreta is diagnosed during delivery when placental removal is either difficult or impossible.

Management

It is clear that placenta accreta is a cause of significant, potentially life-threatening hemorrhage. Therefore, prenatal diagnosis and appropriate management are crucial. It has been shown that attempts to remove the placenta are associated with the worst outcomes [47]. Similarly, in a study of 99 consecutive cases of placenta accreta, Warshak et al. demonstrated that a predelivery diagnosis of placenta accreta was associated with a significantly better maternal outcome [53]. Perhaps the worst outcomes occur when a woman is delivered without any foreknowledge that she might have a placenta accreta, and placental removal is attempted. It is crucial to maintain a high index of suspicion for placenta accreta, particularly in patients with a history of prior cesarean deliveries and a placenta previa in the current pregnancy.

Several studies have demonstrated that outcomes can be optimized by prenatal diagnosis and management by a multidisciplinary team consisting of obstetricians, anesthesiologists, blood bank personnel, neonatology interventional radiologists, and adequately trained and experienced surgeons, which may include those in the fields of gynecological oncology, urology, and/or surgery [46, 47, 62]. Ideally, all cases are managed in centers with these resources available [46]. In addition, protocols for the management of placenta accreta, as well as periodic drills, are desirable.

The ideal approach to the problem is cesarean delivery via a vertical uterine incision in the fundus, taking care to avoid the placenta. Hysterectomy is then performed, leaving the placenta in place. It is desirable to reduce the uterine blood supply prior to performing the hysterectomy. Two main techniques have been used to achieve it. The first is surgical, via ligation of the uterine arteries or the hypogastric arteries. The second, more recent, is embolization or balloon occlusion of either of these vessels, usually performed by the interventional radiologist [63]. Uterine blood flow should be interrupted immediately after the delivery of the fetus. When the interventional radiologist performs uterine artery embolization, the catheters should be inserted before the surgery commences. One approach involves inflating the balloon catheters immediately after delivery of the fetus and keeping them inflated until the hysterectomy is successfully completed. The balloons are then deflated while watching for evidence of hemorrhage. In other cases, the vessels are embolized using gelfoam or other embolizing agents after delivering the fetus.

Although it is intuitive that embolization should lead to reduced blood loss and improved outcomes, studies have varied regarding whether embolization does indeed have this effect [63–67]. Designing a study that would appropriately answer this question is fraught with difficulty. Some data on pregnancies following uterine artery embolization [68] found an increased incidence of problems such as placenta accreta in subsequent pregnancies [68].

Surgery is often difficult in these patients due to adhesions from prior surgery and because of placental invasion. For this reason, it is advisable to have the most experienced surgeon available involved in the surgery and to perform it in a well-equipped operating theater. It is essential to have adequate units of cross-matched blood immediately ready for use. In addition, because there is a high risk of disseminated intravascular coagulopathy (DIC), blood products such as fresh frozen plasma, cryoprecipitate, and platelets should be available.

There is a high rate of urological injury during surgery for placenta accreta. Ideally, a urologist is available to assist with the surgery if needed. Some advocate prophylactic ureteral stent insertion prior to the surgery [47].

Acute normovolemic hemodilution is a technique in which some maternal blood is drawn off using controlled conditions prior to surgery [48]. The blood that is drawn off is replaced with intravenous fluids. During the surgery, as the patient loses blood, the volume is replaced with the blood that was drawn off prior to surgery. This technique has been used in other surgical specialties where a large blood loss is anticipated, such as some orthopedic surgery. More recently, some have used this technique at the time of surgery in patients with placenta accreta [48].

Without a doubt, hysterectomy is a radical solution and removes any chance of fertility. Hence, this option is not appealing to women who desire further childbearing. Some women decline a hysterectomy. To complicate matters further, the false-positive diagnosis rate for placenta accreta is as high as 50%, and some patients have a hysterectomy when they did not have an accreta. More recently, a variety of alternative management strategies have been utilized to avoid hysterectomy with the goal of uterine conservation.

It must be emphasized that these options are associated with significant risk, and any patient who opts not to have a hysterectomy must be fully counseled of the risks associated with conservative management and be willing to undertake these risks.

Several authors have published case reports and series of patients with successful conservative management of placenta accreta where the uterus was conserved [69, 70]. Two major flaws with several of these studies are the questionable diagnosis of placenta accreta and selection bias. When the uterus is not removed, it is difficult in most cases to determine that the diagnosis was truly placenta accreta. Often this diagnosis is made clinically when there is difficulty removing the placenta. However, there may be other reasons, such as uterine contraction that may make placental removal difficult. Furthermore, unsuccessful cases of attempted uterine conservation are much less likely to be reported or published [71]. Consequently, there is a strong publication bias toward cases managed successfully.

Strategies that have been used in these cases include bilateral embolization of the uterine or hypogastric arteries [65], methotrexate injection [72], and compression sutures around the uterus or of the placental bed. Whereas some have advocated the use of methotrexate [72, 73], others have questioned it, arguing that the placental cells are no longer dividing and that therefore methotrexate may be ineffective.

In one of the earliest series, Courbiere et al. from France described 13 cases of attempted conservative management [74], 11 of which were successful. One of the two that failed required a hysterectomy for severe life-threatening hemorrhage, and the other had postembolization necrosis of the uterus. Blood transfusion was the most common morbidity.

In a 2007 review, Timmermans et al. summarized 48 reports published during 1985–2006 describing outcomes of 60 women with placenta accreta in whom uterine conservation was attempted [75]. These women were managed using a variety of strategies. In ten cases, the attempted uterine conservation failed; 4 of the 60 women developed DIC, and 11 women developed infection. Interestingly, negative human chorionic gonadotropin levels did not guarantee complete resorption of the placental tissue. The authors concluded that conservative management should be attempted only in highly selected cases with minimal bleeding in which the women desired further fertility.

Senthiles et al. published the results of a multicenter retrospective study from university medical centers in France in which 167 women were treated conservatively for placenta accreta by attempting uterine conservation [76]. It should be emphasized that this study was based on recall, which itself leads to significant bias. Of the 167 cases in which uterine conservation was attempted, 131 were successful. The other 36 women required hysterectomy: 18 immediately and delayed in the other 18. One woman died from myelosuppression from methotrexate injection. Severe maternal morbidity occurred in ten cases. The placenta underwent spontaneous resorption in 75% of cases with a median interval between delivery and placenta resorption of 13.5 weeks (range 4–60 weeks). Of the 96 women available for long-term follow-up, 8 had severe intrauterine synechiae and were amenorrheic. Only 27 of the women actively tried to have subsequent pregnancies. Among the 24 who succeeded in getting pregnant, there were 34 pregnancies. Altogether, 21 pregnancies resulted in third trimester births; there were also 10 miscarriages, 2 elective terminations, and 1 ectopic pregnancy.

Uterine conservation may be an option with placenta accreta. However, proper patient selection and counseling are crucial. It is important that women who desire uterine conservation also wish for further childbearing and understand the risks of this approach.

Conclusion

Placenta previa and accreta are serious conditions with which the obstetrician will have to contend more often owing to the rising cesarean delivery rate. Familiarity with risk factors, a high index of suspicion, prenatal diagnosis, and predelivery planning have the potential to produce the best outcomes and to avoid the serious complications associated with these conditions.

References

1. Dunn PM. Paul Portal (1630–1703), man-midwife of Paris. Arch Dis Child Fetal Neonatal Ed. 2006;91(5):F385–7.
2. McShane PM, Heyl PS, Epstein MF. Maternal and perinatal morbidity resulting from placenta previa. Obstet Gynecol. 1985;65(2):176–82.
3. Oppenheimer LW, Farine D. A new classification of placenta previa: measuring progress in obstetrics. Am J Obstet Gynecol. 2009;201(3):227–9.

 4. Oyelese Y. Placenta previa and vasa previa: time to leave the Dark Ages. Ultrasound Obstet Gynecol. 2001;18(2):96–9.
 5. Oyelese Y. Placenta previa: the evolving role of ultrasound. Ultrasound Obstet Gynecol. 2009;34(2):123–6.
 6. Sheiner E, Shoham-Vardi I, Hallak M, Hershkowitz R, Katz M, Mazor M. Placenta previa: obstetric risk factors and pregnancy outcome. J Matern Fetal Med. 2001;10(6):414–9.
 7. Faiz AS, Ananth CV. Etiology and risk factors for placenta previa: an overview and meta-analysis of observational studies. J Matern Fetal Neonatal Med. 2003;13(3):175–90.
 8. Crenshaw Jr C, Jones DE, Parker RT. Placenta previa: a survey of twenty years experience with improved perinatal survival by expectant therapy and cesarean delivery. Obstet Gynecol Surv. 1973;28(7):461–70.
 9. Hibbard LT. Placenta previa. Am J Obstet Gynecol. 1969;104(2):172–84.
10. Iyasu S, Saftlas AK, Rowley DL, Koonin LM, Lawson HW, Atrash HK. The epidemiology of placenta previa in the United States, 1979 through 1987. Am J Obstet Gynecol. 1993;168(5):1424–9.
11. Tuzovic L, Djelmis J, Ilijic M. Obstetric risk factors associated with placenta previa development: case-control study. Croat Med J. 2003;44(6):728–33.
12. Oyelese Y, Smulian JC. Placenta previa, placenta accreta, and vasa previa. Obstet Gynecol. 2006;107(4):927–41.
13. O'Brien JM. Placenta previa, placenta accreta, and vasa previa. Obstet Gynecol. 2007;109(1):203–4. author reply 04.
14. Taylor VM, Kramer MD, Vaughan TL, Peacock S. Placenta previa and prior cesarean delivery: how strong is the association? Obstet Gynecol. 1994;84(1):55–7.
15. Bender S. Placenta previa and previous lower segment cesarean section. Surg Gynecol Obstet. 1954;98(5):625–8.
16. McMahon MJ, Li R, Schenck AP, Olshan AF, Royce RA. Previous cesarean birth. A risk factor for placenta previa? J Reprod Med. 1997;42(7):409–12.
17. Barrett JM, Boehm FH, Killam AP. Induced abortion: a risk factor for placenta previa. Am J Obstet Gynecol. 1981;141(7):769–72.
18. Grimes DA, Techman T. Legal abortion and placenta previa. Am J Obstet Gynecol. 1984;149(5):501–4.
19. Abu-Heija AT, El-Jallad F, Ziadeh S. Placenta previa: effect of age, gravidity, parity and previous caesarean section. Gynecol Obstet Invest. 1999;47(1):6–8.
20. Zhang J, Savitz DA. Maternal age and placenta previa: a population-based, case-control study. Am J Obstet Gynecol. 1993;168(2):641–5.
21. Chelmow D, Andrew DE, Baker ER. Maternal cigarette smoking and placenta previa. Obstet Gynecol. 1996;87(5 Pt 1):703–6.
22. Monica G, Lilja C. Placenta previa, maternal smoking and recurrence risk. Acta Obstet Gynecol Scand. 1995;74(5):341–5.
23. Kramer MD, Taylor V, Hickok DE, Daling JR, Vaughan TL, Hollenbach KA. Maternal smoking and placenta previa. Epidemiology. 1991;2(3):221–3.
24. Macones GA, Sehdev HM, Parry S, Morgan MA, Berlin JA. The association between maternal cocaine use and placenta previa. Am J Obstet Gynecol. 1997;177(5):1097–100.
25. Gottesfeld KR, Thompson HE, Holmes JH, Taylor ES. Ultrasonic placentography – a new method for placental localization. Am J Obstet Gynecol. 1966;96(4):538–47.
26. Farine D, Fox HE, Jakobson S, Timor-Tritsch IE. Vaginal ultrasound for diagnosis of placenta previa. Am J Obstet Gynecol. 1988;159(3):566–9.
27. Leerentveld RA, Gilberts EC, Arnold MJ, Wladimiroff JW. Accuracy and safety of transvaginal sonographic placental localization. Obstet Gynecol. 1990;76(5 Pt 1):759–62.
28. Smith RS, Lauria MR, Comstock CH, Treadwell MC, Kirk JS, Lee W, et al. Transvaginal ultrasonography for all placentas that appear to be low-lying or over the internal cervical os. Ultrasound Obstet Gynecol. 1997;9(1):22–4.
29. Lauria MR, Smith RS, Treadwell MC, Comstock CH, Kirk JS, Lee W, et al. The use of second-trimester transvaginal sonography to predict placenta previa. Ultrasound Obstet Gynecol. 1996;8(5):337–40.

30. Becker RH, Vonk R, Mende BC, Ragosch V, Entezami M. The relevance of placental location at 20–23 gestational weeks for prediction of placenta previa at delivery: evaluation of 8650 cases. Ultrasound Obstet Gynecol. 2001;17(6):496–501.
31. Cho JY, Lee YH, Moon MH, Lee JH. Difference in migration of placenta according to the location and type of placenta previa. J Clin Ultrasound. 2008;36(2):79–84.
32. Ancona S, Chatterjee M, Rhee I, Sicurenza B. The mid-trimester placenta previa: a prospective follow-up. Eur J Radiol. 1990;10(3):215–6.
33. Oyelese Y, Catanzarite V, Prefumo F, Lashley S, Schachter M, Tovbin Y, et al. Vasa previa: the impact of prenatal diagnosis on outcomes. Obstet Gynecol. 2004;103(5 Pt 1):937–42.
34. Macafee CH, Phillips LG. Placenta praevia. Lancet. 1945;2:743.
35. D'Angelo LJ, Irwin LF. Conservative management of placenta previa: a cost–benefit analysis. Am J Obstet Gynecol. 1984;149(3):320–6.
36. Rosen DM, Peek MJ. Do women with placenta praevia without antepartum haemorrhage require hospitalization? Aust N Z J Obstet Gynaecol. 1994;34(2):130–4.
37. Mouer JR. Placenta previa: antepartum conservative management, inpatient versus outpatient. Am J Obstet Gynecol. 1994;170(6):1683–5. discussion 85–6.
38. Wing DA, Paul RH, Millar LK. Management of the symptomatic placenta previa: a randomized, controlled trial of inpatient versus outpatient expectant management. Am J Obstet Gynecol. 1996;175(4 Pt 1):806–11.
39. Besinger RE, Moniak CW, Paskiewicz LS, Fisher SG, Tomich PG. The effect of tocolytic use in the management of symptomatic placenta previa. Am J Obstet Gynecol. 1995;172(6):1770–5. discussion 75–8.
40. Cobo E, Conde-Agudelo A, Delgado J, Canaval H, Congote A. Cervical cerclage: an alternative for the management of placenta previa? Am J Obstet Gynecol. 1998;179(1):122–5.
41. Arias F. Cervical cerclage for the temporary treatment of patients with placenta previa. Obstet Gynecol. 1988;71(4):545–8.
42. Oppenheimer LW, Farine D, Ritchie JW, Lewinsky RM, Telford J, Fairbanks LA. What is a low-lying placenta? Am J Obstet Gynecol. 1991;165(4 Pt 1):1036–8.
43. Bhide A, Prefumo F, Moore J, Hollis B, Thilaganathan B. Placental edge to internal os distance in the late third trimester and mode of delivery in placenta praevia. BJOG. 2003;110(9):860–4.
44. Bronsteen R, Valice R, Lee W, Blackwell S, Balasubramaniam M, Comstock C. Effect of a low-lying placenta on delivery outcome. Ultrasound Obstet Gynecol. 2009;33(2):204–8.
45. Vergani P, Ornaghi S, Pozzi I, Beretta P, Russo FM, Follesa I, et al. Placenta previa: distance to internal os and mode of delivery. Am J Obstet Gynecol. 2009;201(3):266.e1–5.
46. Doumouchtsis SK, Arulkumaran S. The morbidly adherent placenta: an overview of management options. Acta Obstet Gynecol Scand. 2010;89(9):1126–33.
47. Eller AG, Porter TF, Soisson P, Silver RM. Optimal management strategies for placenta accreta. BJOG. 2009;116(5):648–54.
48. Hudon L, Belfort MA, Broome DR. Diagnosis and management of placenta percreta: a review. Obstet Gynecol Surv. 1998;53(8):509–17.
49. Roethlisberger M, Womastek I, Posch M, Husslein P, Pateisky N, Lehner R. Early postpartum hysterectomy: incidence and risk factors. Acta Obstet Gynecol Scand. 2010;89(8):1040–4.
50. Miller DA, Chollet JA, Goodwin TM. Clinical risk factors for placenta previa-placenta accreta. Am J Obstet Gynecol. 1997;177(1):210–4.
51. Clark SL, Koonings PP, Phelan JP. Placenta previa/accreta and prior cesarean section. Obstet Gynecol. 1985;66(1):89–92.
52. Comstock CH, Lee W, Vettraino IM, Bronsteen RA. The early sonographic appearance of placenta accreta. J Ultrasound Med. 2003;22(1):19–23. quiz 24–6.
53. Warshak CR, Ramos GA, Eskander R, Benirschke K, Saenz CC, Kelly TF, et al. Effect of predelivery diagnosis in 99 consecutive cases of placenta accreta. Obstet Gynecol. 2010;115(1):65–9.
54. Chou MM, Ho ES. Prenatal diagnosis of placenta previa accreta with power amplitude ultrasonic angiography. Am J Obstet Gynecol. 1997;177(6):1523–5.
55. Chou MM, Ho ES, Lee YH. Prenatal diagnosis of placenta previa accreta by transabdominal color Doppler ultrasound. Ultrasound Obstet Gynecol. 2000;15(1):28–35.

56. Comstock CH, Love Jr JJ, Bronsteen RA, Lee W, Vettraino IM, Huang RR, et al. Sonographic detection of placenta accreta in the second and third trimesters of pregnancy. Am J Obstet Gynecol. 2004;190(4):1135–40.
57. Esakoff TF, Sparks TN, Kaimal AJ, Kim LH, Feldstein VA, Goldstein RB, et al. Diagnosis and morbidity of placenta accreta. Ultrasound Obstet Gynecol. 2011;37(3):324–7.
58. Teo TH, Law YM, Tay KH, Tan BS, Cheah FK. Use of magnetic resonance imaging in evaluation of placental invasion. Clin Radiol. 2009;64(5):511–6.
59. Warshak CR, Eskander R, Hull AD, Scioscia AL, Mattrey RF, Benirschke K, et al. Accuracy of ultrasonography and magnetic resonance imaging in the diagnosis of placenta accreta. Obstet Gynecol. 2006;108(3 Pt 1):573–81.
60. Kupferminc MJ, Tamura RK, Wigton TR, Glassenberg R, Socol ML. Placenta accreta is associated with elevated maternal serum alpha-fetoprotein. Obstet Gynecol. 1993;82(2):266–9.
61. Zelop C, Nadel A, Frigoletto Jr FD, Pauker S, MacMillan M, Benacerraf BR. Placenta accreta/percreta/increta: a cause of elevated maternal serum alpha-fetoprotein. Obstet Gynecol. 1992;80(4):693–4.
62. Ng MK, Jack GS, Bolton DM, Lawrentschuk N. Placenta percreta with urinary tract involvement: the case for a multidisciplinary approach. Urology. 2009;74(4):778–82.
63. Soyer P, Morel O, Fargeaudou Y, Sirol M, Staub F, Boudiaf M, et al. Value of pelvic embolization in the management of severe postpartum hemorrhage due to placenta accreta, increta or percreta. Eur J Radiol. 2010. [Epub ahead of print].
64. Iwata A, Murayama Y, Itakura A, Baba K, Seki H, Takeda S. Limitations of internal iliac artery ligation for the reduction of intraoperative hemorrhage during cesarean hysterectomy in cases of placenta previa accreta. J Obstet Gynaecol Res. 2010;36(2):254–9.
65. Bodner LJ, Nosher JL, Gribbin C, Siegel RL, Beale S, Scorza W. Balloon-assisted occlusion of the internal iliac arteries in patients with placenta accreta/percreta. Cardiovasc Intervent Radiol. 2006;29(3):354–61.
66. Shrivastava V, Nageotte M, Major C, Haydon M, Wing D. Case–control comparison of cesarean hysterectomy with and without prophylactic placement of intravascular balloon catheters for placenta accreta. Am J Obstet Gynecol. 2007;197(4):402.e1–5.
67. Ojala K, Perala J, Kariniemi J, Ranta P, Raudaskoski T, Tekay A. Arterial embolization and prophylactic catheterization for the treatment for severe obstetric hemorrhage*. Acta Obstet Gynecol Scand. 2005;84(11):1075–80.
68. Sentilhes L, Trichot C, Resch B, Sergent F, Roman H, Marpeau L, et al. Fertility and pregnancy outcomes following uterine devascularization for severe postpartum haemorrhage. Hum Reprod. 2008;23(5):1087–92.
69. Sentilhes L, Resch B, Clavier E, Marpeau L. Extirpative or conservative management for placenta percreta? Am J Obstet Gynecol. 2006;195(6):1875–6. author reply 76–7.
70. Sentilhes L, Kayem G, Ambroselli C, Provansal M, Fernandez H, Perrotin F, et al. Fertility and pregnancy outcomes following conservative treatment for placenta accreta. Hum Reprod. 2010;25(11):2803–10.
71. Luo G, Perni SC, Jean-Pierre C, Baergen RN, Predanic M. Failure of conservative management of placenta previa-percreta. J Perinat Med. 2005;33(6):564–8.
72. Gupta D, Sinha R. Management of placenta accreta with oral methotrexate. Int J Gynaecol Obstet. 1998;60(2):171–3.
73. Buckshee K, Dadhwal V. Medical management of placenta accreta. Int J Gynaecol Obstet. 1997;59(1):47–8.
74. Courbiere B, Bretelle F, Porcu G, Gamerre M, Blanc B. Conservative treatment of placenta accreta. J Gynecol Obstet Biol Reprod (Paris). 2003;32(6):549–54.
75. Timmermans S, van Hof AC, Duvekot JJ. Conservative management of abnormally invasive placentation. Obstet Gynecol Surv. 2007;62(8):529–39.
76. Sentilhes L, Ambroselli C, Kayem G, Provansal M, Fernandez H, Perrotin F, et al. Maternal outcome after conservative treatment of placenta accreta. Obstet Gynecol. 2010;115(3):526–34.

Chapter 9
Vasa Previa

Ashwin R. Jadhav and Eran Bornstein

Introduction

Vasa previa is characterized by the presence of a blood vessel or vessels that are not supported by the umbilical cord or placenta and traverse the fetal membranes, which are covering the internal cervical os, in front of presenting fetal part [1]. Vasa previa remains a challenging obstetrical complication with a significant risk of both fetal morbidity and mortality due to fetal exsanguination secondary to rupture of these vessels with the onset of labor or rupture of the membranes [2]. These complications, however, can be minimized if an appropriate and timely prenatal diagnosis is obtained.

Two variants of vasa previa have been reported [3]: type I vasa previa, which is associated with a velamentous cord insertion; and type II vasa previa, which is found in cases of a succenturiate placental lobe or a bilobed placenta.

Incidence and Risk Factors

Vasa previa is a rare condition with a reported incidence of approximately 1:2,500 pregnancies [1]. A report from a single center reported a slightly lower incidence of 1.7:10,000 pregnancies [4].

Various obstetrical conditions increase the risk of vasa previa [1]. They include velamentous cord insertion (Fig. 9.1), in vitro fertilization (IVF) [5], second trimester low-lying placenta, the presence of a succenturiate lobe or bilobed placenta,

E. Bornstein (✉)
Department of Obstetrics and Gynecology,
Lenox Hill Hospital, New York, NY, USA
e-mail: eranbor@yahoo.com

E. Sheiner (ed.), *Bleeding During Pregnancy: A Comprehensive Guide*,
DOI 10.1007/978-1-4419-9810-1_9, © Springer Science+Business Media, LLC 2011

Fig. 9.1 Placenta delivered by a cesarean section owing to vasa previa. Note the velamentous cord insertion, where the umbilical cord (UC) inserts into the membranes and then travels within the membranes (*arrows*) to the placenta (PL). The exposed vessels are not protected by Wharton's jelly and hence are vulnerable to rupture

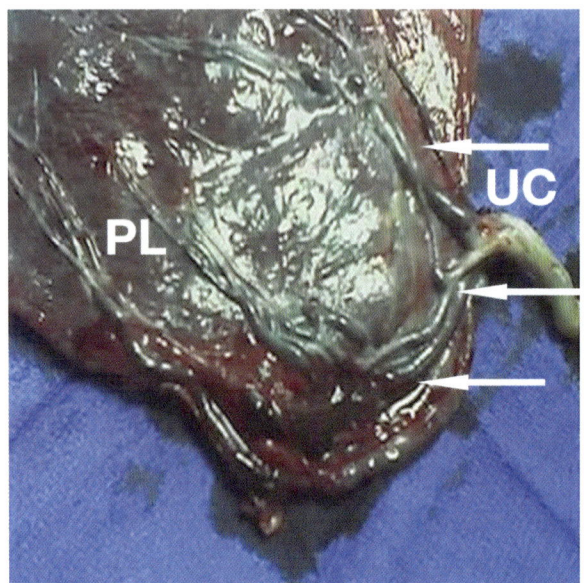

and multiple pregnancies. In a study that analyzed risk factors for vasa previa, the odds ratios (ORs) with IVF pregnancies, bilobed or succenturiate placenta, and second trimester placenta previa were 7.75, 22.11, and 22.86, respectively [6]. Umbilical cord insertion to the lower segment has also been described as a potential risk factor [7].

Diagnosis

In the past, the diagnosis of vasa previa was based on the clinical presentation of vaginal bleeding with rupture of the membranes, nonreassuring fetal heart rate tracing after artificial rupture of the membranes, palpation of pulsating vessels on digital examination during labor, and a positive test for fetal hemoglobin in cases of antepartum vaginal bleeding [8, 9]. The classic teaching at that time was to maintain a high index of suspicion and manage such cases with an emergent delivery by cesarean section [10].

With the advancements in ultrasound (US) technology and the introduction of the sonographic evaluation of the cervix during the late 1980s, multiple groups [11–21] reported high degree of success in diagnosing vasa previa using transvaginal ultrasonography (TVUS) supplemented by either power or color Doppler imaging. This has led to a paradigm change in our approach to the prenatal diagnosis of vasa previa. Substantial evidence has accumulated showing the high specificity (up to 91% in one center) [22] of US for detecting vasa previa, making it the standard diagnostic approach for this condition. This approach also resulted in a substantial minimization of both the morbidity and mortality that have been associated with it. In an authoritative multicenter review of outcomes of patients with vasa previa with or without prenatal diagnosis, Oyelese and colleagues [23] found vastly improved outcomes with a prenatal diagnosis, with survival of 97% in cases with a prenatal diagnosis vs. 44% survival without a prenatal diagnosis. It is important to note that the authors concluded that prenatal diagnosis and gestational age at delivery were the only significant predictors of neonatal survival.

The current standard clinical practice in pregnancies with obstetrical risk factors for vasa previa involves careful evaluation of the lower uterine segment and the cervix using TVUS and power/color Doppler imaging for the presence of vasa previa (Figs. 9.2–9.4).

Recently, investigators have utilized three-dimensional (3D) US for accurate diagnosing vasa previa [24]. This technology permits the reconstruction of the coronal plane of the cervix, which can demonstrate the cervical os and its relation to any traversing abnormal blood vessels.

In our practice, we perform vaginal sonographic evaluation with power Doppler as a screening test for vasa previa in selected high-risk patients. It is performed mainly on the basis of the presence of risk factors for vasa previa and on the evaluation of the placenta and cord insertion. We evaluate the placenta for the presence of a succenturiate or a bilobed placenta. In addition, we evaluate the placental cord insertion and the cervix for the presence of blood vessels that are adjacent to the internal os. 3D US has become an important adjunct to our evaluation in cases in

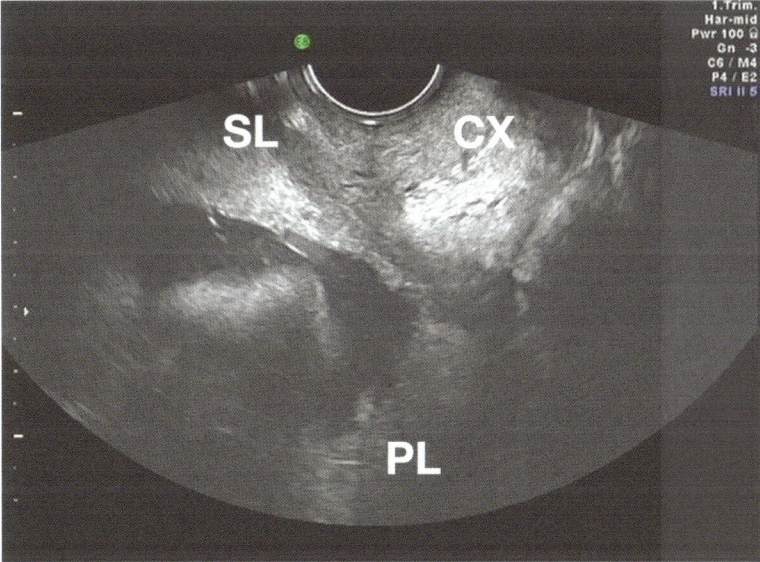

Fig. 9.2 Transvaginal gray scale evaluation of the cervix (CX) and lower uterine segment at 20 weeks' gestation. In addition to the posterior placenta (PL), which was noted, an anterior succenturiate lobe (SL) was visualized. This finding warranted further evaluation to rule out vasa previa

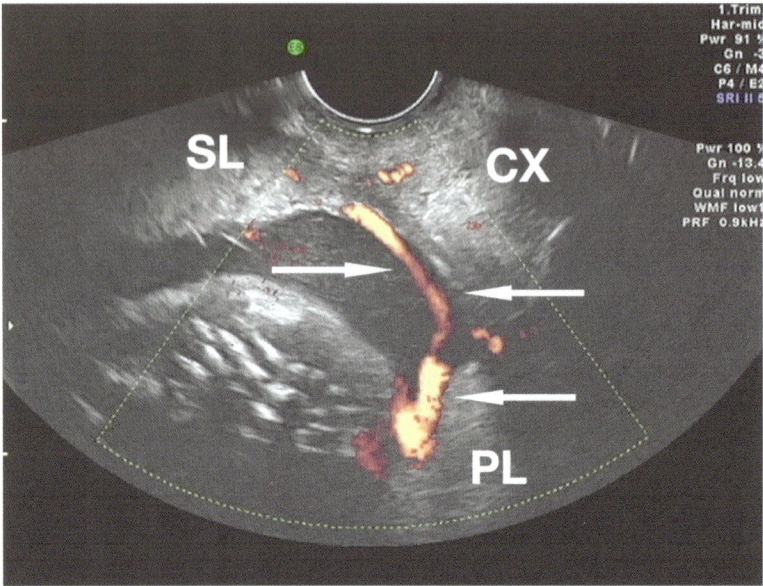

Fig. 9.3 Power Doppler was used to scrutinize the lower uterine segment for abnormal vessels. It enabled the diagnosis of vasa previa (*arrows*), which is seen as a vessel adjacent to the uterine cervix (CX), connecting the placenta (PL) and the succenturiate lobe (SL)

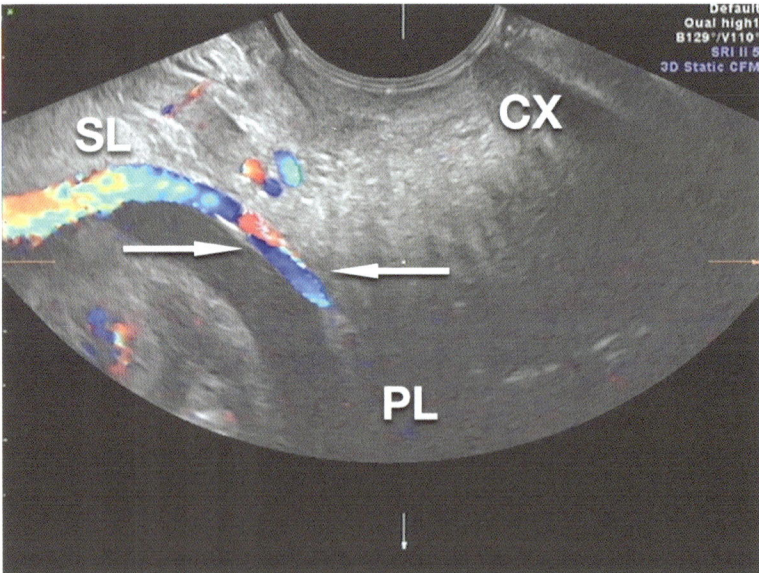

Fig. 9.4 Color Doppler is helpful in the diagnosis of vasa previa by demonstrating the abnormal vessel (*arrows*) adjacent to the uterine cervix (CX), connecting the placenta (PL) and the succenturiate lobe (SL)

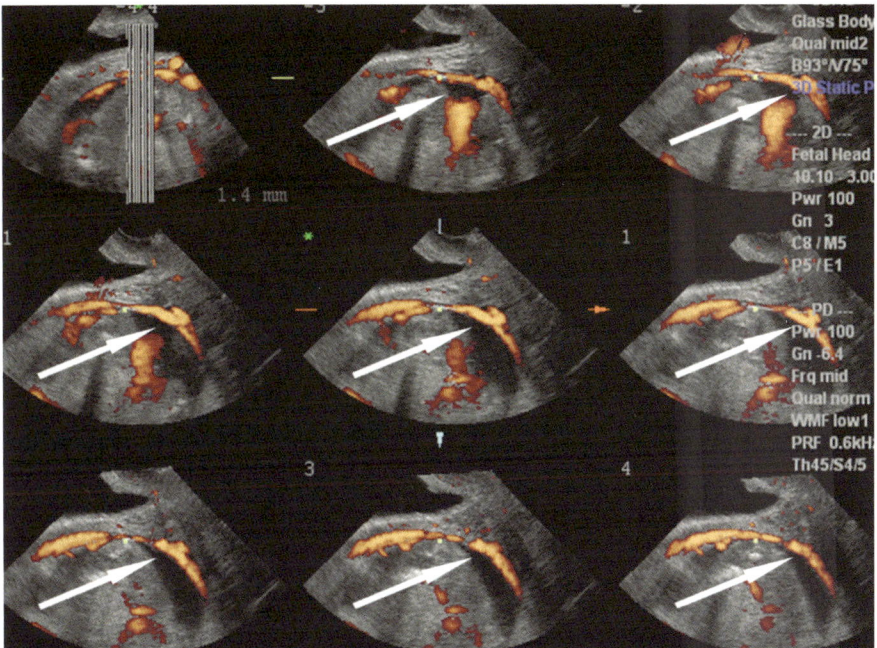

Fig. 9.5 Tomographic ultrasonography imaging (TUI) mode was used to display multiple successive sagittal sections through the cervix and lower uterine segment. It enables evaluation of the abnormal exposed vessel (*arrows*) and its relation to the cervix and fetal presenting part

which the diagnosis is difficult because it has the additive value of demonstrating the coronal plane of the cervix and the relation of the abnormal vasculature to the internal cervical os. We have found that the multiple display modalities, especially the tomographic US imaging (TUI) mode, have improved our diagnostic ability by displaying successive images that depict the relation between the abnormal vasculature and the internal cervical os (Figs. 9.2–9.5). Nevertheless, in most cases, two-dimensional US with Doppler evaluation is sufficient for the diagnosis of vasa previa.

Differential Diagnosis

The sonographic evaluation of vasa previa is difficult in some cases. Owing to significant management implications, it is important to differentiate it from other benign conditions in which vasculature may be found adjacent to the cervix.

1. Umbilical cord funic presentation: A free loop of umbilical cord is sometimes detected over the internal cervical os. Further evaluation with the mother in the trendelenberg position might be helpful to obtain an accurate diagnosis in such cases. Furthermore, imaging the placental cord insertion is important and is

expected to be normal in cases of funic presentation, whereas vellamentous insertion and a bilobed placenta are more common in cases of vasa previa.

2. Maternal uterine or cervical vessels near internal cervical os: A power Doppler evaluation to assess the pulsatility of the vessel is useful in such cases. In addition, the placenta and placental cord insertion are expected to be normal in these women.

Management

The management of vasa previa is challenging and focuses on minimizing the risk of rapid fetal exsanguination with spontaneous rupture of membranes or labor. Even when emergency cesarean section is performed in these cases, the risk of fetal exsanguination prior to delivery is substantial and has been associated with a mortality rate over 56% by some authors [23]. Therefore, the mainstays of treatment are an accurate, timely prenatal diagnosis and early intervention with cesarean delivery prior to initiation of labor or membrane rupture. This approach has significantly improved the fetal outcome among women with this potentially lethal condition.

There is a paucity of evidence comparing the management strategies. The current practice is based on expert opinion and collective clinical experience.

Our management strategy once vasa previa has been diagnosed is performed by a maternal fetal medicine specialist and includes several steps.

1. The patient is instructed to avoid vaginal intercourse, and vaginal digital examinations are deferred.
2. Serial sonographic evaluation of fetal growth is performed as some cases are associated with fetal growth restriction.
3. Antenatal fetal testing is initiated during the third trimester to detect possible cord compression.
4. Patient is admitted to the hospital at 32 weeks' gestation for continuous monitoring of fetal well-being and maternal signs of labor. In addition, we administer antenatal corticosteroids to accelerate fetal lung maturity.
5. Daily antenatal surveillance is practiced in the hospital until the date of delivery.
6. The delivery mode is cesarean section optimally prior to the initiation of labor or rupture of membranes.
7. Some clinicians opt for delivery after amniocentesis for documentation of fetal lung maturity at 35–36 weeks' gestation. However, third trimester amniocentesis in itself has been associated with a small risk of rupture of the membranes, initiation of labor, or the need for emergency delivery [25]. Moreover, postponing delivery due to immature results at this gestational age may not be appropriate. We therefore offer delivery to patients with vasa previa at 35–36 weeks' gestation without documentation of fetal lung maturity (after administration of antenatal corticosteroids at 32 weeks' gestation). We believe that the benefit from early delivery with minimal risk of rupture of membranes or labor outweighs the potential risk of fetal respiratory distress syndrome at this late preterm gestational age.

Caution Box

Evaluation of the placenta, cord insertion, and their relation to the uterine cervix can minimize the risk of fetal demise due to vasa previa.

References

1. Oyelese KO, Turner M, Lees CC, Campbell S. Vasa previa: an avoidable obstetric tragedy [review]. Obstet Gynecol Surv. 1999;54:138–45.
2. Oyelese Y, Smulian JC. Placenta previa, placenta accreta, and vasa previa. Obstet Gynecol. 2006;107(4):927–41.
3. Catanzarite V, Maida C, Thomas W, Mendoza A, Stanco L, Piacquadio KM. Prenatal sonographic diagnosis of vasa previa: ultrasound findings and obstetric outcome in ten cases. Ultrasound Obstet Gynecol. 2001;17:109–15.
4. Smorgick N, Tovbin Y, Ushakov F, Vaknin Z, Barzilay B, Herman A, et al. Is neonatal risk from vasa previa preventable? The 20-year experience from a single medical center. J Clin Ultrasound. 2010;38(3):118–22.
5. Schachter M, Tovbin Y, Arieli S, Friedler S, Ron-El R, Sherman D. In vitro fertilization is a risk factor for vasa previa. Fertil Steril. 2002;78(3):642–3.
6. Baulies S, Maiz N, Muñoz A, Torrents M, Echevarría M, Serra B. Prenatal ultrasound diagnosis of vasa praevia and analysis of risk factors. Prenat Diagn. 2007;27(7):595–9.
7. Hasegawa J, Matsuoka R, Ichizuka K, Fujikawa H, Sekizawa A, Okai T. Umbilical cord insertion to the lower uterine segment is a risk factor for vasa previa. Fetal Diagn Ther. 2007;22(5):358–60. Epub 2007 Jun 5.
8. Pent D. Vasa previa. Am J Obstet Gynecol. 1979;134(2):151–5.
9. Carp HJ, Mashiach S, Serr DM. Vasa previa: a major complication and its management. Obstet Gynecol. 1979;53(2):273–5.
10. Tollison SB, Huang PH. Vasa previa. A case report. J Reprod Med. 1988;33(3):329–30.
11. Gianopoulos J, Carver T, Tomich PG, Karlman R, Gadwood K. Diagnosis of vasa previa with ultrasonography. Obstet Gynecol. 1987;69(3 Pt 2):488–91.
12. Nelson LH, Melone PJ, King M. Diagnosis of vasa previa with transvaginal and color flow Doppler ultrasound. Obstet Gynecol. 1990;76(3 Pt 2):506–9.
13. Harding JA, Lewis DF, Major CA, Crade M, Patel J, Nageotte MP. Color flow Doppler–a useful instrument in the diagnosis of vasa previa. Am J Obstet Gynecol. 1990;163(5 Pt 1): 1566–8.
14. Hsieh FJ, Chen HF, Ko TM, Hsieh CY, Chen HY. Antenatal diagnosis of vasa previa by color-flow mapping. J Ultrasound Med. 1991;10(7):397–9.
15. Arts H, Van Eyck J. Antenatal diagnosis of vasa previa by transvaginal color Doppler sonography. Ultrasound Obstet Gynecol. 1993;3(4):276–8.
16. Meyer WJ, Blumenthal L, Cadkin A, Gauthier DW, Rotmensch S. Vasa previa: prenatal diagnosis with transvaginal color Doppler flow imaging. Am J Obstet Gynecol. 1993;169(6): 1627–9.
17. Hata K, Hata T, Fujiwaki R, Ariyuki Y, Manabe A, Kitao M. An accurate antenatal diagnosis of vasa previa with transvaginal color Doppler ultrasonography. Am J Obstet Gynecol. 1994;171(1):265–7.
18. Raga F, Ballester MJ, Osborne NG, Bonilla-Musoles F. Role of color flow Doppler ultrasonography in diagnosing velamentous insertion of the umbilical cord and vasa previa. A report of two cases. J Reprod Med. 1995;40(11):804–8.
19. Fleming AD, Johnson C, Targy M. Diagnosis of vasa previa with ultrasound and color flow Doppler: a case report. Nebr Med J. 1996;81(7):191–3.

20. Devesa R, Muñoz A, Torrents M, Carrera JM. Prenatal diagnosis of vasa previa with transvaginal color Doppler ultrasound. Ultrasound Obstet Gynecol. 1996;8(2):139–41.
21. Chen KH, Konchak P. Use of transvaginal color Doppler ultrasound to diagnose vasa previa. J Am Osteopath Assoc. 1998;98(2):116–7.
22. Catanzarite V, Maida C, Thomas W, Mendoza A, Stanco L, Piacquadio KM. Prenatal sonographic diagnosis of vasa previa: ultrasound findings and obstetric outcome in ten cases. Ultrasound Obstet Gynecol. 2001;18(2):109–15.
23. Oyelese Y, Catanzarite V, Prefumo F, Lashley S, Schachter M, Tovbin Y, et al. Vasa Previa: the impact of prenatal diagnosis on outcomes. Obstet Gynecol. 2004;103(5 Pt 1):937–42.
24. Canterino JC, Mondestin-Sorrentino M, Muench MV, et al. Vasa previa: prenatal diagnosis and evaluation with 3-dimensional sonography and power angiography. J Ultrasound Med. 2005;24:721.
25. Stark CM, Smith RS, Lagrandeur RM, Batton DG, Lorenz RP. Need for urgent delivery after third-trimester amniocentesis. Obstet Gynecol. 2000;95:48–50.

Chapter 10
Uterine Rupture

Sharon R. Sheehan and Deirdre J. Murphy

Introduction

Uterine rupture may be defined as a disruption of the uterine muscle extending to and involving the uterine serosa or disruption of the uterine muscle with extension to the bladder or broad ligament [1]. Uterine dehiscence is defined as disruption of the uterine muscle with intact uterine serosa [1]. Uterine rupture is associated with severe maternal and perinatal morbidity and mortality, and it remains one of the most catastrophic obstetrical emergencies. It has consequences not only for the index pregnancy but also, if it is possible to conserve the uterus, for further fertility and pregnancy outcomes. In the developed world, most cases occur in women with a uterine scar [2–4]. In less and least developed countries, cephalopelvic disproportion causing obstructed labor is the major cause of uterine rupture [5–7]. The prevalence of uterine rupture is likely to increase in the developed world reflecting increasing rates of cesarean section, and it continues to contribute significantly to maternal mortality among women giving birth in the developing world.

This chapter evaluates recent publications addressing the diagnosis, etiology, and management of uterine rupture. It explores aspects of maternal and neonatal morbidity and mortality from an international perspective.

International Perspective

Uterine rupture occurs most commonly during labor and is a devastating complication. Most cases in the developed world result from rupture of a previous cesarean section scar and are diagnosed in a hospital setting. Although intrapartum fetal death

D.J. Murphy (✉)
Department of Obstetrics and Gynaecology, Trinity College Dublin and
Coombe Women and Infants University Hospital, Dublin 8, Ireland
e-mail: deirdre.j.murphy@tcd.ie

E. Sheiner (ed.), *Bleeding During Pregnancy: A Comprehensive Guide*,
DOI 10.1007/978-1-4419-9810-1_10, © Springer Science+Business Media, LLC 2011

or early neonatal death may occur, the life of the mother is usually saved. Timely laparotomy may result in safe delivery of the baby and repair of the uterus. The optimal management of major obstetrical hemorrhage with the availability of surgical, anesthetic, and hematological expertise and ready access to blood products results in few maternal deaths. In the developing world this is not the case, with uterine rupture contributing significantly to maternal mortality. A major factor among black African women is obstructed labor, in part explained by the high incidence of contracted pelvis. Limited access to medical expertise and blood products results in a suboptimal response to major obstetrical hemorrhage.

The World Health Organization commissioned a systematic review of maternal morbidity and mortality with a focus on the prevalence of uterine rupture [4]. Prevalence figures were available for 86 groups of women, mainly hospital-based, from secondary and tertiary institutions. For unselected pregnant women, the prevalence was considerably lower for community-based studies (median 0.05%, range 0.02–0.30%) than for hospital-based studies (median 0.31%, range 0.01–2.90%) studies. For women with a history of previous cesarean section, the prevalence of uterine rupture was in the region of 1%. Only one report gave a prevalence from a developed country for women without a history of previous cesarean section; it was extremely low (0.006%). The prevalence of uterine rupture tended to be lower for countries defined by the United Nations as developed than the less or least developed countries. Reports from Nigeria, Ghana, Ethiopia, and Bangladesh indicated that about 75% of cases are associated with an unscarred uterus. Maternal mortality was 1–13% and perinatal mortality 74–92%.

Studies from the less and least developed countries continue to emerge with perinatal mortality rates in excess of 90% [7–9]. A report from a university teaching hospital in Nigeria described the incidence of uterine rupture as 1 in 81 deliveries, with a perinatal mortality rate of 97.1%; it contributed to 13.8% of maternal mortality in this center [9]. An earlier report from a Nigerian center cited uterine rupture as the most common cause of maternal mortality with a case fatality rate for the year 2001 of 47% [10].

Emergency obstetrical care in many countries is not free, resulting in delays in receiving care for patients with limited resources. A loan scheme was initiated in a Nigerian hospital for indigent patients with uterine rupture. The case fatality rate was reduced from 38 to 11%; and of the 17 patients who benefited from the scheme, 16 repaid the loan ($40 US) before discharge [10]. Another study described the practice of abdominal massage in southern Nigeria [11]. This practice was associated with a maternal mortality rate of 5% and perinatal mortality rate of 14%. Uterine rupture was implicated in 10% of cases. Abdominal massage has been described as a silent killer that has added to maternal and perinatal mortality and morbidity. Clearly, there are social and cultural issues that need to be addressed in preventing and managing uterine rupture in developing countries. A concerted effort is required when addressing unwanted pregnancies especially among women of high parity, accessibility of obstetrical services, innovative solutions such as symphysiotomy or cesarean section with local analgesia where conventional cesarean section facilities are not available, and guidelines to ensure that agents such as misoprostol for labor induction are used in safe dosages [4].

In developed countries, uterine rupture is among the four most common clinical causes of medical litigation in obstetrics and gynecology [12]. Litigation, in most cases, is driven by bad outcomes and not by malpractice. High standards of clinical care, clear communication, and careful documentation are of paramount importance if obstetricians are to be in a position to offer a balanced approach to patient care without fear of litigation.

Diagnosis

The initial symptoms and signs of uterine rupture are typically nonspecific, which makes the diagnosis difficult and may delay definitive treatment. It requires a high index of diagnostic suspicion. There is no single pathognomonic feature indicative of uterine rupture, but the presence of any of the following conditions peripartum should raise concern about the possibility of rupture: [13].

- Abnormal cardiotocography (CTG)
- Severe abdominal pain, especially if persisting between contractions
- Chest pain or shoulder tip pain; sudden onset of shortness of breath
- Acute onset of scar tenderness
- Abnormal vaginal bleeding or hematuria
- Cessation of previously efficient uterine activity
- Maternal tachycardia, hypotension, or shock
- Loss of station of the presenting part

Caution Box

The initial symptoms and signs of uterine rupture are typically nonspecific, which makes the diagnosis difficult and may delay definitive treatment. It requires a high index of diagnostic suspicion.

Recent attention has focused on antenatal imaging techniques but during labor the main indicator continues to be the fetal heart rate pattern on CTG. The diagnosis is ultimately confirmed at emergency cesarean section or postpartum laparotomy (Fig. 10.1).

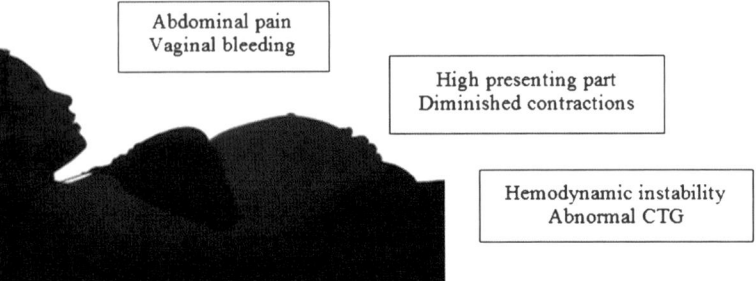

Fig. 10.1 Diagnosis of uterine rupture. *CTG* cardiotocography

Imaging Techniques

Ultrasonographic (US) examination was performed in 236 pregnant women with one or more previous cesarean sections at 35–38 weeks' gestation to assess thickness of the lower uterine segment (LUS) and to assess the validity of this measurement for predicting the risk of uterine rupture [14]. The median full LUS thickness was 2.8 mm (interquartile range 2.2–3.5 mm). A thickness of <2.3 mm was linked with a high rate of uterine rupture (9.1%). It has previously been shown that women with a history of a low transverse cesarean section have an LUS thickness at term that is approximately 0.9 mm thinner than women without a cesarean delivery [15, 16]. Several authors have suggested that the degree of LUS thinning, when measured sonographically near term, may be related to the functional status of the scarred LUS and thus to the risk of uterine rupture [17–19]. Nevertheless, no ideal cutoff value for thickness could be recommended in a recent review; and, accordingly, further replication of this approach is required [20]. The use of magnetic resonance imaging (MRI) has been described as an alternative approach when US findings of dehiscence are inconclusive [21–23], but expertise in this approach is still limited.

Fetal Heart Rate Patterns

Continuous electronic fetal heart rate monitoring is recommended for women with a previous cesarean section as it may prove useful in heralding the imminent rupture of the uterus, although in most cases it merely reflects the fact that uterine rupture has already occurred. Two studies report on fetal heart rate changes associated with uterine rupture. One study compared 36 patients with uterine rupture with 100 controls, all of whom had had one previous cesarean section [24]. Fetal bradycardia during the first and second stages of labor was the only finding to differentiate uterine rupture from successful vaginal birth among vaginal birth after cesarean section (VBAC) patients. This suggests that the CTG may change only after rupture has already occurred. A second study compared tracings from 50 patients with uterine rupture with 601 controls without scarred uteri [25]. Using two backward, stepwise multiple logistic regression models, severe fetal bradycardia [OR 8.2, 95% confidence interval (CI) 2.2–31.0, $P=0.002$] and uterine tachysystole (OR 8.0, 95% CI 1.7–37.9, $P=0.008$) were found to be independent patterns preceding uterine rupture during the first stage of labor; and reduced baseline variability (OR 4.2, 95% CI 1.4–12.3, $P=0.009$) and uterine tachysystole (OR 42.3, 95% CI 10.6–168.3, $P<0.001$) were independently associated with uterine rupture during the second stage. The problem with using reduced variability as a warning sign for uterine rupture is that it is nonspecific and could easily be explained by a fetus with an inherent physiological tendency to long sleep cycles; or it could reflect the use of opiate analgesia.

Epidural Analgesia

Pain as a symptom may or may not be helpful in the diagnosis of uterine rupture. It may occur in association with the rupture but also may reflect difficult labor, malposition, or cephalopelvic disproportion, which could all be on the causal pathway. One study challenged the notion that pain and scar tenderness associated with uterine rupture may be masked by epidural analgesia. Cahill and colleagues investigated the association between epidural dosage and the risk of uterine rupture in women undergoing a trial of labor after a previous cesarean section [26]. Women who experienced a uterine rupture required 4.1 doses compared to 3.5 doses in women who did not have a uterine rupture ($P=0.4$) In the final 90 min of labor, women who experienced a rupture were 8.1 times more likely than controls to have required four or more additional epidural doses. The authors recommended a high index of suspicion of rupture in women requiring frequent epidural dosages [26].

Etiology

The key to preventing uterine rupture is understanding the etiological factors and high-risk clinical situations. Although uterine rupture occurs most commonly during labor by women who have had a previous cesarean section, it can occur subsequently after any type of uterine instrumentation, including dilatation and curettage, hysteroscopy, and forceps delivery [27]. Risk factors for rupture of an unscarred uterus include grand multiparity, cephalopelvic disproportion, malpresentation, administration of oxytocin, fetal macrosomia, placenta previa, placenta percreta, external cephalic version, and uterine abnormalities and trauma [28].

Previous Cesarean Section

For women with one previous cesarean section, the overall chances of a successful planned VBAC are 72–76% [1, 29, 30]. In the USA, the National Institutes of Health (NIH) issued a consensus statement stating that the overall risk for perinatal mortality and morbidity with trial of labor after a previous cesarean section (TOLAC) is similar to that for any primiparous women in labor [31]. A systematic review prepared to inform the 2010 NIH Consensus Development Conference: Vaginal Birth After Cesarean: New Insights [32] determined from studies conducted in the developed world that VBAC is a reasonable and safe choice for most women with a prior cesarean section. Many studies assessing the safety of VBAC have compared it to elective repeat cesarean section; however, comparing first VBAC to labor in women who have not undergone a previous vaginal delivery may be far more appropriate [33].

A Norwegian population-based registry study of more than 18,000 women with a prior cesarean delivery assessed the effects of trial of labor and repeat cesarean on maternal and perinatal outcomes [34]. The overall incidence of uterine rupture was 0.5%, with an eightfold increase in the odds of rupture with a trial of labor compared to an elective prelabor cesarean delivery. The risk was greatest in trials of labor associated with prostaglandin induction [34]. Uterine rupture was associated with dramatic increases in the rates of postpartum hemorrhage, exposure to general anesthesia, and peripartum hysterectomy; and these morbidities significantly increased if rupture occurred after a trial of labor. There were no maternal deaths in this study. A serious perinatal outcome following uterine rupture occurred in 9 (9.3%) infants after a trial of labor compared to no cases after cesarean section.

A prospective 4-year observational study of more than 33,000 women with a singleton pregnancy and a prior cesarean delivery had previously provided robust information on maternal and perinatal outcomes associated with a trial of labor [1]. Symptomatic uterine rupture occurred in 0.7% of women and hypoxic ischemic encephalopathy (including neonatal death) occurred in 0.46:1,000 women undergoing a trial of labor vs. no cases delivered by elective cesarean delivery. The frequency of hysterectomy and maternal death did not differ significantly between the groups.

A retrospective study in a large Scottish population reported a higher rate of rupture in association with prostaglandin for induction of labor (OR 2.9, 95% CI 2.0–4.3) [35]. Perinatal death was associated with uterine rupture and use of prostaglandins for induction. Interestingly, the risk of perinatal death was higher in units with lower annual numbers of births (1:1,300 for units with <3,000 births vs. 1:4,700 for units with ≥3,000 births). While relative risks are increased for women attempting VBAC, absolute risks are low.

Induction of Labor with a Previous Cesarean Section

The safety of induction of labor for women with a previous cesarean section has been evaluated with inconsistent findings. Kayani and Alfirevic concluded that induction of labor carries a relatively high risk of uterine rupture/dehiscence despite precautions including intrauterine pressure monitoring [36]. In contrast, Locatelli et al. reported a similar rate of uterine rupture (0.3%) for each group and suggested that induction of labor can be considered within the context of a consistent protocol with strict criteria for intervention [37]. Nonetheless, the more robust evidence suggests an increased risk of uterine rupture for induction of labor following a previous cesarean delivery, particularly with the use of prostaglandins, and it needs to be addressed during patient consultations [35, 38].

VBAC with a Previous Vaginal Birth

A previous vaginal birth appears to offer some protection. A prior vaginal delivery was associated with a lower risk of uterine rupture for the Scottish cohort, and similar results were reported in a case–control study from the USA (adjusted OR 0.40, 95% CI 0.20–0.81) [35, 39]. Another study confirmed the higher rate of successful trials of labor among women with a prior vaginal delivery; however, in this population a prior VBAC was associated with an increased rate of uterine scar dehiscence [40].

VBAC After Multiple Previous Cesarean Sections

The risk in relation to multiple previous cesarean sections has been explored. The likelihood of major complications was higher with a VBAC attempt after two prior cesarean deliveries compared with a single cesarean delivery in a U.S. study (adjusted OR 2.3, 95% CI 1.4–3.9 for uterine rupture) [41]. A study from Turkey addressed the maternal and neonatal outcomes in relation to multiple repeat cesarean sections and reported little difference in adverse outcomes for women with two or more cesarean sections compared to one previous cesarean section. The women were delivered by elective cesarean section, and the findings only provide reassurance for the antenatal period [42]. Tahseen and Griffiths conducted a systematic review of the success rate of vaginal birth after two cesarean sections and concluded that it was 71.1%; the uterine rupture rate was 1.36% with a comparative maternal morbidity with the repeat cesarean delivery choice [43]. The conclusion of the Royal College of Obstetricians and Gynaecologists (RCOG) green top guideline that women with two uncomplicated low transverse cesarean sections may be considered suitable for a planned VBAC is very different from current practice in the USA [38].

Uterine Closure at Cesarean Section

The role of uterine closure in the risk of uterine rupture has been the subject of recent interest. A multicenter case–control study examined the effects of prior single-layer vs. double-layer uterine closure. The risk of uterine rupture during a trial of labor with a prior single-layer closure was more than twice that compared with double-layer closure (OR 2.69; 95% CI 1.37–5.28) [44]. We await the results of the CORONIS trial, a multicenter, fractional factorial randomized controlled trial, which examines the effects of five aspects of cesarean section, including uterine closure [45].

Gestational Age at VBAC

The timing of birth after a previous cesarean has also received much attention recently. Preterm patients have higher success rates when compared with term patients undergoing a VBAC (adjusted OR 1.54, 95% CI 1.27–1.86) and may even have lower rates of uterine rupture (adjusted OR 0.28, 95% CI 0.07–1.17) [46]. The corollary has been reported with a study showing that the risk of uterine rupture is significantly higher among patients with advanced gestational age (≥41 weeks vs. 24–36 weeks and 37–40 weeks, $P = 0.006$) [47].

VBAC and Multiple Pregnancy

The success rate and risks for women with a twin pregnancy who attempt VBAC have been explored within a U.S. network cesarean registry. A trial of labor with twins did not appear to increase maternal morbidity, and perinatal morbidity was uncommon at ≥34 weeks of gestation [48]. The findings in relation to maternal morbidity were confirmed in a retrospective study in Israel. Trial of labor was noted, however, as a risk factor for perinatal mortality, although the authors did note that confounding may be responsible for this finding [49].

Interdelivery Interval

It has been suggested that a short interdelivery interval may be associated with incomplete healing of the uterine scar, thus predisposing it to rupture. A study of 1,768 women has shown that an interdelivery interval shorter than 18 months (OR 3.0, 95% CI 1.3–7.2), but not between 18 and 24 months (OR 1.1, 95% CI 0.4–3.2), may be a risk factor for uterine rupture [50].

New evidence suggests that gestational age, maternal obesity, underlying medical conditions, and hospital factors such as delivery volume and a tertiary compared with a nontertiary care setting may affect maternal and neonatal outcomes. These emerging data highlight the need for future research [51]. Vaginal birth after a previous cesarean section and the risk of uterine rupture is clearly a complex area that requires careful patient counseling.

Previous Uterine Surgery

The term vaginal birth after laparoscopic myomectomy (VBALM) has been coined to take account of the increasing number of women who undergo minimal access uterine surgery prior to childbirth [52]. In all, 47 pregnancies in 40 patients were reviewed. Vaginal birth was attempted in 72% and achieved in 83% of these women, with no case of uterine rupture. The authors advised that vaginal birth can be achieved safely following laparoscopic myomectomy provided the delivery is managed as for VBAC. A detailed review of the literature confirms that the risk of uterine rupture is low when the myometrium is repaired appropriately [53].

The reproductive outcomes for women who have experienced a pregnancy complicated by maternofetal surgery were explored in a retrospective review of 93 women from a single institution [54]. The pregnancy rate was 50.5%, and complications included uterine rupture (14%) and dehiscence (14%). The uterine rupture rate compares with that of "classic" cesarean section (4–9%), and therefore similar caution is required when planning delivery.

Misoprostol

Misoprostol, a synthetic prostaglandin E_1 analog is effective for cervical ripening and labor induction. More recently it has been evaluated for use in first and second trimester terminations of pregnancy.

Priming with mifepristone prior to misprostol administration for the management of intrauterine death has been shown to shorten the time needed for induction [55]. A Cochrane review explored the use of misoprostol for termination of pregnancy during the second or third trimester for women with a fetal anomaly or after intrauterine fetal death [56]. A total of 38 studies were included in the review, with vaginal misoprostol proving as effective as other prostaglandin preparations and more effective than oral misoprostol preparations. Berghella et al. conducted a systematic review of cases of second trimester misoprostol termination and found it to be safe among women with one prior low transverse cesarean birth [57]. It was associated with an incidence of uterine rupture of 0.4% (95% CI 0.08–1.67%) and of transfusion of 0.2%. There were no cases of hysterectomy in this review. They concluded that there are insufficient data on risk with more than one prior cesarean birth or with prior classic cesarean birth. Uterine ruptures following misoprostol induction of labor in patients with and without previous cesarean sections have been described. The risk of uterine rupture with the use of misoprostol in women attempting a VBAC is reported at 6–12% and for this reason misoprostol is contraindicated for induction of labor in women with a uterine scar [58, 59].

Numerous protocols are in existence for misoprostol use, employing different dosing regimens and methods of administration, thus making it difficult to compare studies and reach definitive conclusions about its safety. It appears however, to have a reasonable safety profile in women with a previous cesarean section. The International Federation of Gynecology and Obstetrics (FIGO) and the World Health Organization (WHO) have issued recommended dosing schedules following an expert meeting in Bellagio, Italy [60]. Care has been advised in the use of misoprostol in women with a previous uterine scar. Its use has been contraindicated in certain situations, and halving the dose has been recommended for other situations. There remains a paucity of data on maternal safety and the risks of uterine rupture, thus highlighting the need for further research.

Trauma

Maternal and neonatal outcomes of pregnancy have been evaluated within a retrospective cohort study of women hospitalized for trauma in California [61]. A total of 10,316 deliveries were identified from a cohort of almost five million births. Women who delivered at the time of trauma hospitalization had serious adverse outcomes compared to nontrauma controls, with a marked increase in uterine rupture (OR 43, 95% CI 19–97). The study highlighted the need to optimize education in trauma prevention during pregnancy. A further study from the same cohort focused on pregnancy outcomes among women hospitalized for assault [62]. The incidence of uterine rupture was 0.71%, markedly higher than that in women with no history of assault (OR 46, 95% CI 6.5–337.8). Women experiencing an assault during pregnancy experience both immediate and long-term sequelae.

Uterine Malformation

Several case reports have described rupture of a rudimentary uterine horn. In one case the clinicians achieved a live birth following rupture of a noncommunicating horn of a bicornuate uterus at 30 weeks' gestation, but a hysterectomy was required [63]. In another case there was rupture of a noncommunicating horn at 27 weeks' gestation with neonatal and maternal survival. It was possible to resect the rudimentary horn and conserve the uterus [64]. Another series of two cases described a rudimentary horn pregnancy diagnosed by US ultrasound and confirmed by MRI during the first trimester of pregnancy [65]. Both were resected without complications. Congenital uterine anomalies occur in 0.5% of women. A review of the literature advises that the key to successful management is early detection [66]. A total of 156 obstetric cases of rudimentary uterine horn were found, with noncommunicating horns accounting for 92% of cases. Many functional noncommunicating horns present during or after the third decade of life with acute obstetrical uterine rupture. Surgical removal before pregnancy is recommended. Prerupture diagnosis rates remain disappointingly low; it is mainly diagnosed from an incidental finding during investigations for infertility.

Mechanisms of Rupture

The underlying pathophysiology behind rupture of the uterus has received little attention to date. The incidence of uterine rupture for women in labor with a uterine scar increases two- to threefold and the risk of cesarean section rises 1.5-fold in induced or augmented labors compared with spontaneous labors [1]. Previous cesarean section was associated with an OR of 6.0 (95% CI 3.2–11.4) for uterine rupture in a study investigating risk factors for uterine rupture [67]. Accordingly, the authors in another study attempted to define differences among patients with a scarred uterus vs. an unscarred uterus [68]. Their hypothesis was that more risk factors would be required to rupture an unscarred uterus. However, although factors such as higher birth order, uterine tachysystole, and fetal macrosomia were found in higher rates in the unscarred group, the small number of cases precluded achieving statistical significance [68].

Induction with prostaglandin further increases the risk of uterine rupture [35]. A study of 26 women with a prior cesarean section experiencing uterine rupture in active labor explored whether prostaglandins induce biochemical changes in the uterine scar similar to changes in the cervix by examining the site of rupture [69]. Women treated with prostaglandins experienced rupture at the site of their old scar more frequently than women in the oxytocin-only group, whose rupture tended to be remote from their old scar. The authors proposed that prostaglandins induce local biochemical modifications that weaken the scar, predisposing it to rupture. This provides further support for the need to be cautious in the use of prostaglandins for women with a previous cesarean scar (Fig. 10.2).

Risk factors for uterine rupture

- Previous caesarean section
- Previous uterine rupture
- Previous uterine surgery
- Excessive uterine stimulation –
- e.g. oxytocin, prostaglandin E1 and E2
- Trauma
- Uterine malformation
- Malpresentation
- Obstructed labor
- Fetal anomaly

Fig. 10.2 Risk factors for uterine rupture

Management

The management of acute intrapartum rupture of the uterus requires an urgent response in keeping with any obstetrical emergency. Senior staff should be summoned, and a multidisciplinary team approach should address immediate resuscitation followed by specific care. The aim is to stabilize the maternal condition and achieve delivery of a live-born, healthy infant where possible [70]. Airway, breathing, and circulation (ABC) must be remembered. Two large-bore intravenous cannulas should be on site, and blood is obtained for a full blood count, coagulation screen, and blood group and cross-match. Intravenous crystalloid and colloid should be given to replace volume loss, with transfusion of blood and blood products where necessary. Closer inspection of the uterus at laparotomy determines whether the uterus can be conserved, but early recourse to hysterectomy should be considered if there is any immediate threat to the life of the mother (e.g., unavailability of blood products or patient refusal of transfusion). Massive blood loss is likely, and the local major obstetric hemorrhage protocol should be implemented. Advanced resuscitation of the newborn is likely to be required, and sometimes difficult end-of-life decisions need to be made during the neonatal period [71]. The parents require careful debriefing at a later stage about the nature of these dramatic events and any adverse outcomes.

Much of the management around uterine rupture is now focused on counseling about risk in the context of a previous cesarean section. Uterine rupture has a marked impact on the medical staff that can limit their ability to counsel in a well-informed nondirective manner (Fig. 10.3).

Counseling

Women who have had a cesarean section should see a consultant obstetrician early during the antenatal period and have a frank discussion about the problems that may arise in relation to the mode of delivery. Written materials for reflection should be

Management of the mother with uterine rupture

- Airway, Breathing, Circulation
- Institute major obstetric hemorrhage protocol
- 2 large bore IV cannulae
- Full blood count, coagulation screen, group & cross-match
- Replenish volume loss
- Transfusion
- Laparotomy – uterine conservation or hysterectomy
- Counsel & debrief

Fig. 10.3 Management of the mother with uterine rupture

provided in an appropriate format. The DiAMOND study examined the effects of two computer-based decision aids on decisional conflict and mode of delivery among pregnant women with a previous cesarean section and demonstrated that such aids can help these women decide on the mode of delivery in a subsequent pregnancy [72]. The Royal College of Obstetricians and Gynaecologists and the Society of Obstetricians and Gynaecologists of Canada have produced useful clinical practice guidelines and supporting patient information that addresses vaginal birth after previous cesarean birth [38, 73, 74].

The literature has been extensively reviewed, and clear recommendations are provided. It is recommended that a woman with a history of one uncomplicated lower segment transverse cesarean section, in an otherwise uncomplicated pregnancy at term, with no contraindication to vaginal birth, should be able to discuss the option of planned VBAC and the alternative of a repeat cesarean section (ERCS). Risks and benefits should cover success rates, uterine rupture, perinatal mortality, and surgical complications. Written information or decision aids should supplement the discussions [38, 72]. In the event of an adverse outcome, many of these cases result in litigation. Clear documentation of all discussions and decisions is essential.

The operative notes from the previous delivery should be reviewed (or a summary requested if performed elsewhere) and should help inform the advice given. A US scan should be performed to document the placental location. The final decision on mode of delivery should be agreed on before the expected date of delivery (ideally by 36 weeks' gestation) [38]. If the woman decides on an elective cesarean section, it should be performed at 39 weeks' gestation, with a contingency plan in place in the event of spontaneous labor before this date [38]. Infants born by elective cesarean section before 39 weeks' gestation are at increased risk of neonatal respiratory morbidity [75].

Women with a previous cesarean delivery should also be advised about induction of labor and oxytocin augmentation. If induction or augmentation is proposed, discussion with the consultant obstetrician is essential [38].

Numerous international guidelines for VBAC exist, although they vary widely regarding their recommendations. Caution should be exercised in their interpretation [76]. One must be wary when considering VBAC in women with a twin gestation, fetal macrosomia, and/or a short interdelivery interval, as there is limited knowledge on the safety and efficacy of planned VBAC in such circumstances [38].

Summary

Uterine rupture is a devastating complication for the mother, her partner, and her family; and it is distressing for the staff involved. Uterine rupture due to obstructed labor is a tragedy almost exclusively limited to less developed and least developed countries. It requires a comprehensive approach to health care provision spanning family planning services to acute management of obstetrical emergencies. In the developed world, the emphasis is on the risks of labor for the woman with a previous cesarean section. The unrelenting increase in primary cesarean sections is creating a high-risk population of parous women. Balanced counseling is required on the place of birth, time of birth, and mode of delivery. Maternal and infant safety must be addressed alongside the maternal preferences for the birth experience. Future developments in imaging may allow us to predict with greater accuracy women at highest risk of uterine rupture and so to plan preventive measures accordingly. A high index of suspicion prompting a multidisciplinary response and regular drills can achieve optimal outcomes.

References

1. Landon MB, Hauth JC, Leveno KJ, et al. Maternal and perinatal outcomes associated with a trial of labor after prior cesarean delivery. N Engl J Med. 2004;351:2581–9.
2. Gardeil F, Daly S, Turner MJ. Uterine rupture in pregnancy reviewed. Eur J Obstet Gynecol Reprod Biol. 1994;56:107–10.
3. Yap OW, Kim ES, Laros Jr RK. Maternal and neonatal outcomes after uterine rupture in labor. Am J Obstet Gynecol. 2001;184(7):1576–81.
4. Hofmeyr GJ, Say L, Gulmezoglu AM. WHO systematic review of maternal mortality and morbidity; the prevalence of uterine rupture. BJOG. 2005;112:1221–5.
5. Ola ER, Olamijulo JA. Rupture of the uterus at the Lagos University Teaching Hospital, Lagos, Nigeria. West Afr J Med. 1998;17:188–93.
6. Gessessew A, Melese MM. Ruptured uterus – eight year retrospective analysis of causes and management outcome in Adigrat Hospital, Tigray region, Ethiopia. Ethiop J Health Dev. 2002;16:241–5.
7. Gupta A, Nanda S. Uterine rupture in pregnancy: a five-year study. Arch Gynecol Obstet. 2010;283(3):437–41.
8. Esike CO, Umeora OU, Eze JN, Igberasse GO. Ruptured uterus: the unabating obstetric catastrophe in South eastern Nigeria. Arch Gynecol Obstet. 2011;283(5):993–7.
9. Fabamwo A, Akinola O, Tayo A, Akpan E. Rupture of the gravid uterus: a never-ending obstetric disaster! The Ikeja experience. J Gynecol Obstet. 2009;10.
10. Ahmed Y, Shehu CE, Nwobodo EI, Ekele BA. Reducing maternal mortality from ruptured uterus – the Sokoto initiative. Afr J Med Sci. 2004;33:135–8.
11. Ugboma HA, Akani CI. Abdominal massage: another cause of maternal mortality. Niger J Med. 2004;13:259–62.
12. Mavroforou A, Koumantakis E, Michalodimitrakis E. Physicians' liability in obstetric and gynecology practice. Med Law. 2005;24:1–9.
13. Turner MJ. Uterine rupture. Best Prac Res Clin Obstet Gynaecol. 2002;16:69–79.
14. Bujold E, Jastrow N, Simoneau J, Brunet S, Gauthier RJ. Prediction of complete uterine rupture by sonographic evaluation of the lower uterine segment. Am J Obstet Gynecol. 2009;201:320.e1–6.
15. Gotoh H, Masuzaki H, Yoshida A, Yoshimura S, Miyamura T, Ishimaru T. Predicting incomplete uterine rupture with vaginal sonography during the late second trimester in women with prior cesarean. Obstet Gynecol. 2000;95:596–600.
16. Cheung VY. Sonographic measurement of the lower uterine segment thickness in women with previous caesarean section. J Obstet Gynaecol Can. 2005;27:674–81.
17. Rozenberg P, Goffinet F, Phillippe HJ, Nisand I. Ultrasonographic measurement of lower uterine segment to assess risk of defects of scarred uterus. Lancet. 1996;347:281–4.
18. Fukuda M, Fukuda K, Mochizuki M. Examination of previous caesarean section scars by ultrasound. Arch Gynecol Obstet. 1988;243:221–4.

19. Sen S, Malik S, Salhan S. Ultrasonographic evaluation of lower uterine segment thickness in patients of previous cesarean section. Int J Gynaecol Obstet. 2004;87:215–9.
20. Jastrow N, Chaillet N, Roberge S, Morency AM, Lacasse Y, Bujold E. Sonographic lower uterine segment thickness and risk of uterine scar defect: a systematic review. J Obstet Gynaecol Can. 2010;32(4):321–7.
21. Leyendecker JR, Gorengaut V, Brown JJ. MR imaging of maternal diseases of the abdomen and pelvis during pregnancy and the immediate postpartum period. Radiographics. 2004;24: 1301–16.
22. Vadnais M, Awtrey C, Pedrosa I. Breaking point: magnetic resonance imaging evaluation of an obstetric emergency. Am J Obstet Gynecol. 2009;200(3):344.e1–3.
23. Kamaya A, Ro K, Benedetti NJ, Chang PL, Desser TS. Imaging and diagnosis of postpartum complications: sonography and other imaging modalities. Ultrasound Q. 2009;3:151–62.
24. Ridgeway JJ, Weyrich DL, Benedetti TJ. Fetal heart rate changes associated with uterine rupture. Obstet Gynecol. 2004;103:506–12.
25. Sheiner E, Levy A, Ofir K, et al. Changes in fetal heart rate and uterine patterns associated with uterine rupture. J Reprod Med. 2004;49:373–8.
26. Cahill AG, Odibo AO, Allsworth JE, Macones GA. Frequent epidural dosing as a marker for impending uterine rupture in patients who attempt vaginal birth after caesarean delivery. Am J Obstet Gynecol. 2010;202(4):355.e1–5.
27. Fedorkow DM, Nimrod CA, Taylor PJ. Ruptured uterus in pregnancy: a Canadian hospital's experience. CMAJ. 1987;137:27–9.
28. Sweeten KM, Graves WK, Athanassiou A. Spontaneous rupture of the unscarred uterus. Am J Obstet Gynecol. 1995;172:1851–6.
29. Smith GCS, Pell JP, Cameron AD, Dobbie R. Risk of perinatal death associated with labor after previous caesarean delivery in uncomplicated term pregnancies. JAMA. 2002;287: 2684–90.
30. Wen SW, Rusen ID, Walker M, Liston R, Kramer MS, Baskett T, et al. Comparison of maternal mortality and morbidity between trial of labor and elective cesarean section among women with previous caesarean delivery. Am J Obstet Gynecol. 2004;191:1263–9.
31. National Institutes of Health Consensus Development Conference Statement. Vaginal birth after cesarean: new insights. Obstet Gynecol. 2010;115:1279–95.
32. Guise JM, Eden K, Emeis C, Denman MA, Marshall N, Fu R, et al. Vaginal birth after caesarean: new insights. Evidence report/technology assessment No 191. Rockvile (MD): Agency for Healthcare Research and Quality; 2010. http://www.arhq.gov/downloads/pub/evidence/pdf/vbacup.pdf.
33. Rozen G, Ugoni AM, Sheehan PM. A new perspective on VBAC: a retrospective cohort study. Women Birth 2010; May 4. [Epub ahead of print].
34. Al-Zirqi I, Stray-Pedersen B, Forsen L, Vangen S. Uterine rupture after previous caesarean section. BJOG. 2010;117:809–20.
35. Smith GC, Pell JP, Pasupathy D, Dobbie R. Factors predisposing to perinatal death related to uterine rupture during attempted vaginal birth after caesarean section: retrospective cohort study. BMJ. 2004;329:375.
36. Kayani SI, Alfirevic Z. Uterine rupture after induction of labour in women with previous caesarean section. BJOG. 2005;112:451–5.
37. Locatelli A, Regalia AL, Ghidini A, et al. Risks of induction of labour in women with a uterine scar from previous low transverse caesarean section. BJOG. 2004;111:1394–9.
38. Royal College of Obstetricians and Gynaecologists. Birth after previous caesarean birth. Green-top guideline no 45, 2007. http://www.rcog.org.uk/files/rcog-corp/uploaded-files/GT45BirthAfterPreviousCeasarean.pdf.
39. Macones GA, Peipert J, Nelson DB, et al. Maternal complications with vaginal birth after caesarean delivery: a multicentre study. Am J Obstet Gynecol. 2005;193:1656–62.
40. Hendler I, Bujold E. Effect of prior vaginal delivery or prior vaginal birth after cesarean delivery on obstetric outcomes in women undergoing trial of labor. Obstet Gynecol. 2004;104:273–7.

41. Macones GA, Cahill A, Pare E, et al. Obstetric outcomes in women with two prior cesarean deliveries: is vaginal birth after cesarean delivery a viable option? Am J Obstet Gynecol. 2005;192:1223–8.
42. Uygur D, Tapisiz OL, Mungan T. Multiple repeat cesarean sections: maternal and neonatal outcomes. Int J Gynaecol Obstet. 2005;89:284–5.
43. Tahseen S, Griffiths M. Vaginal birth after two caesarean sections (VBAC-2) – a systematic review with meta-analysis of success rate and adverse outcomes of VBAC-2 versus VBAC-1 and repeat (third) caesarean sections. BJOG. 2010;117:5–19.
44. Bujold E, Goyet M, Marcoux S, Brassard N, Cormier B, Hamilton E, et al. The role of uterine closure in the risk of uterine rupture. Obstet Gynecol. 2010;116:43–50.
45. CORONIS Trial Collaborative Group. The CORONIS Trial. International study of caesarean section surgical techniques: a randomised fractional, factorial trial. BMC Pregnancy Childbirth. 2007;7:24.
46. Quinones JN, Stamilio DM, Pare E, et al. The effect of prematurity on vaginal birth after cesarean delivery: success and maternal morbidity. Obstet Gynecol. 2005;105:519–24.
47. Hammoud A, Hendler I, Gauthier RJ, et al. The effect of gestational age on trial of labor after Cesarean section. J Matern Fetal Neonatal Med. 2004;15:202–6.
48. Varner MW, Leindecker S, Spong CY, et al. The Maternal-Fetal Medicine Unit caesarean registry: trial of labor with twin gestation. Am J Obstet Gynecol. 2005;193:135–40.
49. Aaronson D, Harlev A, Sheiner E, Levy A. Trial of labor after caesarean section in twin pregnancies: maternal and neonatal safety. J Matern Fetal Neonatal Med. 2010;23:550–4.
50. Bujold E, Gauthier RJ. Risk of uterine rupture associated with an interdelivery interval between 18 and 24 months. Obstet Gynecol. 2010;115:1003–6.
51. Guise JM, Denman MA, Emeis C, Marshall N, Walker M, Fu R, et al. Vaginal birth after caesarean. New insights on maternal and neonatal outcomes. Obstet Gynecol. 2010;115:1267–78.
52. Kumakiri J, Takeuchi H, Kitade M, et al. Pregnancy and delivery after laparoscopic myomectomy. J Minim Invasive Gynecol. 2005;12:241–6.
53. Hurst BS, Matthews ML, Marshburn PB. Laparoscopic myomectomy for symptomatic uterine myomas. Fertil Steril. 2005;83:1–23.
54. Wilson RD, Johnson MP, Flake AW, et al. Reproductive outcomes after pregnancy complicated by maternal-fetal surgery. Am J Obstet Gynecol. 2004;191(4):1430–6.
55. Fairley TE, Mackenzie M, Owen P, Mackenzie F. Management of late intrauterine death using a combination of mifepristone and misoprostol; experience of two regimens. Eur J Obstet Gynecol Reprod Biol. 2005;118:28–31.
56. Dodd JM, Crowther CA. Misoprostol for induction of labour to terminate pregnancy in the second or third trimester for women with a fetal anomaly or after intrauterine fetal death. Cochrane Database Syst Rev. 2010 Apr 14;4:CD004901.
57. Berghella V, Airoldi J, O'Neill AM, Einhorn K, Hoffman M. Misoprostol for second trimester pregnancy termination in women with prior caesarean: a systematic review. BJOG. 2009;116:1151–7.
58. Plaut MM, Schwartz ML, Lubarsky SL. Uterine rupture associated with the use of misoprostol in the gravid patient with a previous caesarean section. Am J Obstet Gynecol. 1999;180:1535–42.
59. Wing DA, Lovett K, Paul RH. Disruption of prior uterine incision following misoprostol for labor induction in women with previous caesarean delivery. Obstet Gynecol. 1998;91:828–30.
60. Weeks A, Faundes A. Misoprostol in obstetrics and gynecology. Int J Gynecol Obstet. 2007;99(s2):S156–9.
61. El-Kady D, Gilbert WM, Anderson J, et al. Trauma during pregnancy: an analysis of maternal and fetal outcomes in a large population. Am J Obstet Gynecol. 2004;190:1661–8.
62. El Kady D, Gilbert WM, Xing G, Smith LH. Maternal and neonatal outcomes of assaults during pregnancy. Obstet Gynecol. 2005;105:357–63.
63. Ashelby L, Toll G, Patel RR, et al. Live birth after rupture of a non-communicating horn of a bicornuate uterus. BJOG. 2005;112:1576–7.

64. Shinohara A, Yamada A, Imai A. Rupture of non-communicating rudimentary uterine horn at 27 weeks' gestations with neonatal and maternal survival. Int J Gynaecol Obstet. 2005;88: 316–7.
65. Tsafrir A, Rojansky N, Sela HY, et al. Rudimentary horn pregnancy: first-trimester prerupture sonographic diagnosis and confirmation by magnetic resonance imaging. J Ultrasound Med. 2005;24:219–23.
66. Jayasinghe Y, Rane A, Stalewski H, Grover S. The presentation and early diagnosis of the rudimentary uterine horn. Obstet Gynecol. 2005;105:1456–67.
67. Ofir K, Sheiner E, Levy A, Katz M, Mazor M. Uterine rupture: risk factors and pregnancy outcome. Am J Obstet Gynecol. 2003;189(4):1042–6.
68. Ofir K, Sheiner E, Levy A, Katz M, Mazor M. Uterine rupture: differences between a scarred and an unscarred uterus. Am J Obstet Gynecol. 2004;191(2):425–9.
69. Buhimschi CS, Buhimschi IA, Patel S, et al. Rupture of the uterine scar during term labour: contractility or biochemistry? BJOG. 2005;112:38–42.
70. Murphy DJ. Uterine rupture. Curr Opin Obstet Gynaecol. 2006;18:135–40.
71. Pradhan P. Ruptured uterus. In: Grady K, Howell C, Cox C, editors. Managing obstetric emergencies and trauma: the MOET course manual. London: RCOG Press; 2007. p. 257–61.
72. Montgomery AA, Emmett CL, Fahey T, Jones C, Ricketts I, Patel RR, et al. Two decision aids for mode of delivery among women with previous caesarean section: randomised controlled trial. BMJ. 2007;334:1305.
73. Royal College of Obstetricians and Gynaecologists. Birth after previous caesarean. Information for you.2008.http://www.rcog.org.uk/files/rcog-corp/uploaded-files/PIVaginalBirthAfterCaesarean 2008.pdf.
74. Society of Obstetricians and Gynaecologists of Canada. SOGC clinical practice guidelines. Guidelines for vaginal birth after previous caesarean birth. Number 155. February 2005. Int J Gynaecol Obstet. 2005;89:319–31.
75. Morrison JJ, Rennie JM, Milton PJ. Neonatal respiratory morbidity and mode of delivery at term: influence of timing of elective caesarean section. BJOG. 1995;102:101–6.
76. Foureur M, Ryan CL, Nicholl M, Homer C. Inconsistent evidence: analysis of six national guidelines for vaginal birth after caesarean section. Birth. 2010;37:3–10.

Part IV
Bleeding After Delivery

Chapter 11
Postpartum Hemorrhage

Rachel Pope, Iris Ohel, Gershon Holcberg, and Eyal Sheiner

Introduction

Simply put, postpartum hemorrhage (PPH) is excessive bleeding after childbirth. It is a leading cause of maternal mortality worldwide, but most of the deaths occur in low-income countries. Specifically, PPH is defined as blood loss of >500 ml after vaginal delivery or >1,000 ml after cesarean delivery. "Early" PPH occurs within 24 h after delivery, and "late" PPH occurs between 24 h and 6 weeks after delivery. In most parts of the world, PPH accounts for 35–55% of maternal deaths. In rural regions and low-income countries, where access to quick medical attendance is limited, it is a major health concern. Even in industrialized countries, what may be considered a low-risk birth can rapidly deteriorate into hypovolemic shock and death through PPH. Therefore, although it is considered a treatable obstetrical emergency, delayed treatment results in significant morbidity and mortality [1].

Clinically recognizing PPH is critical and requires skill and experience. It is usually agreed that objective evaluation and estimation of the amount of blood loss after labor is difficult, especially when bleeding is slow and continuous, or in the presence of concomitant intraabdominal bleeding or concealed bleeding, as in the case of a hematoma in the retroperitoneum. The clinical signs of blood loss (decreased blood pressure, increased heart rate) tend to appear late, when the quantity of blood loss reaches 1,500 ml, mainly due to the high blood volume of the pregnant state. Hence, practitioners generally underestimate the amount of blood loss surrounding labor and delivery. Therefore, a decreased hematocrit is considered a more precise description; a drop of 10% of the blood volume and the need for blood transfusion are considered signs of PPH.

R. Pope (✉)
Department of Obstetrics and Gynecology,
Soroka University Medical Center, Ben-Gurion University of the Negev, Beer-Sheva, Israel
e-mail: rachel.pope@gmail.com

E. Sheiner (ed.), *Bleeding During Pregnancy: A Comprehensive Guide*,
DOI 10.1007/978-1-4419-9810-1_11, © Springer Science+Business Media, LLC 2011

The literature [2–4] has documented a rise in PPH across countries of various economic levels and has spurred formal inquiries in effort to understand the cause. Research and innovations are assisting clinicians to find better ways to assess, prevent, and treat hemorrhage in the hope of reducing maternal mortality worldwide. The goal is to reach Millennium Development Goal number five, which is to reduce the maternal mortality ratio (MMR) by three-fourths by 2015 [5].

Incidence

The incidence of PPH is estimated to be 1–5% of deliveries. However as evident in a retrospective review after delivery, PPH is vaguely defined [6]. Clinicians use varying criteria, and estimating the amount of bleeding is imprecise and sometimes even not recorded, making it difficult to evaluate the incidence. Variations in the incidence of PPH are enormous because of the inconsistencies in definition and lack of reporting, especially in low-income countries [7] and rural areas where out-of-hospital deliveries, with their associated increased risk for adverse maternal outcomes, specifically hemorrhage, are more frequent [8].

To address the discrepancies in clinical estimation of blood loss, several teams have suggested improvements. Bose et al. developed tools to standardize the estimation of blood loss using pictorial algorithms; they also trained staff in simulated hemorrhage scenarios to improve the accuracy of estimated blood loss [9]. Maslovitz et al. suggested estimating blood loss periodically throughout delivery to improve accuracy [10]. The EUPHRATES group use a plastic collector bag to estimate blood loss [11]. The Modified Obstetric Early Warning Scoring System (MOEWS) is gaining popularity because it facilitates tracking the hemodynamic status from the moment a woman is admitted to the hospital [12].

The problems presented by PPH take on an epidemiological form once the significance of maternal mortality related to PPH is understood. A comprehensive summary of the magnitude and distribution of the causes of maternal deaths elucidates this relation and is critical to designing and conducting programs for treating and reducing the incidence of maternal mortality. The World Health Organization (WHO) has analyzed the causes of maternal death for this purpose [5, 13]. The American College of Obstetricians and Gynecologists estimates that 140,000 maternal deaths each year are attributable to PPH [14]. However, for developing countries without routine registration of the cause of death, measuring demographics and etiology is almost impossible. Roughly two-thirds of the world's nations do not have the means to count their populations, making epidemiological measures incalculable [15].

In the analysis done by the WHO on the causes of death, data confirmed the prominent role played by hemorrhage in maternal death in developing countries. Hemorrhage is the leading cause of maternal death in Africa and Asia, causing >30% of deaths. Hypertensive disorders represent the highest cause of maternal mortality in Latin America and the Caribbean, accounting for 25% of the total number, followed by hemorrhage with 21%. As expected, the rate of reported PPH

Table 11.1 Maternal mortality rate in various countries

Country of study	Maternal mortality rate (per 100,000 live births)	Year
Sweden [54]	2	2000
UK [20]	17	2000–2002
Israel [55]	7	2000–2007
USA [54]	11	2000
Venezuela [54]	64	2000
Nigeria [19]	454	1996–2000
Malawi [17]	1,027	1999–2000

Counting techniques vary among countries

was ranged from 1.4 to 9.6%, both across and within geographical regions. This review highlights the need for increased emphasis on programs relevant to specific settings, such as the prevention and treatment of hemorrhage antepartum and postpartum. The authors emphasized that "at the very least, most PPH deaths should be avoidable by appropriate diagnosis and management" [15].

Sadly, PPH is a much more severe public health problem in the developing world. Whereas the average overall MMR per 100,000 live births is 13 in industrialized countries and reported to be 2 in Sweden [16], MMR can be as high as 1,027 per 100,000 live births in low-resource countries, as found in a study from Malawi, East Africa [17] (Table 11.1). In the study, obstetrical hemorrhage comprised 10.6% of the total deaths and was the fourth leading cause of maternal mortality after puerperal sepsis, postabortion complications, and other infectious conditions. In similar low-resource settings, PPH has been attributed to poor management of the third stage of labor, anemia, lack of sufficient resources and access to health care and medicines, delays in transferring women to a hospital, and infectious diseases such as malaria [18].

Despite the dearth of accurate statistics, efforts are being made around the world to collect data, and as a result some figures do exist. An example from Nigeria is a 5-year (1996–2000) review of the causes of maternal mortality in a centrally located mission hospital in Benin City [19]. A total of 7,055 women gave birth during the 5-year period, with 32 maternal deaths, producing an MMR of 454 per 100,000 live births. Eclampsia (34.4%), hemorrhage (25.0%), infections (18.8%), and abortions (12.5%) were the four leading causes of death.

Women suffer complications of pregnancy even when they live in an environment of national prosperity as maternal death can occur within a short period of time due to irreversible shock. The reduced mortality rates in these developed countries is the result of specific improvements in pregnancy care, including confidential inquiries into maternal death cases. For example, in the UK there were 17 deaths from obstetric hemorrhage during 2000–2002 among almost two million births [20].

Among approximately 6,000 cases of major obstetric hemorrhage, more than 99% of cases of life-threatening bleeding were treated successfully. In any country, a reduction in maternal mortality is attained by ensuring that high-quality care is available and accessible.

Trends in Rates of PPH Over Time

There are reports of increasing rates of PPH in both high- and low-income countries. Although it may be due to increased documentation, the trends have spurred inquiry. In the USA, Callaghan and colleagues found that there has been an overall 26% increase in PPH from 1994 to 2006. The increase is primarily seen in the incidence of uterine atony. Although the age of parturients has increased during that time, cesarean sections have become more common, and risk factors such as multiple gestations, hypertension, and diabetes mellitus have increasingly compounded pregnancy, the authors were unable to explain, statistically or conclusively, the overall increase inuterine atony [21].

As an example from our institution, Soroka University Medical Center, in Beer-Sheva, Israel, we found that there has been a gradual rise in the incidence of reported PPH from all births, from 3.3% in 1988 to 9.2% in 2010 (Fig. 11.1) [22]. Soroka University Medical Center serves as a referral (and only) hospital for the entire population of the Negev region in Israel (approximately 630,000 people). The maternity ward and delivery room are active, with more than 12,000 births a year; and many of our patients are multiparous or grandmultiparous [23]. Among the total cesarean deliveries (CDs) and vaginal births, there were 0.33 and 0.55% cases of PPH, respectively. Multiple operations increase the risk for PPH. These figures imply that perhaps the rising rates of CDs resulting in repeat CDs and associated complications, such as adherent placenta, may be one of the causes for the general rise in PPH over the years. The increase in risk factors for PPH (e.g., multiple gestations) [8] might be another contributor to the gradual rise in the incidence of PPH.

A population-based study from Australia of 752,374 women giving birth during 1994–2002 was aimed at determining whether changes in risk factors for PPH over

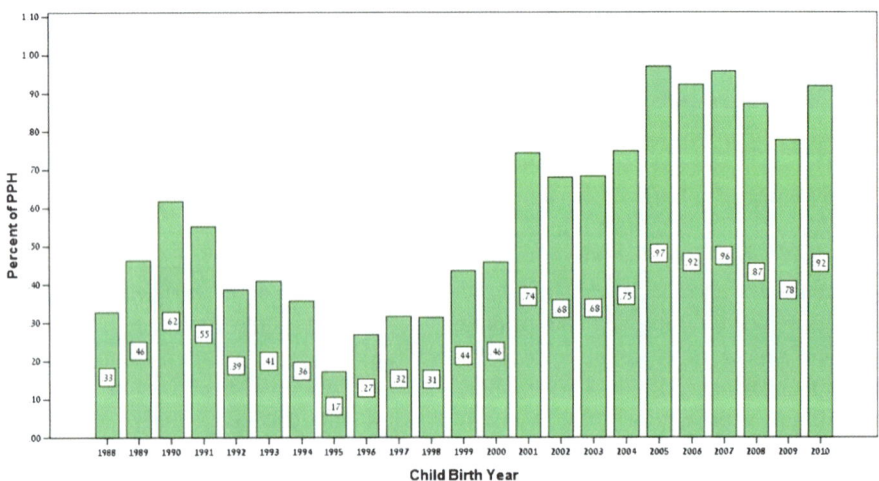

Fig. 11.1 Incidence of postpartum hemorrhage (PPH) during the years 1988–2006. Data from Soroka University Medical Center, Beer-Sheva, Israel [22]

time are associated with a rise in PPH rates [2]. In this population, there was also an increased proportion of women >35 years of age and more nulliparous and cesarean deliveries. Observed PPH rates increased from 4.7 to 6.0%. The authors concluded that this increase was not explained by the changing risk profile of the women but, rather, by a rise in the reporting of PPH. A study in Canada found an unexplained increase in the frequency, and possibly severity, of atonic PPH, leading to higher rates of hysterectomy [3].

To address such factors in high-income countries, the International Postpartum Hemorrhage Collaborative Group was formed. The Group found that the increase in the rates of PPH in the USA, Australia, and Canada was due to the presence of uterine atony. Some associated factors in their studied populations were an older maternal age at childbirth, cesarean delivery, multiple pregnancies, and a higher proportion of induced labor. The group has since called for more specific and unified coding for atonic PPH and PPH of other causes as well as the severity of PPH (the use of blood transfusions and procedures to control bleeding). They recommended further investigation in the areas of potential risk factors, including increased duration of labor, obesity, and changes in second- and third-stage management practices [24]. Similarly, Walker called for in-depth, careful investigations into national causes of maternal morbidity and mortality with the aim of developing country-specific interventions [25].

Etiologies and Risk Factors

Etiologies of and risk factors for PPH are presented in Table 11.2. It is known that any woman can experience PPH at any point without obvious risk factors; however, several etiologies have been elucidated. The leading cause of PPH is uterine atony.

Table 11.2 Predisposing factors and causes of postpartum hemorrhage, by the site of bleeding

Uterus
1. Uterine atony
   • Problems with perfusion of the uterine muscle
   • Hemorrhage resulting in hypotensive shock
   • Some anesthetics used in conduction anesthesia
   • Overdistended uterus
     – Large fetus
     – Multifetal pregnancy
     – Polyhydramnios
   • Prolonged or precipitous labor
   • Chorioamnionitis
2. Retained placental fragments or pathological adherence (e.g., placenta accreta)
3. Uterine rupture
Genital tract
Laceration of the cervix, vagina, or perineum

Note: Bleeding disorders, which may present for the first time during labor or delivery, could intensify any of the above

With this condition, upon palpation, the uterus is "boggy" and lacks its original musculature. Although idiopathic atony can occur, there are several predispositions: lack of uterine perfusion; a large, distended uterus as might be present with a multifetal gestation, polyhydramnios, or fetal macrosomia; prolonged labor; rapid forceful labor; uterine inversion; chorioamnionitis. An overstimulated uterus due to induction of labor and prolonged use of oxytocin are also risk factors for PPH [26, 27].

Other causes of PPH include retention of the placenta, which is more common in atypical placental development or cord insertion. In a Dutch population-based cohort study on PPH, the incidence and risk factors were evaluated among vaginally delivering nulliparous women [28]. Cases were divided into standard and severe PPH based on the amount of blood lost. The incidence of standard PPH ($\geq$500 ml) and severe PPH ($\geq$1,000 ml) were 19.0% and 4.2%, respectively. The most important risk factors for standard and severe PPH were related to a prolonged third stage of labor ($\geq$30 min) and retained placenta, which occurred in 1.8%. High birth weight and perineal damage were also independent, significant risk factors. These data show higher values than those in other studies in the literature. Naturally formed and iatrogenic genital lacerations of the cervix, vagina, or perineum also can lead to PPH. Therefore, avoiding unnecessary episiotomy could reduce morbidity. Obviously, an underlying bleeding disorder could increase the risk of any of the aforementioned situations, especially if it is undiagnosed at the time of delivery.

Parity is also thought to influence the risk of PPH. Primiparity is associated with increased risk [6]. Although once thought as a risk factor, grand multiparity has been questioned [29]. Other attributed risks of PPH include Asian and Hispanic races, and medications such as halogenated anesthetic agents [27].

Caution Box

Women who have experienced postpartum hemorrhage during a previous delivery are at increased risk of recurrence.

Recurrent PPH

Women who have survived PPH are at greater risk of PPH during subsequent deliveries. This finding was supported by a study examining the risk of recurrence of PPH as determined by following the records of pregnancies from 1994 through 2002 [30]. Among 125,295 women with consecutive pregnancies, the rate of PPH during their first pregnancy was 5.8%. Risk of recurrent PPH was 3.3 times greater than for women without a history of PPH [relative risk (RR) 3.3; 95% confidence interval (CI) 3.1–3.5] and for women who experienced prior PPH twice it was even higher (RR 5.0, 95% CI 3.8–6.5). Furthermore, the risk of PPH during the third pregnancy rose from 4.4% when there was no PPH during the first two pregnancies to 10.2% when there was PPH during the first pregnancy but not in the second, 14.3% when the PPH event occurred during the second delivery only, and 21.7% for women who had experienced prior PPH twice.

The study showed that the risk of a first PPH during any pregnancy was 1:20 (risk of about 5%), and the risk of recurrent PPH increased to 1:7 for a second pregnancy and 1:5 for a third. As suspected in other studies, the increased risk of recurrence was also evident when the mode of delivery was taken into account. Medical staff should be prepared to act immediately and use measures of prevention and quick management in the face of recurrent PPH.

A population-based study of risk factors for early PPH at our institution included 154,311 women with singleton gestations [26]. Early PPH complicated 0.43% of all singleton deliveries included in this study and highlighted several risk factors. Independent risk factors for early PPH using multivariate analysis included retained placenta [odds ratio (OR) 3.5, 95% CI 2.1–5.8], failure to progress during the second stage of labor (OR 3.4, 95% CI 2.4–4.7), placenta accreta (OR 3.3, 95% CI 1.7–6.4), perineal lacerations (OR 2.4, 95% CI 2.0–2.8), instrumental delivery (OR 2.3, 95% CI 1.6–3.4), large for gestational age (LGA) newborn (OR 1.9, 95% CI 1.6–2.4), hypertensive disorder (OR 1.7, 95% CI 1.2–2.1), induction of labor (OR 1.4, 95% CI 1.1–1.7), and augmentation of labor with oxytocin (OR 1.4, 95% CI 1.2–1.7).

Caution Box

More women *without* risk factors have atonic PPH compared to those with risk factors. To prevent uterine atony, the leading cause of PPH, interventions should be targeted at all women during childbirth [1].

To examine the severity of PPH, women were than assigned to one of three groups. Those in Group 1 did not require revision of the birth canal or a blood transfusion (n=137), women in Group 2 required uterine revision (n=330), and those in Group 3 required a blood transfusion due to significant bleeding and/or both uterine revision and a blood transfusion (n=199) (Fig. 11.2). A statistically significant linear association was found between the severity of bleeding and the following factors: vacuum extraction ($P < 0.001$), oxytocin augmentation ($P < 0.001$), hypertensive disorders ($P < 0.001$), uterine rupture ($P < 0.001$), peripartum hysterectomy ($P < 0.001$), and uterine or internal iliac artery ligation ($P < 0.001$). Most of these cases of PPH occur at term: at 37–42 weeks' gestation, with a peak at 40 weeks.

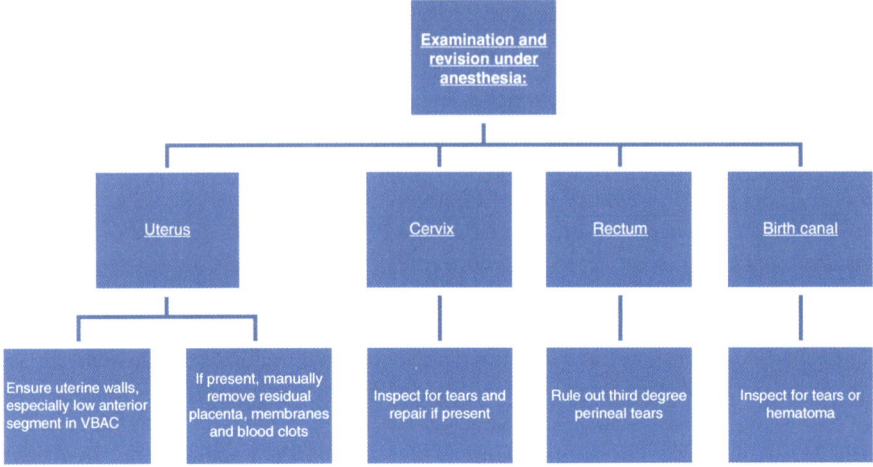

Fig. 11.2 Examination algorithm. *VBAC* vaginal birth after cesarean section

Treatment

Throughout the world, interventions are taking place to train medical personnel to manage PPH emergently. Before treatment, however, is the prevention of a disease state. Today, the active management of labor and routine prophylactic administration of uterotonic drugs to reduce the risk of PPH has become an integral part of the management of labor and delivery [31]. Active management of labor includes, especially in this context, active management of the third stage of labor, which is the period of time starting after the delivery of the baby and ending after delivery of the placenta. The incidence of PPH >500 ml is estimated to be only 5% when active management of the third stage of labor is implemented compared to 13% when it is not [31].

At this phase, the most important mechanism for reducing blood loss from the placental site and thus avoiding uterine atony is vasoconstriction of blood vessels produced by the firm and steady contraction of the uterine myometrium. Drugs used during this stage stimulate uterine contractions and enhance vasoconstriction. If given immediately after delivery of the baby, they also enhance placental detachment. These drugs, which are considered first line, are "uterotonic." They include oxytocin, ergometrine, or a regimen of the two (Table 11.3). Other options are oxytocin agonists and misoprostol (discussed later). The timing of administration of the drug is varied, depending on the institution. Some prefer administering them immediately after birth of the fetal shoulders and others only after the placenta is delivered. Other measures of active management of the third stage of labor include clamping the umbilical cord, exercising controlled cord traction, and guiding the parturient to bear down. (Recent debate concerning the timing of cord clamping has resulted in discouragement of immediate clamping).

An intervention to improve obstetrical care, demonstrating the difficulties of these interventions and their rewards, has been published [32]. A total of 19 hospitals in

Table 11.3 Medications used during the third stage of labor

- Oxytocin: 10–40 U IV saline or 10 U IM
- Ergometrine: 500 µg IM; often used in combination with oxytocin as syntometrine. Caution with patients with sepsis or Raynaud's disease
- Methergine/methylergonervine: 0.2 mg IM every 2–4 h if not hypertensive, Raynaud's phenomenon, or scleroderma. Repeat every 2–4 h if good response
- Carboprost tromethamine: 15-methyl-prostaglandin $F_2\alpha$ 250 µg IM every 15–90 min until 2 mg if no history of asthma
- Misoprostol (Cytotec, prostaglandin E_1): 800–1,000 µg rectally. Less effective than oxytocin at preventing PPH, but it can be administered to women with asthma and does not require refrigeration – therefore may be more practical for low-income areas [35]

Argentina and Uruguay were randomized to be introduced to an intervention aimed at developing guidelines for managing the third stage of labor and carrying them out or not to participate in the intervention (the controls). Primary outcomes were the rates of prophylactic use of oxytocin during the third stage of labor. The main secondary outcome was the rate of PPH. The use of prophylactic oxytocin increased from 2.1% at baseline to 83.6% after the end of the intervention at the participating hospitals compared to a rise from 2.6 to 12.3% at the control hospitals ($P = 0.01$ for the difference in changes). There was also an associated reduction in the incidence of PPH of ≥500 ml [relative rate reduction (RRR) 45%, 95% CI 9–71] and for ≥1,000 ml (RRR 70%, 95% CI 16–78).

Once PPH is diagnosed, the situation should be considered an emergency that requires the coordinated functioning of multidisciplinary practitioners: an obstetrician, midwife, anesthesiologist, hematologist, and laboratory team with functioning blood bank services. The treatment is a dynamic one built on basic actions to treat and simultaneously identify the cause of bleeding, provide treatment, prevent deterioration, and facilitate life support and invasive procedures as necessary (Fig. 11.3).

Medical Treatment

Fluid Resuscitation

Fluid resuscitation should not be delayed, as this simple medical intervention can stabilize the situation promptly. Intravascular normal saline or lactated Ringer's solution is recommended (dextrose solutions can lead to peripheral edema). The Cochrane Review indicates that crystalloids had better outcomes than colloids [33]. If blood loss continues or is >2,000 ml, blood transfusion is necessary.

Uterotonics

Much debate surrounds the merit of any medical treatment over oxytocin for managing PPH. The WHO recommends that active management of the third stage of

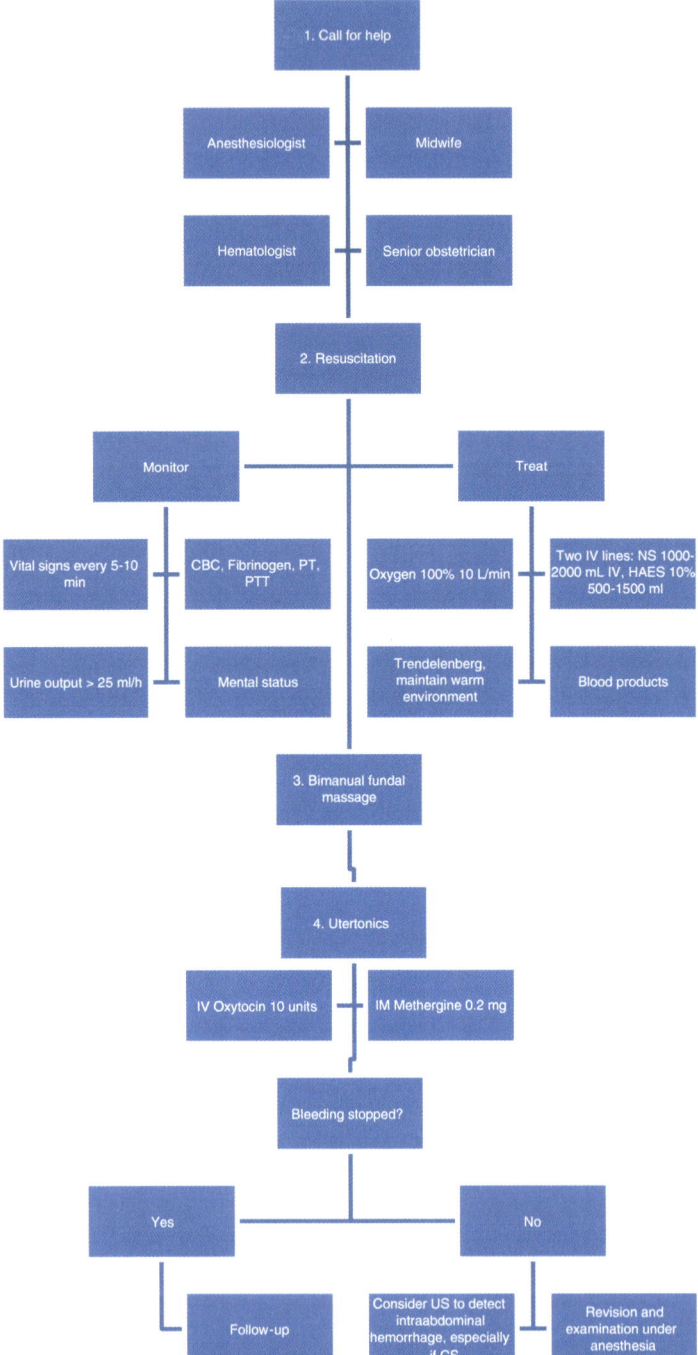

Fig. 11.3 Postpartum hemorrhage: diagnosis to treatment algorithm. *CBC* complete blood count, *PT* prothrombin time, *PTT* partial thromboplastin time, *NS* normal saline, *CS* cesarean section

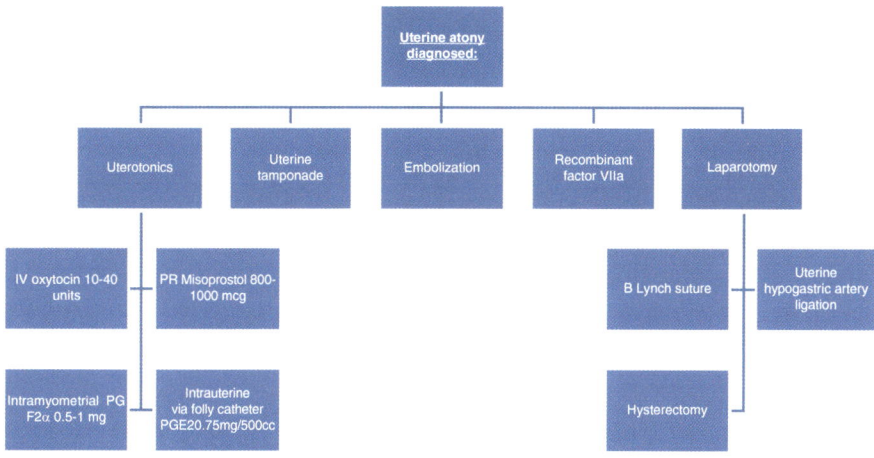

Fig. 11.4   Uterine atony. *IV* intravenous, *PGF2α* prostaglandin $F_{2α}$, *PR* per rectum

labor be offered to all women delivered by skilled birth attendants to prevent PPH, including administering 10 IU oxytocin, clamping and cutting the cord around 3 min after birth, and delivering the placenta by controlled cord traction. In settings where it is not possible to use oxytocin or ergometrine, the WHO recommends the use of misoprostol 600 μg orally immediately after the birth of the baby by trained health workers. They specify that health workers who administer misoprostol must be trained in its correct use after birth of the baby, avoiding its administration before birth or at incorrect doses, and in identifying and managing its side effects [34]. If an oxytocin infusion is already being maintained, the dosage may be increased. Thereafter, it is common to administer methylergonovine followed by carboprost tromethamine 15 min later [34]. Implementing uterotonics early is helpful as atony is the most common cause of PPH (Fig. 11.4).

Misoprostol (Prostaglandin E₁)

Evidence supporting the use of misoprostol (prostaglandin E_1, PGE_1) is unclear. It has been shown to be less effective than oxytocin for preventing PPH. However, it does not require refrigeration and therefore may be more practical for use in low-income areas [35].

A thorough review of PPH treatment was done for the Cochrane Library (2007) that included all randomized controlled trials (RCTs) dealing with the treatment of primary PPH. The review identified only three trials that met all the requirements [6]. These three trials examined the place of misoprostol in the management of primary PPH in a total of 462 women. In one trial examining misoprostol vs. oxytocin/ergometrine, the use of misoprostol was noted to be superior to oxytocin/ergometrine regarding the subjective cessation of hemorrhage within 20 min, and there was a significant reduction in the number of women who required additional uterotonics.

The two other trials had a different design; they examined misoprostol vs. placebo after failure of first-line treatment with oxytocin/ergometrine. Misoprostol use was associated with a significant reduction in blood loss of ≥500 ml; however, the additional use of uterotonics, blood transfusion, and evacuation of retained products did not differ between the two groups. The number of subjects was too small, though, to evaluate the effect on maternal mortality. Therefore, at present there are insufficient data to draw any conclusions about the effectiveness and safety for either first- or second-line therapy with misoprostol in the setting of primary PPH.

Nevertheless, the importance of misoprostol is now beyond clinical trials. Having shown that it does work to control excessive bleeding after delivery, its impact is enormous and could save thousands of lives in areas in the world where there is no option of administering injectable uterotonics because they are not available or manageable. Misoprostol tablets are administered either by mouth or rectally and are stable in extreme climates. A Cochrane review included 46 trials involving 42,621 women after delivery; among them, 37 trials evaluated misoprostol use [36]. Most trials were conducted in hospital settings where deliveries are performed by skilled caregivers, but still the results are encouraging for implementing strategies that make use of misoprostol as a modality to prevent PPH in remote areas where out-of-hospital deliveries are the rule. Trials comparing misoprostol with other uterotonics are designed to evaluate whether misoprostol is as effective as the gold standard drugs, given its advantage of an oral or rectal route of administration.

Recombinant Activated Factor VIIa

A recent advance in the treatment of bleeding disorders is the introduction of recombinant activated factor VIIa (rFVIIa). rFVIIa was initially approved in 1998 for surgery prophylaxis or to treat bleeding in patients with hemophilia who have acquired antibodies to factors VIII or IX, in Glanzmann thrombasthenia, and patients with factor VII deficiency. The drug's "off-label" use was first reported for trauma and surgical life-threatening hemorrhage. The rationale was that no matter what the cause of bleeding is, the clotting system should be maintained and kept from compromise. Recombinant activated factor VII initiates coagulation when tissue factor (TF) has been exposed at the site of injury. They comprise a complex that activates factor X and subsequently converts prothrombin into thrombin. This restriction to the local site of damage makes the use of the drug specific.

At this stage, mainly only case descriptions have been published of the use of rFVIIa for PPH, with guidelines based on specialist opinions and local experience [37]. There are currently no RCTs. The drug was reported in some case series to save lives – as well as a last resort to save fertility before hysterectomy. The two major concerns with its use are life-threatening thromboembolism in obstetrical patients known to be already in a hypercoagulable state and its cost [38]. Thus, improvements in conventional and surgical management are necessary before introducing routine use of rFVIIa [39].

Surgical Treatment

Examination and Revision Under Anesthesia

One must always consider examination and surgical revision under anesthesia in the following cases: (1) PPH is not responding to the first steps of resuscitation; or (2) the uterus remains atonic or contracts in response to massage but becomes atonic again immediately when not held contracted. Revision must also be considered when, after routine inspection of the placenta, it is suspected that placental tissue or membranes remain in the uterus. Commonly, retained placenta is not obvious on ultrasonography, although trained personnel can identify the echogenic mass as the cause for hemorrhage. The decision is usually clinical.

Embolization

If there is medical capacity for embolization and the woman is otherwise stable, arterial embolization is a promising solution. For women with placenta accreta, a study has shown that prophylactic embolization of the pelvic artery can prevent the need for hysterectomy [40]. This is especially significant for women who wish to preserve their fertility.

B-Lynch

When other methods fail, the B-lynch technique may be effective in providing adequate tension to the uterus [41]. A suture is applied in two longitudinal segments of the uterus via a loop, which conveys enough compression to cause bleeding cessation [42]. Modifications to this technique have been developed over the years and have proved effective [43, 44]. Unfortunately, complications such as uterine necrosis and erosion have been documented [42], and several individuals have expressed concern over the lack of evidence of long-term effects on fertility [45].

Ligation

The uterine arteries supply most of the vascular supply to the uterus. Therefore, when PPH is not resolved with medication and other less invasive procedures, ligation of the uterine arteries or internal iliac arteries, may prove necessary and effective [46]. By interrupting the blood flow to the broad ligament, pulse pressure is decreased in the distal artery. Blanching is noted, and the hemorrhage is controlled. Ovarian artery ligation is also an option [46]. PPH after a cesarean section also has been shown to be resolvable in 95% of cases with artery ligation [47].

Table 11.4 Balloon tamponade

Type of balloon	Notes
Bakri tamponade	Silicone balloon, 500 ml saline
BT-Cath	Silicone with two lumens: one to infuse saline and the other to drain blood
Segstaken-Blakemore tube	Tamponade and drain
Foley catheter (no. 24)	30-ml balloon inflated with 60–80 ml
Condom catheter	
Rusch	

With severe cases of PPH in which hemorrhage persists after a hysterectomy that was the first surgical step, internal iliac artery ligation may be done [48], although it is difficult to perform.

Other Modalities

Balloon tamponade is another, less invasive approach that is both quick and effective (Table 11.4). It was recommended as the first step in a large systematic review [49]. Several variations of balloons have been designed and may be used in combination with other treatments generally conferring low risk.

The patient's vital signs and response to resuscitation should be closely monitored. If in place, the Modified Obstetric Early Warning Scoring System (MOEWS) could help follow the hemodynamic status [12]. Treatment of the underlying cause of PPH is clearly the best way to resolve the situation. Therefore, surgical intervention such as laparotomy, arterial ligation (uterine, ovarian, or internal iliac artery), arterial embolization, or hysterectomy may become necessary. Arterial embolization is an important option for preserving fertility and in case of a hematoma; however, not all facilities are able to provide the equipment and staff for emergency availability. A hysterectomy may be inevitable if these measures fail to achieve hemostasis.

Innovations

PPH is rarely foreseeable; therefore, several new innovations for dealing with obstetrical emergencies, especially in low-income countries, are being developed. The Program for Appropriate Technology in Health (PATH) has created a sterile, prefilled injection of oxytocin, known as Uniject. This user-friendly, convenient injection has been tested by village midwives in Indonesia and Angola, with positive clinician reviews [50, 51]. Another community-based innovation is a noninflatable antishock garment (NI-ASG). Composed of neoprene, the garment can apply 30–50 mmHg of pressure to the lower body to facilitate hemostasis during hypovolemic shock. This device not only provides rapidity and ease of use, it extends the period of stabilization while awaiting blood transfusion, another problematic element of coping with PPH. Although only modest studies have been conducted, it is possible that injecting a saline solution containing oxytocin or prostaglandin may reduce the need for manual removal of the retained placenta [52]. Lastly, the balloon condom catheter, modeled after hydrostatic balloon catheters, offers a potentially inexpensive and improvised way to reduce blood loss when the original models are not affordable. More research is necessary to prove the safety and efficacy of these innovations, and more low-cost innovations are needed for low-income communities [53].

Summary

PPH is a treatable emergency with profound consequences. In many parts of the world, it accounts for up to 55% of the total maternal deaths, which presents a major health problem. Clinicians use different definitions of PPH, and estimates of the amount of bleeding are often imprecise or missing, making variations in the incidence of PPH enormous. In the presence of PPH, maternal death can occur within a short time due to irreversible shock [54, 55].

Active management of labor, especially the third stage of labor, and routine prophylactic administration of uterotonic drugs to reduce the risk of PPH have become an integral part of the management of labor and delivery. Treatment once PPH is diagnosed as an emergency requires coordinated functioning of multidisciplinary practitioners – midwife, obstetrician, anesthesiologist, hematologist, and laboratory team including blood bank services. The treatment progresses in steps, from basic actions to treat the problem and simultaneously identify the cause of bleeding, prevent deterioration, and provide life support and invasive procedures as necessary. The importance of misoprostol is now beyond clinical trials. As a simply administered drug that has been shown to control excessive bleeding after delivery, it could save thousands of lives in areas where there is no option for advanced treatment. Implementation of these strategies is part of the United Nations' Millennium Development Goals to reduce the maternal mortality rate by 75% by 2015.

References

1. Mathai M, Gülmezoglu A, Hill S. WHO Department of Making Pregnancy Safer. Recommendations for the prevention of postpartum hemorrhage. 2007. WHO/MPS/07.06.
2. Ford J, Roberts C, Simpson J, Vaughan J, Cameron C. Increased postpartum hemorrhage rates in Australia. Int J Gynaecol Obstet. 2007;98(3):237–43.
3. Joseph K, Rouleau J, Kramer M, et al. Investigation of an increase in postpartum haemorrhage in Canada. BJOG. 2007;114(6):751–9.
4. Schutte J, Steegers E, Schuitemaker N, et al. Rise in maternal mortality in the Netherlands. BJOG. 2010;117(4):399–406.
5. World Health Organization. Health and the millennium development goals. Geneva: World Health Organization; 2005.

6. Mousa H, Alfirevic Z. Treatment for primary postpartum haemorrhage. Cochrane Database Syst Rev. 2007;(1):CD003249.
7. Carroli G, Cuesta C, Abalos E, Gulmezoglu A. Epidemiology of postpartum haemorrhage: a systematic review. Best Pract Res Clin Obstet Gynaecol. 2008;22(6):999–1012.
8. Sheiner E, Ohel I, Hadar A. Out of hospital deliveries and post partum hemorrhage. In: Lynch CB, Keith L, Lalonde A, Karoshi M, editors. A textbook of post-partum hemorrhage. Dumfries, Scotland: Sapiens Publishing; 2006.
9. Bose P, Regan F, Paterson-Brown S. Improving the accuracy of estimated blood loss at obstetric haemorrhage using clinical reconstructions. BJOG. 2006;113(8):919–24.
10. Maslovitz S, Barkai G, Lessing J, Ziv A, Many A. Improved accuracy of postpartum blood loss estimation as assessed by simulation. Acta Obstet Gynecol Scand. 2008;87(9):929–34.
11. Zhang W, Deneux-Tharaux C, Brocklehurst P, et al. Effect of a collector bag for measurement of postpartum blood loss after vaginal delivery: cluster randomised trial in 13 European countries. BMJ. 2010;340:c293.
12. Smith G, Prytherch D, Schmidt P, et al. Hospital-wide physiological surveillance – a new approach to the early identification and management of the sick patient. Resuscitation. 2006;71(1):19–28.
13. Khan K, Wojdyla D, Say L, Gülmezoglu A, Van Look P. WHO analysis of causes of maternal death: a systematic review. Lancet. 2006;367(9516):1066–74.
14. American College of Obstetricians and Gynecologists. ACOG Practice Bulletin: Clinical Management Guidelines for Obstetrician-Gynecologists Number 76, October 2006: postpartum hemorrhage. Obstet Gynecol. 2006;108(4):1039–47.
15. Hill K. Making deaths count. Bull World Health Organ. 2006;84(3):162.
16. Drife J. Maternal mortality in well-resourced countries: is there still a need for confidential enquiries? Best Pract Res Clin Obstet Gynaecol. 2008;22(3):501–15.
17. Lema V, Changole J, Kanyighe C, Malunga E. Maternal mortality at the Queen Elizabeth Central Teaching Hospital, Blantyre, Malawi. East Afr Med J. 2005;82(1):3–9.
18. Soltani H. Uterine massage for preventing postpartum hemorrhage: RHL commentary. Geneva: The WHO Reproductive Health Library; last updated April 2010.
19. Onakewhor J, Gharoro E. Changing trends in maternal mortality in a developing country. Niger J Clin Pract. 2008;11(2):111–20.
20. Lewis G. Why mothers die 2000–2002: the sixth report of the confidential enquiries into maternal deaths in the United Kingdom. London: RCOG; 2004.
21. Callaghan W, Kuklina E, Berg C. Trends in postpartum hemorrhage: United States, 1994–2006. Am J Obstet Gynecol. 2010;202(4):353.e1–6.
22. Ohel I, Holcberg G, Sheiner E. Epidemiology of post-partum hemorrhage. In: Sheiner E, editor. Textbook of Perinatal Epidemiology. Nova Science Publishers; 2010.
23. Shechter Y, Levy A, Wiznitzer A, Zlotnik A, Sheiner E. Obstetric complications in grand and great grand multiparous women. J Matern Fetal Neonatal Med. 2010;23(10):1211–7.
24. Knight M, Callaghan W, Berg C, Alexander S, Bouvier-Colle M, Ford J, Joseph KS, Lewis G, Liston R, Roberts C, Oats J, and Walker J. Trends in postpartum hemorrhage in high resource countries: a review and recommendations from the International Postpartum Hemorrhage Collaborative Group. BMC Pregnancy Childbirth. 2009;9(1):55.
25. Walker J. Confidential enquiries into maternal mortality. BJOG. 2010;117(4):379–81.
26. Sheiner E, Sarid L, Levy A, Seidman D, Hallak M. Obstetric risk factors and outcome of pregnancies complicated with early postpartum hemorrhage: a population-based study. J Matern Fetal Neonatal Med. 2005;18(3):149–54.
27. Combs C, Murphy E, Laros RJ. Factors associated with postpartum hemorrhage with vaginal birth. Obstet Gynecol. 1991;77(1):69–76.
28. Bais J, Eskes M, Pel M, Bonsel G, Bleker O. Postpartum haemorrhage in nulliparous women: incidence and risk factors in low and high risk women. A Dutch population-based cohort study on standard (> or = 500 ml) and severe (> or = 1000 ml) postpartum haemorrhage. Eur J Obstet Gynecol Reprod Biol. 2004;115(2):166–72.
29. Stones R, Paterson C, Saunders N. Risk factors for major obstetric haemorrhage. Eur J Obstet Gynecol Reprod Biol. 1993;48(1):15–8.

30. Ford J, Roberts C, Bell J, Algert C, Morris J. Postpartum haemorrhage occurrence and recurrence: a population-based study. Med J Aust. 2007;187(7):391–3.
31. Prendiville WJ, Elbourne D, McDonald S. Active versus expectant management in the third stage of labour. Cochrane Database Syst Rev. 2000;(3):CD000007.
32. Althabe F, Buekens P, Bergel E, et al. A behavioral intervention to improve obstetrical care. N Engl J Med. 2008;358(18):1929–40.
33. Roberts I, Alderson P, Bunn F, Chinnock P, Ker K, Schierhout G. Colloids versus crystalloids for fluid resuscitation in critically ill patients. Cochrane Database Syst Rev. 2004;(4):CD000567.
34. World Health Organization DoRHaR, Department of Making Pregnancy Safer, Department of Essential Medicines and Pharmaceutical Policy. WHO Statement regarding the use of misoprostol for postpartum hemorrhage prevention and treatment. 2009.
35. Kundodyiwa T, Majoko F, Rusakaniko S. Misoprostol versus oxytocin in the third stage of labor. Int J Gynaecol Obstet. 2001;75(3):235–41.
36. Gülmezoglu A, Forna F, Villar J, Hofmeyr G. Prostaglandins for preventing postpartum haemorrhage. Cochrane Database Syst Rev. The Cochrane Library. 2007;(4):CD000494.
37. Alfirevic Z, Elbourne D, Pavord S, et al. Use of recombinant activated factor VII in primary postpartum hemorrhage: the Northern European registry 2000–2004. Obstet Gynecol. 2007;110(6):1270–8.
38. Welsh A, McLintock C, Gatt S, Somerset D, Popham P, Ogle R. Guidelines for the use of recombinant activated factor VII in massive obstetric haemorrhage. Aust N Z J Obstet Gynaecol. 2008;48(1):12–6.
39. Ahonen J, Jokela R, Korttila K. An open non-randomized study of recombinant activated factor VII in major postpartum haemorrhage. Acta Anaesthesiol Scand. 2007;51(7):929–36.
40. Sivan E, Spira M, Achiron R, et al. Prophylactic pelvic artery catheterization and embolization in women with placenta accreta: can it prevent cesarean hysterectomy? Am J Perinatol. 2010;27(6):455–61.
41. Elhassan E, Mirghani O, Adam I. The B-Lynch surgical technique for control of postpartum haemorrhage. J Obstet Gynaecol. 2010;30(1):94.
42. El-Hamamy E, Wright A, B-Lynch C. The B-Lynch suture technique for postpartum haemorrhage: a decade of experience and outcome. J Obstet Gynaecol. 2009;29(4):278–83.
43. Cho J, Jun H, Lee C. Hemostatic suturing technique for uterine bleeding during cesarean delivery. Obstet Gynecol. 2000;96(1):129–31.
44. Hayman R, Arulkumaran S, Steer P. Uterine compression sutures: surgical management of postpartum hemorrhage. Obstet Gynecol. 2002;99(3):502–6.
45. Sentilhes L, Descamps P, Marpeau L. Has B-Lynch suture hidden long-term effects? Fertil Steril. 2010;94(4):e62.
46. AbdRabbo S. Stepwise uterine devascularization: a novel technique for management of uncontrolled postpartum hemorrhage with preservation of the uterus. Am J Obstet Gynecol. 1994;171(3):694–700.
47. O'Leary J. Uterine artery ligation in the control of postcesarean hemorrhage. J Reprod Med. 1995;40(3):189–93.
48. Camuzcuoglu H, Toy H, Vural M, Yildiz F, Aydin H. Internal iliac artery ligation for severe postpartum hemorrhage and severe hemorrhage after postpartum hysterectomy. J Obstet Gynaecol Res. 2010;36(3):538–43.
49. Doumouchtsis S, Papageorghiou A, Arulkumaran S. Systematic review of conservative management of postpartum hemorrhage: what to do when medical treatment fails. Obstet Gynecol Surv. 2007;62(8):540–7.
50. Tsu V, Sutanto A, Vaidya K, Coffey P, Widjaya A. Oxytocin in prefilled Uniject injection devices for managing third-stage labor in Indonesia. Int J Gynaecol Obstet. 2003;83(1):103–11.
51. Strand R, Da Silva F, Jangsten E, Bergström S. Postpartum hemorrhage: a prospective, comparative study in Angola using a new disposable device for oxytocin administration. Acta Obstet Gynecol Scand. 2005;84(3):260–5.
52. Carroli G, Belizan J, Grant A, Gonzalez L, Campodonico L, Bergel E. Intra-umbilical vein injection and retained placenta: evidence from a collaborative large randomised controlled

trial. Grupo Argentino de Estudio de Placenta Retenida. Br J Obstet Gynaecol. 1998;105(2): 179–85.

53. Akther S. Innovations in the treatment of PPH. Proceedings of preventing postpartum hemorrhage: from research to practice. Bangkok, Thailand; 2004.

54. AbouZahr C, Wardlaw T. Maternal mortality in 2000: estimates developed by WHO, UNICEF and UNFPA. Geneva: World Health Organization Department of Reproductive Health and Research; 2004.

55. Schneid-Kofman N, Sheiner E. Frustration from not achieving the expected reduction in maternal mortality. Arch Gynecol Obstet. 2008;277(4):283–4.

Part V
Coagulopathy and Intensive Care

Chapter 12
Coagulopathy and Pregnancy

Scott Dunkley

Introduction

Women may have disordered hemostasis associated with pregnancy due to an underlying congenital bleeding disorder or to acquired thrombocytopenia or coagulopathy arising from problems in the pregnancy itself. Bleeding associated with these disorders remains an important cause of maternal death worldwide [1].

Pregnancy-Associated Thrombocytopenia

A physiological decrease in platelet count of approximately 10% is typically seen by the end of the third trimester. Thrombocytopenia is common, affecting up to 10% of all pregnancies [2]. Thrombocytopenia during pregnancy may be secondary to a variety of situations (Table 12.1).

Common Thrombocytopenias

Congenital thrombocytopenia is uncommon, but the patient may be aware of a preexisting personal or family history. Some rare congenital thrombocytopenias are associated with platelet dysfunction and so have a more severe bleeding phenotype [3]. It should be remembered that acquired platelet dysfunction is common and may be seen in the presence of a normal platelet count. Common causes include

S. Dunkley (✉)
Institute of Haematology, Royal Prince Alfred Hospital,
Sydney, NSW, Australia
e-mail: Scott.Dunkley@sswahs.nsw.gov.au

E. Sheiner (ed.), *Bleeding During Pregnancy: A Comprehensive Guide*, 199
DOI 10.1007/978-1-4419-9810-1_12, © Springer Science+Business Media, LLC 2011

Table 12.1 Causes of thrombocytopenia in pregnancy

Isolated thrombocytopenia
  Gestational
  Idiopathic thrombocytopenia (ITP)
  Congenital
  Drug-induced
  Viral
Thrombocytopenia associated with other laboratory abnormalities or systemic disease
  Pregnancy related
    Preeclampsia
    HELLP (hemolysis, elevated liver function tests, low platelet syndrome)
    Acute fatty liver
    Thrombotic thrombocytopenic purpura/hemolytic uremic syndrome (TTP/HUS)
    Disseminated intravascular coagulopathy (DIC)
  Not pregnancy specific
    Vitamin B_{12}/folate deficiency
    Bone marrow dysfunction (primary or secondary)
    Hypersplenism

the consumption of aspirin, nonsteroidal antiinflammatory drugs (NSAIDs), and some herbal preparations.

Gestational, or incidental, thrombocytopenia is the most common form of thrombocytopenia during pregnancy (>75% of cases), affecting more than 5% of pregnant women [4]. It is generally benign, not leading to an increased risk of bleeding. Most patients with gestational thrombocytopenia have platelet counts $>100 \times 10^9$/L. Generally there are no features of preeclampsia and no associated liver function test abnormalities, coagulopathy, or another cytopenia. No specific therapy is required.

Immune thrombocytopenic purpura (ITP), is the most common cause of significant thrombocytopenia during pregnancy, occurring in 1 in 1,000 pregnancies and accounting for 5% of thrombocytopenia in pregnant women [5]. It can occur during early pregnancy, often with platelet counts of $<50 \times 10^9$/L; otherwise, it may be difficult to distinguish from gestational thrombocytopenia. Specific laboratory investigations, such as platelet-associated immunoglobulin G (IgG), are unhelpful owing to the poor specificity of these tests. Some patients have an associated autoimmune disorder such as systemic lupus erythematosus (SLE) or antiphospholipid syndrome. A response to steroids or intravenous immunoglobulin (IVIG) secures the diagnosis.

Often the mother with ITP does not require therapy during the pregnancy. However, if the platelet count is $<20-30 \times 10^9$/L, steroid therapy (prednisone, initially 1 mg/kg/day) is often effective and safe (except for an elevated risk of gestational diabetes). Women who are not responsive to steroids or in whom steroids are contraindicated, can be treated with IVIG (typically 0.4 g/kg/day for 3–5 consecutive days). Rh(D)-positive patients can be given intravenous anti-D (available in Europe and North America) [2, 5]. Platelet transfusion is typically not helpful due to short half-life of transfused platelets in the presence of active anti-platelet antibodies. Nevertheless, platelet transfusion is indicated in patients with inadequate platelet counts at the time of delivery or bleeding.

It is generally accepted that a platelet count $>50 \times 10^9/L$ is safe for normal vaginal delivery and a count $>80 \times 10^9/L$ for cesarean section with epidural anesthesia [2, 5, 6]. If this platelet count cannot be achieved prior to cesarean section, epidural anesthetic should not be risked and the operation is performed under general anesthesia.

Despite the fact that platelet autoantibodies can cross the placenta in maternal ITP, fewer than 5% of babies have platelet counts $<20 \times 10^9/L$ and require treatment [5]. Nonetheless, the platelet counts of neonates should be determined and monitored. Maternal ITP is not an indication for cesarean section unless there is a history of a prior child with severe ITP [2, 4, 5]. Some patients require planned induction of labor.

Other Causes of Thrombocytopenia

In addition to the thrombocytopenias already reviewed, there are many other serious causes for thrombocytopenia during pregnancy, including preeclampsia, HELLP (hemolysis, elevated liver enzymes, low platelets) syndrome, thrombotic thrombocytopenic purpura (TTP), hemolytic uremic syndrome (HUS), disseminated intravascular coagulation (DIC), drugs, infections, and bone marrow infiltration. The presence of hemolysis or fragmented red cells on the blood film [microangiopathic hemolytic anemia (MAHA)], renal impairment, abnormal liver function tests, coagulopathy, or hypertension should prompt urgent investigation for other causes of thrombocytopenia. Clinical and laboratory features help distinguish these conditions (Table 12.2).

Up to 50% of women with preeclampsia develop a degree of thrombocytopenia, but often it is minimal and proportional to the severity of the underlying disease [7]. Coagulation studies are generally normal, although DIC can develop with severe preeclampsia.

The *HELLP syndrome* is associated with severe preeclampsia. It is characterized by MAHA, elevated liver enzymes [aspartate aminotransferase (AST)>70 U/L], and thrombocytopenia $<100 \times 10^9/L$. Abnormal coagulation studies and evidence of DIC are often present, although the degree of thrombocytopenia is more profound [7, 8]. Conversely, the coagulopathy associated with *acute fatty liver of pregnancy (AFLP)* is more severe than the thrombocytopenia and MAHA typically seen with HELLP. DIC is very common with AFLP [7].

Prompt delivery is the most important therapeutic modality in the presence of severe preeclampsia, HELLP, or AFLP, although reversal of the coagulopathy may be delayed in those with AFLP. Platelets should be transfused to elevate the platelet count $>50 \times 10^9/L$ and the coagulopathy corrected by transfusing fresh frozen plasma (FFP) and fibrinogen-containing concentrates.

TTP and HUS represent a clinical spectrum of the same disorder where deficiency (congenital or autoantibody/acquired) of the von Willebrand factor (VWF)-cleaving protease called ADAMTS13 (*a d*isintegrin *a*nd *m*etalloprotease with *t*hrombospondin family) allows VWF and platelets to accumulate unchecked in microvascular thrombi, which leads to platelet consumption, hemolysis, and microvascular occlusion with associated organ damage [9]. TTP is characterized

Table 12.2 Clinical and laboratory features of conditions associated with thrombocytopenia during pregnancy

Condition	Thrombocytopenia	Timing	Coagulopathy	Low fibrinogen	MAHA	Liver dysfunction	Renal	Specific therapy
Gestation	+	Third TM	−	−	−	−	−	−
ITP	+ to +++	Anytime	−	−	−	−	−	Steroids IVIG
Preeclampsia	+	Third TM	±	±	±	−	+	Delivery
HELLP	++	Third TM	+	+	++	++ to +++	+	Delivery
AFLP	+	Third TM	+++	+++	+	+++	±	Delivery
TTP	+++	Second TM	−	−	+++	−	±	Plasmapheresis
HUS	++	Postpartum	−	−	+++	−	+++	Trial plasmapheresis
DIC	++	Postpartum	+++	+++	+	±	+ to ++	Underlying cause

TM trimester, *ITP* immune thrombocytopenia, *HELLP* hemolysis elevated liver enzymes low platelet syndrome, *AFLP* acute fatty liver of pregnancy, *TTP* thrombotic thrombocytopenic purpure, *HUS* hemolytic uremic syndrome, *DIC* disseminated intravascular coagulopathy, *MAHA* blood film features of microangiopathic hemolytic anemia, *IVIG* intravenous immunoglobulin by the pentad of MAHA, thrombocytopenia, neurological abnormalities (confusion, headache, seizures, stroke), renal dysfunction (typically HUS), and fever. Often only the first two features are seen. There is no coagulopathy and no DIC. Obstetrical cases account for 10% of all cases of TTP. TTP is seen during the second trimester, whereas HUS is generally a postpartum disorder [8, 9].

Plasma exchange is effective because it removes the pathogenic autoantibodies and replenishes the missing ADAMTS13 protease, restoring normal regulation of VWF-dependent platelet adhesion. It is highly efficacious for TTP, but the response and prognosis of postpartum HUS is poor, with many patients being left with renal failure. Unlike preeclampsia and HELLP, the course of TTP is not ameliorated by delivery.

Acquired Coagulopathy During Pregnancy

Massive blood loss from postpartum hemorrhage, with or without secondary DIC, is the most common cause of severe acquired coagulopathy during pregnancy. Other causes of acquired coagulopathy include DIC from severe obstetrical disorders and liver dysfunction associated with AFLP. Iatrogenic coagulopathy from the administration of "heparins" for thromboembolic disease is relatively common today. Rarely also, autoantibodies to coagulation factors develop during and immediately after pregnancy, leading to acquired hemophilia.

Physiological Changes in Coagulation During Pregnancy

Normal pregnancy is accompanied by increased concentrations of factors VII, VIII, X, and VWF and pronounced increases in fibrinogen. Free protein S, an inhibitor of coagulation, is decreased during pregnancy. Plasminogen activator inhibitor type 1 (PAI-1) levels are significantly increased as is PAI-2, produced by the placenta, which increases dramatically during the third trimester. Both inhibit fibrinolysis. Markers of thrombin generation such as thrombin–antithrombin (TAT) complexes and the D-dimer are also increased [10]. These changes, which may not completely return to baseline until more than 8 weeks postpartum, begin with conception and result in the hypercoagulable state of pregnancy that presumably has evolved to protect women from hemorrhage at the time of miscarriage or childbirth. In developed countries, however, this situation has evolved so that now, thromboembolic disease represents a leading cause of maternal death.

Disseminated Intravascular Coagulopathy

Disseminated intravascular coagulopathy is characterized by widespread ongoing activation of coagulation, leading to vascular or microvascular fibrin deposition, which compromises the blood supply to various organs, contributing to organ failure. Ongoing activation of the coagulation system, impaired synthesis, and increased degradation of coagulation factors frequently results in decreased levels of procoagulant proteins, protease inhibitors, and platelets (as well as platelet dysfunction), which can cause bleeding [11]. Causes of obstetrical DIC include massive hemorrhage, placental abruption, amniotic fluid embolism, severe preeclampsia/HELLP syndrome, intrauterine fetal demise, and sepsis [8, 11, 12].

Acute DIC is associated with placental abruption and amniotic fluid emboli. Amniotic fluid can directly activate coagulation in vitro, and placental separation releases thromboplastin-like material from the placental system, activating the coagulation pathway and resulting in DIC [11].

Although the coagulation system may be activated in patients with preeclampsia and HELLP syndrome, it is subclinical. Overt DIC occurs in only a small percentage of patients, usually those with abruptio placentae or some other complication of preeclampsia [8].

Disseminated intravascular coagulopathy is diagnosed by identifying thrombocytopenia in the presence of coagulopathy – elevated activated partial thromboplastin time (aPTT) and prothrombin time, international normalized ratio (PT/INR) – and particularly evidence of fibrinogen consumption (low fibrinogen and elevated fibrin degradation products such as D-dimer). Protein C, protein S, and antithrombin levels are decreased but are less important for the initial diagnosis [11].

Therapy is aimed at reversal of the underlying cause and supporting the coagulopathy with transfusion. Depending on the circumstance, this may involve immediate delivery, evacuation of the uterus, and/or hysterectomy.

Transfusional support is similar to that for massive hemorrhage with similar hemostatic targets (Table 12.3). There is no evidence that administration of blood components

Table 12.3 Example of a massive transfusion protocol

"*Activate*" *massive transfusion protocol if:*
1. Life-threatening bleeding
2. Expected transfusion > one blood volume in 24 h
3. Four units of packed cell transfusion within 4 h

↓

Blood products

First: 4 U packed cells (PC) + 4 U fresh frozen plasma (FFP)

Second: 4 U PC + 4 U FFP + platelets (4 U equivalent)

Third: 4 U PC + 4 U FFP + 10 U cryoprecipitate

Thereafter, alternate second and third treatments

↕

rFVIIa

Give 90 µg/kg if ongoing bleeding with or after second treatment with blood products

Repeat after 20 min if no response or every 2 h if a partial response

↕

Targets of transfusion therapy
1. Hemorrhage control (surgical/medical)
2. Platelets > 50×10^9/L
3. Fibrinogen > 1–2 g/L
4. Prevent hypothermia
5. Correct hypocalcemia
6. Monitor coagulation studies, fibrinogen, platelets, and hemoglobin

might "add fuel to the fire" – indeed aggressive support of the coagulopathy is paramount. Conversely, the use of heparin to minimize microthrombi-induced organ dysfunction has not been shown to be effective and worsens bleeding [13].

Massive Hemorrhage

Massive postpartum hemorrhage is an important cause of acquired coagulopathy during pregnancy and still accounts for around one-fourth of direct maternal deaths in developed countries such as Australia [14].

The coagulopathy that develops is multifactorial. The major cause is blood loss and hemodilution of clotting factors and platelets. However, DIC is common as a result of the massive blood loss itself as well as any underlying obstetrical disorder (e.g., placental abruption, HELLP) [15]. Consumption of clotting factors, fibrinogen, and platelets not only occurs systemically in DIC but also at sites of local injury and bleeding [16, 17]. Hypothermia and acidosis cause reduced coagulation factor activation/activity, resulting in hypothermia-induced platelet dysfunction [16]. In addition, massive blood loss causes an increased fibrinolytic state [16]. Indeed, changes in the fibrinogen level, even in the normal range, have been shown to be an important predictor of the risk and severity of postpartum hemorrhage [18]. Hyperfibrinolysis and the released fibrin degradation products also inhibit uterine contractions, exacerbating postpartum blood loss [15].

The principles of therapy are (1) restoration and maintenance of circulating blood volume to maintain organ perfusion and oxygenation, and (2) cessation of bleeding by either correcting a surgical bleeding diathesis or reversing the coagulopathy.

Blood banks use component therapy rather than whole blood concentrates. Common blood products are packed red blood cell concentrates, FFP (rich in all clotting factors but proportionally low in fibrinogen), cryoprecipitate (high levels of fibrinogen), and platelets (Table 12.4). These products are virally screened but generally not virally inactivated/treated, so they carry a risk of blood pathogen transmission. Blood product concentrates rarely transmit viruses, but bacterial contamination of platelet concentrates (which are stored at room temperature) is not uncommon. Febrile transfusion reactions are common and are due to transfused cytokines. The risk of alloimmunization, the formation of antibodies to mismatched red blood cell antigens (e.g., anti-Kell), is diminished by cross-matching and phenotyping the patients red blood cells. Other transfusion-related problems, such as transfusion-associated lung injury (TRALI) and posttransfusion purpura (PTP), are rare but serious complications. Although access may be limited, there are also specific fibrinogen concentrates available that can elevate fibrinogen levels to a greater degree in a much more predictable fashion.

There have been changes in massive transfusion practice, with the view that early, aggressive administration of plasma and platelets can break the "bloody vicious cycle" of hemorrhage, resuscitation, hemodilution, and further coagulopathy – leading to more hemorrhage [16]. Thus current dogma is to identify massive hemorrhage early and commence immediate plasma replacement in a ratio of 1:1 packed cells to FFP [19, 20].

Table 12.4 Content of common blood products[a]

Product	Contents	Use, dose, effect
Packed RBCs (1 U = 200–300 ml)	RBCs only	Consider if Hb < 70 g/L or "massive hemorrhage"
	ABO and RhD compatible	
	Specific phenotype (e.g., Kell) available	One unit increases hemoglobin by 10 g/L
	Group O-negative for emergency	
Fresh frozen plasma (1 U = 200–300 ml)	All clotting factors, no platelets	Correct deficiencies of multiple coagulation factors such as in DIC or to prevent coagulopathy in massive transfusion
	Relatively low in fibrinogen	
	ABO group specific	
	Group A in emergency	
		Adequate dose 15–30 ml/kg
Cryoprecipitate (1 U = approximately 25 ml) (typically administered in lots of 10 U)	Fibrinogen, factors V, VIII, XIII, VWF	Ten bags of cryoprecipitate increase plasma fibrinogen by 0.5–1.0 g/L
Platelets (typically administered in 4-U lots = one "pooled" platelets)	Platelets	Four-unit equivalent increases the platelet count by approximately > 30–50 × 10⁹/L
	Best platelet survival if group specific	
Recombinant factor VIIa	rFVIIa	Standard dose 90 µg/kg

RBCs red blood cells

[a]For all blood products, the response is highly independent and is dependent on the clinical situation

Hence, many units have "massive transfusion protocols." In our unit, patients are identified as having life-threatening hemorrhage if there is an expected blood replacement in excess of one blood volume and/or ongoing bleeding after four units of packed cell transfusion within 4 h. The blood bank then provides blood products in "shipments," which allow and encourage clinicians to maintain adequate transfusion of plasma, fibrinogen, and platelets. For example, in our unit the "first shipment" contains four units of packed cells (PC) and four units of FFP (1:1 ratio). If bleeding is ongoing, the second shipment contains platelets (one "pooled unit" or four conventional units) plus four PC units and four FFP units. The third shipment contains cryoprecipitate (10 U) in addition to the four PC and four FFP units. This regimen then alternates between platelets and cryoprecipitate with ongoing shipments. Recombinant factor VIIa should also be considered (see below).

If there is inadequate time for an initial cross-match, group O-negative red blood cells are released and group A FFP. Non-cross-matched blood carries the risk of alloimmunization and a delayed hemolytic transfusion reaction.

Targets of transfusion therapy are the following.

1. Hemorrhage control
2. Platelets >50 × 10⁹/L[a]
3. Fibrinogen >1–2 g/L[b]
4. Prevent hypothermia
5. Correct hypocalcemia
6. Monitor coagulation studies, fibrinogen, platelets, and hemoglobin

[a]Coagulation targets such as PT/INR <1.5 may represent an ideal but come second to clinical efficacy and are often difficult to achieve.
[b]A fibrinogen target of >2 g/L (rather than the usual 1 g/L) may be more applicable to obstetrical patients with bleeding.

It should be noted that such an aggressive plasma replacement regimen is not required for nonmassive transfusion. Indeed, in other situations associated with anemia, transfusion and exposure to the accompanying risks should be avoided whenever possible in this young population group, who can tolerate significant levels of anemia and recover quickly with simple therapy such as iron replacement.

Recombinant Factor VIIa for Obstetrical Bleeding

Recombinant factor VIIa (rFVIIa) was developed for the prevention or treatment of bleeding in patients with hemophilia who develop inhibitors to exogenous factor concentrates. It enhances coagulation at the site of bleeding, where tissue factor (TF) and platelets localize. Recombinant FVIIa works by directly binding to TF and initiating the coagulation cascade, but it can also act independent of TF by directly activating platelet-bound factor X [21]. Thus, rFVIIa ultimately augments the thrombin burst leading to the formation of a stable fibrin clot.

The use of rVIIa (Novoseven) for "off-label" indications, including obstetrical use, has been reported [22]. A recent update to the original published cohort documented its use in 110 obstetrical patients with bleeding and showed impressive efficacy (stopped or reduced bleeding in 76% of patients) [23].

Although the role of rFVIIa in controlling life-threatening hemorrhage is the most important indication, several other potential reasons for its use are unique to the obstetrical population. They include avoidance of hysterectomy and of exposure to blood products in these young women who are likely to desire more pregnancies. A group of Australian and New Zealand clinicians formulated guidelines for the use of rFVIIa in massive obstetrical hemorrhage and proposed that rFVIIa always be considered/used prior to considering hysterectomy for ongoing postpartum hemorrhage [24]. Ultimately, however, the decision for an immediate hysterectomy should be driven by clinical factors.

The efficacy of rFVIIa in the face of massive bleeding drops with the volume of blood transfused and the degree of coagulopathy, hypothermia, and acidosis [24, 25]. Thus, it is important not to delay the decision to use rFVIIa until it is too late. Obstetrical data from the Australian and New Zealand Haemostasis Registry revealed that 83% of patients had received more than five units of packed cells prior to receiving rFVIIa, with a median transfusion quantity of 11 U [23].

The standard treatment dose is 90 μg/kg, and a second dose should be considered after 20 min in nonresponders or after 2 h in responders who have some ongoing bleeding. Adjuvant coagulation therapy is critical, and special attention should be made to coadministering fibrinogen and platelets. In addition, the use of antifibrinolytics, such as tranexamic acid, should be considered.

The major concern with the use of rFVIIa, apart from the issue of its high cost, is an increased risk of thromboembolism. Of the 110 obstetrical cases recorded in the Haemostasis Registry, three had thromboembolic events that were thought to be "probably or possibly" linked to the use of rFVIIa [23]. Fortunately, our experience overall has been that the rate of thromboembolic events does not appear significantly increased in similarly matched patient groups who did or did not receive rFVIIa, even in patients with DIC [24, 25].

Bleeding in Patients on Low-Molecular-Weight Heparin

Heparin – standard unfractionated and low-molecular-weight heparin (LMWH) – works by binding to antithrombin and potentiating its anticoagulant effect on clotting factors IIa, Xa, IXa, XIa, and XIIa. Thrombin and factor Xa are most sensitive to the heparin/antithrombin effect. Unfractionated heparin (UFH) also inhibits thrombin by direct binding, and it is largely this effect that is reflected, and monitored, in changes seen in the aPTT. In contrast, the aPTT is insensitive to the anticoagulant effect of LMWH, and a specific anti-Xa assay must be performed to gauge the level of anticoagulation [26].

Obstetrical patients are not infrequently treated with LMWH for thrombotic disorders. Some may be on a prophylactic dose and others on a full anticoagulant dose. and thus the bleeding risk is significantly higher.

The LMWHs have a long half-life (4–6 h) and accumulate in the presence of renal dysfunction. A planned labor is required for patients on these agents so adequate time can elapse to minimize the risk of bleeding with delivery and an epidural anesthetic. In patients on treatment doses, this interval is in excess of 24 h. Specific guidelines are available [27].

Protamine sulfate neutralizes the effect of UFH but only 60% of the anti-Xa effect of LMWH. Nonetheless, in patients who are on LMWH and are bleeding, it can be used to attenuate the bleeding. It has been suggested that if LMWH was given within 8 h, protamine sulfate should be administered at a dose of 1 mg per 100 anti-Xa units of LMWH (1 mg enoxaparin equals approximately 100 anti-Xa units). A second dose of 0.5 mg protamine sulfate per 100 anti-Xa units should be administered if bleeding continues. Smaller doses of protamine sulfate can be given if the time since LMWH administration is longer than 8 h [26]. Data on the safety of protamine during pregnancy are limited, but in this instance it would most commonly be given during the postpartum setting [28]. Transfusional support is appropriate, but transfused clotting factors can be subsequently inactivated by residual heparin.

Caution Box

Protamine sulphate neutralises the effect of UFH but only 60% of the anti-Xa effect of LMWH.

Management of Pregnancy and Delivery in Women with Congenital Bleeding Disorders

Women with inherited bleeding disorders (Table 12.5) are at risk of bleeding complications from hemostatic challenges during pregnancy and childbirth. The Australian Haemophilia Centre Directors' Organisation (AHCDO), as well as many other international hemophilia organizations, have developed and published practical guidelines for the management of pregnancy and delivery in women with bleeding disorders (Table 12.6) [29, 30].

Expected Physiological Response During Pregnancy

Factor VIII levels increase significantly in carriers of hemophilia A during pregnancy, reaching a peak at 29–35 weeks [29]. Although most of the women develop levels within the normal range, the rise is variable and some may still have insufficient levels for safe hemostasis at term. Similarly, factor VIII and VWF antigen (VWFAg) usually increase during pregnancy in women with type 1 von Willebrand's disease (VWD) but not type 3 VWD. [29] Factor IX levels in carriers of hemophilia B and factor XI levels in deficient states usually do not change significantly during pregnancy [10, 29].

Table 12.5 Bleeding disorders that may increase the risk of bleeding in pregnant women

Disorder	Factor affected	Bleeding phenotype in women
Hemophilia A	Factor VIII levels decreased[a]	Mild to moderate when levels <40 IU/dl[b]
Hemophilia B	Factor IX levels decreased	Mild to moderate with levels <40 IU/dl[b]
Factor XI deficiency	Factor XI levels decreased	Highly variable; risk increased with levels <15 IU/dl
Von Willebrand disease		
Type 1	VWF levels decreased	Mild to moderate
Type 2	Dysfunctional VWF	Variable, usually moderate
Type 3	VWF absent	Severe (VWFAg undetectable, factor VIII <10 IU/dl)
Rare coagulation factor deficiencies	Afibrinogenemia; deficiencies in factors II, V, V + VIII, VII, X, and XIII	Highly variable, mild to severe, not always predictable on factor levels
		Recurrent fetal loss associated with factor II and factor XIII deficiency

VWFAg von Willebrand factor antigen
[a]May normalize throughout the pregnancy
[b]Women with factor VIII or IX >40% but below the lower limit of the normal reference range (laboratory normal values vary based on methodology) may also have increased bleeding tendencies

Table 12.6 AHCDO consensus statement on the management of pregnancy and delivery in women who are either carriers or affected with bleeding disorders [29]

During pregnancy
- Usually no specific therapy is required for most inherited bleeding disorders antenatally
- Factor levels should be measured at presentation and repeated during the third trimester (usually at 32–34 weeks)

Labor and delivery
- Spontaneous vaginal delivery is preferred. An inherited bleeding disorder, in the mother or fetus, by itself is not an indication for delivery by cesarean section. The mode of delivery should be chosen based on obstetrical indications
- Patients with severe bleeding disorders or who are at risk of delivering a hemophiliac boy ideally should be managed by a high-risk obstetrical unit and hemophilia treatment center
- A normal factor level in the mother (or quantitative/functional von Willebrand's studies for VWD) is desirable for delivery
- Vacuum extraction is contraindicated. Forceps, fetal scalp blood sampling, and scalp electrodes should be avoided where possible
- DDAVP has poor efficacy for types 2 and 3 VWD but may be used in carriers of hemophilia A. DDAVP may cause fluid retention with hyponatremia, hypotension, uterine contractions, and premature labor

Obstetrical anesthesia
- No guidelines adequately cover epidural/spinal anesthesia in patients with bleeding disorders
- Epidural anesthesia should only be considered in close consultation with an anesthetist and hematology team
- Coagulation factor levels should be maintained in the normal range (>50 U/dl) for the duration of catheter placement and for 12 h (mild bleeding disorder) to 24 h (moderate-to-severe bleeding disorder) after catheter removal

Postpartum care
- In general, factor levels should be maintained in the normal range for 3–4 days after a vaginal delivery and up to 7 days after cesarean section

Postpartum hemorrhage
- Active management of third stage of labor should be practiced
- Early postpartum hemorrhage, associated with low factor levels, should be managed by factor replacement therapy or DDAVP in carriers of hemophilia A or women with type 1 VWD
- Should late postpartum hemorrhage occur, first-line management includes tranexamic acid, oral contraceptives, and in the longer term a levonorgestrel-releasing intrauterine device

Management of neonates at risk of a severe bleeding disorder
- If the baby is at risk of having a severe bleeding disorder, blood samples should be taken for factor levels
- In general, intramuscular injections should be avoided
- Vitamin K is often given orally or subcutaneously to avoid the risk of intramuscular hematoma
- Trans-fontanel ultrasonography should be considered soon after birth in babies "known to be affected" with a severe bleeding disorder to check for intracranial hemorrhage. The baby is then observed for symptoms of ICH such as poor feeding
- Even in neonates known to be affected with a severe bleeding disorder, prophylactic factor replacement should not be given owing to the potential risk of inhibitor development

Because the rise in factor levels is unpredictable during pregnancy, they should be checked at presentation, prior to any invasive procedure, and during the third trimester. After delivery, factor levels usually return to baseline after days to weeks but may drop earlier. It should be noted that women with normal factor levels may still be hemophilia carriers.

Management During Pregnancy

Women who are carriers of the genes for factor VIII or factor IX deficiency, (hemophilia A and B, respectively) may have plasma factor levels outside the normal range. When they are <30% (classified as mild hemophilia), the patient may be at increased risk of bleeding [31]. Most carriers of hemophilia A develop "normal" factor levels as the pregnancy progresses and thus do not require replacement therapy [29]. However, in carriers with a moderate-to-severe deficiency, factor levels may not correct adequately during pregnancy. Rare bleeding disorders, such as fibrinogen or factor XIII deficiency, may require antenatal treatment to prevent fetal loss. Genetic counseling is desirable, optimally before conception, if the mother is a hemophilia carrier or if there is a family history of hemophilia.

Women with type 1 VWD also experience increased levels of factor VIII and VWFAg during pregnancy, with normal levels in most women by delivery. Women with type 2 VWD may also show an increase in factor VIII and VWFAg during pregnancy, but measures of VWF function [ristocetin cofactor (RCoF) and the collagen binding assay (CBA)] usually remain low [29, 32]. In addition, the thrombocytopenia associated with type 2B VWD can worsen during pregnancy. Type 3 VWD patients do not show any change in factor levels during pregnancy, and all require replacement therapy for delivery [31].

Factors level assays should be repeated during the third trimester (32–34 weeks) to allow planning of the appropriate management of labor and delivery and the need for prophylactic therapy [29].

Factor Levels for Delivery and Invasive Procedures

The mother's factor levels should be checked before any invasive procedure; if they are below the normal range, replacement therapy must be provided [29, 30]. In general, normal levels of factor VIII, factor IX, and VWFAg are >50 IU/dl for hemophilia A, hemophilia B, and type 1 VWD, respectively. Bleeding in those with factor XI deficiency is highly variable, and therapy should be individualized; replacement therapy is required if the factor XI level is <15 IU/dl [29, 32]. Treatment of rare bleeding disorders (e.g., factor II, V, VII, X, or XIII deficiency) should be individualized.

Desmopressin (1-desamino-8-D-arginine vasopressin, abbreviated DDAVP) is a synthetic analog of vasopressin that increases plasma VWF and factor VIII levels. DDAVP has been used in the treatment of women with hemophilia A and type 1 VWD during pregnancy; although the data are limited data, it is thought to be safe during pregnancy [28]. However, DDAVP can stimulate uterine contraction and cause premature labor and hyponatremia [33]. Importantly, most patients with type 1 VWD, who would respond to DDAVP, have already corrected their factor levels during pregnancy. In patients with type 2 and 3 VWD, in whom elevation of VWF is most required, the response to DDAVP is generally poor. Thus, the AHCDO recommends VWF containing concentrates for antenatal treatment of VWD, although DDAVP may be a suitable alternative in carriers of hemophilia A [29].

Management During Labor and Delivery

Mode of Delivery

Normal vaginal delivery is recommended for women with inherited bleeding disorders [29–31]. Cesarean section does not eliminate the risk of cranial hemorrhage in the neonate and elevates the risk of bleeding and the factor replacement requirements in the mother [29–31]. In some series, the risk of cranial bleeding was in fact higher with cesarean section than with vaginal delivery. However, the use of vacuum extraction should be avoided because of the unacceptably high risk of cranial hemorrhage (~60%). Also, forceps and prolonged labor should be avoided. The mode of delivery should ultimately be determined based on obstetrical factors.

Caution Box

Instrumental delivery (vacuum extraction is completely contraindicated) in women with congenital bleeding disorders should be avoided due to high risk of cranial hemorrhage.

Epidural Analgesia

There are no comprehensive guidelines that cover epidural/spinal anesthesia in patients with bleeding disorders, and studies are lacking. Patients with inherited bleeding disorders are at an increased risk of spinal hematoma [29, 34]. However, if the coagulation factors are in the normal range or supported and maintained in the normal range, regional anesthesia is not contraindicated [29, 30, 34]. Epidural anesthesia is generally not recommended for use in patients with severe type 2 or 3 VWD, but the decision should be individualized [30].

Factor levels should be maintained in the normal range for the duration of catheter placement and for 12 h (mild bleeding disorder) to 24 h (moderate-to-severe bleeding disorder) after catheter removal [29].

Postpartum Management

Factor levels that may have normalized during pregnancy tend to return to baseline by 7–21 days after delivery, although they may drop earlier and should be closely monitored [10, 31]. Women who have low baseline factor VIII or VWFAg levels are at continuing risk of postpartum hemorrhage for this time and should be advised to report symptoms. To reduce the risk of postpartum hemorrhage and surgical bleeding, factors levels should be maintained in the normal range for at least 3–5 days after vaginal delivery and up to 7 days following cesarean section [29–31].

Carriers of hemophilia, women with VWD, and those with factor XI deficiency have a significantly higher risk of both primary and secondary postpartum hemorrhage [30–32]. The risk of postpartum hemorrhage can be reduced by active management of labor [35].

Early postpartum hemorrhage, associated with low factor levels, should be managed by factor replacement therapy or DDAVP in women with type 1 VWD or hemophilia A [29, 30]. Desmopressin acetate has been detected in the breast milk of lactating women and so is not recommended for use in lactating women [28, 29]. Tranexamic acid, which is safe in breast-feeding mothers [28], can be used to control secondary postpartum hemorrhage [29, 30]. Tranexamic acid also does not increase the risk of venous thromboembolism [36]. An oral contraceptive pill and, in the longer term, a levonorgestrel-releasing intrauterine device are alternative therapies [37].

Management of Neonates at Risk of a Severe Bleeding Disorder

Cord blood testing is recommended in the UK's Haemophilia Doctors' Organisation guidelines and is useful for excluding severe disease [30]. However, its value regarding milder disease (particularly hemophilia B) is controversial, and results should be confirmed with peripheral blood testing. In addition, adult levels of vitamin K-dependent clotting factors and factor XI may not be present until after 6 months of age [29].

The risk of intracranial hemorrhage is around 4% in newborns with severe hemophilia [30, 31]. In the case of hemophilia, predelivery "sexing" of the fetus by ultrasonography is useful because female infants do not ordinarily have an elevated risk of cranial hemorrhage. The risk of cranial hemorrhage is also increased in neonates with severe forms of VWD but is rare in infants with factor XI deficiency [29, 31, 32].

The AHCDO recommended that neonates with a bleeding disorder undergo trans-fontanel ultrasonography soon after birth to check for intracranial hemorrhage. Because intracranial hemorrhage may be delayed (median time after delivery is 4.5 days), mothers should be made aware of potential symptoms, such as vomiting, seizures, and poor feeding [29].

Prophylactic factor replacement therapy should not be given routinely as it may be associated with an increased risk of inhibitor development in children with hemophilia [38]. Similarly, the use of prophylactic recombinant factor VIIa has not been shown to improve clinical outcomes [39]. Vitamin K should be given orally or subcutaneously to neonates with hemophilia or severe VWD subtypes [29, 30].

Learning points

- Seek specialist advice.
- An accurate diagnosis enables specific therapy and estimation of risk.
- DIC is associated with severe disorder of pregnancy and massive transfusion.
- Blood loss is frequently underestimated.
- Address coagulopathy early and aggressively.
- Treat the mother.

Conclusion

Acquired and congenital coagulopathy during pregnancy are major contributors to the risk of bleeding. An understanding of the causes and management is critical for safe obstetrical practice. Coagulopathy is due to disorders of platelets or coagulation factors. Although some types of thrombocytopenia in pregnancy, such as gestational thrombocytopenia, are common and benign, others such as ITP or TTP are moderate-to-severe disorders that pose a threat to the mother and child. These disorders require specific interventions. It is important to recognize them and seek specific hematological advice and therapy.

Suspicion of an acquired coagulopathy during pregnancy is often obvious owing to the poor health of the mother. The coagulopathy, often DIC, presents not so much as a diagnostic challenge (though identifying the underlying cause that may require specific intervention such as delivery is important) but a therapeutic one with management of coagulation factor replacement and massive transfusion. Finally, although hereditary coagulopathy is rare and often self-corrects during the pregnancy, its identification and monitoring is paramount for preventing complications for both mother and baby.

Caution Box

Neonates with a bleeding disorder should be monitored for intracranial hemorrhage. Many centres perform routine trans-fontanel ultrasonography.

References

1. Ronsmans C. Lancet Maternal Survival Series steering group. Maternal mortality: who, when, where, and why. Lancet. 2006;368:1189–200.
2. Provan D, Stasi R, Newland AC, et al. International consensus report on the investigation and management of primary immune thrombocytopenia. Blood. 2010;115:168–86.
3. Dunkley S, Arthur JF, Evans S, Gardiner EE, Shen Y, Andrews RK. A familial platelet function disorder associated with abnormal signalling through the glycoprotein VI pathway. Br J Haematol. 2007;137:569–77.
4. Crowther MA, Burrows RF, Ginsberg J, Kelton JG. Thrombocytopenia in pregnancy: diagnosis, pathogenesis and management. Blood Rev. 1996;10:8–16.
5. Choi PY, Dunkley S, Rasko J. Investigating the patient with thrombocytopenia – ITP. Medicine Today. 2011;12(3):41–6.
6. Beilin Y, Zahn J, Comerford M. Safe epidural analgesia in thirty parturients with platelet counts between 69,000 and 98,000 mm(−3). Anesth Analg. 1997;85:385–8.
7. McRae KR, Samuels P, Schrieder AD. Pregnancy associated thrombocytopenia: pathogenesis and management. Blood. 1992;80:2697–714.
8. Norwitz ER, Hsu CD, Repke JT. Acute complications of preeclampsia. Clin Obstet Gynaecol. 2002;45:308–29.
9. George JN. The association of pregnancy with thrombotic thrombocytopenic purpura-hemolytic uremic syndrome. Curr Opin Hematol. 2003;10:339–44.
10. Bremme KA. Haemostatic changes in pregnancy. Best Pract Res Clin Haematol. 2003;16:153–68.
11. Levi M, ten Cate H. Disseminated intravascular coagulation. N Engl J Med. 1999;341: 586–92.
12. Silver RM, Major H. Maternal coagulation disorders and postpartum hemorrhage. Clin Obstet Gynaecol. 2010;53:252–64.
13. Feinstein DI. Diagnosis and management of disseminated intravascular coagulation: the role of heparin therapy. Blood. 1982;60:284–7.
14. Sullivan EA, King JF. Maternal deaths in Australia 2000–2002. Maternal death series no 2. Sydney: AIHW National Perinatal Statistic Unit; 2006.
15. McLintock C. Obstetric haemorrhage. Thromb Res. 2009;123 Suppl 2:S30–4.
16. Hess JR. Blood and coagulation support in trauma care. Haematology Am Soc Haematol Educ Program. 2007;1:187–191.
17. Hirsh J, Bauer KA, Donati MB, Gould M, Samana MM, Weitz JI. Parenteral anticoagulants: American College of Chest Physicians Evidence-Based Clinical Practice Guidelines (8th Edition). Chest. 2008;133:141S–59.
18. Charbit B, Mandelbrot L, Samain E, Baron G, Haddaoui B, Keita H, et al. The decrease of fibrinogen is an early predictor of the severity of postpartum hemorrhage. J Thromb Haemost. 2007;5:266–73.
19. Kashuk JL, Moore EE, Johnson JL, et al. Postinjury life threatening coagulopathy: is 1:1 fresh frozen plasma:packed cells the answer? J Trauma. 2008;65:261–70.
20. Gunter OL, Au BK, Isabell JM, et al. Optimizing outcomes in damage control resuscitation: identifying blood product ratios associated with improved survival. J Trauma. 2008;65(2): 261–70.
21. Hoffman M, Monroe 3rd DM, Roberts HR. Activated factor VII activates factors IX and X on the surface of activated platelets: thoughts on the mechanism of action of high-dose activated VII. Blood Coagul Fibrinolysis. 1998;9:S61–5.
22. Isbister J, Phillips L, Dunkley S, Janklelowitz G, McNeil J, Cameron P. Recombinant activated factor VII in critical bleeding: experience from the Australian and New Zealand haemostasis registry. Intern Med. 2008;38:156–65.
23. Phillips LE, McLintock C, Pollock W, et al. Recombinant activated factor VII in Obstetric hemorrhage: experience form the Australian and New Zealand Haemostasis Registry. Anesth Analg. 2009;109:1908–15.

24. Welsh A, McLintock C, Gatt S, et al. Guidelines for the use of recombinant factor VII in massive obstetric haemorrhage. Aust NZ J Obstet Gynaecol. 2008;48:12–6.
25. Dunkley S, Phillips L, McCall P, et al. Recombinant Activated Factor VII in cardiac surgery: experience from the Australian and New Zealand Haemostasis Register. Ann Thorac Surg. 2008;85:836–44.
26. Hirsh J, Raschke R. Heparin and low molecular weight heparin: the seventh ACCP conference on antithrombotic and thrombolytic therapy. Chest. 2004;126:188S–203.
27. Bates SM, Greer IA, Pabinger I, Sofaer S, Hirsh J. Venous thromboembolism, thrombophilia, antithrombotic therapy, and pregnancy: American College of Chest Physicians Evidence-Based Clinical Practice Guidelines (8th Edition). Chest. 2008;133:844S–66.
28. Australian Drug Evaluation Committee. Prescribing medicines in pregnancy. 4th ed. 1999 and updates [Internet]. http://www.tga.gov.au/DOCS/HTML/medpreg.htm. Accessed September 2008.
29. Dunkley S, Russell S, Rowell J, Barnes C, Baker R, Street A. A consensus statement on the management of pregnancy and delivery in women who are either carriers or affected with bleeding disorders. Med J Aust. 2009;191:460–3.
30. Lee CA, Chi C, Pavord SR, et al. The obstetric and gynaecological management of women with inherited bleeding disorders – review with guidelines produced by a taskforce of UK Haemophila Doctors' Organisation. Haemophilia. 2006;12:301–36.
31. Street AM, Ljung R, Lavery SA. Management of carriers and babies with haemophilia. Haemophilia. 2008;14 Suppl 3:181–7.
32. Kadir RA, Lee CA, Sabin CA, et al. Pregnancy in women with von Willebrand's disease or factor XI deficiency. Br J Obstet Gynaecol. 1998;105:314–21.
33. Kouides PA. Obstetric and gynaecological aspects of von Willebrand disease. Best Pract Res Clin Haematol. 2001;14:381–99.
34. Haljamäe H. Thromboprophylaxis, coagulation disorders, and regional anaesthesia. Acta Anaesthesiol Scand. 1996;40:1024–40.
35. Hoveyda F, MacKenzie IZ. Secondary postpartum haemorrhage: incidence, morbidity, and current management. Br J Obset Gynaecol. 2001;108:927–30.
36. Rybo G. Tranexamic acid therapy: effective treatment in heavy menstrual bleeding: clinical update on safety. Ther Adv. 1991;4:1–8.
37. Demers C, Derzko C, David M, Douglas J. Gynaecological and obstetric management of women with inherited bleeding disorders. J Obstet Gynaecol Can. 2005;27:707–32.
38. Gouw SC, van der Bom JG, van den Berg HM, et al. Treatment-related risk factors of inhibitor development in previously untreated patients with hemophilia A: the CANAL cohort study. Blood. 2007;109:4648–54.
39. Veldman A, Josef J, Fischer D, Volk WR. A prospective pilot study of prophylactic treatment of preterm neonates with recombinant activated factor VII during the first 72 hours of life. Pediatr Crit Care Med. 2006;7:34–9.

Chapter 13
Anesthesia and Intensive Care Management of Bleeding During Pregnancy

Jennifer A. Taylor and Felicity Plaat

Introduction

Obstetrical hemorrhage can be defined in many ways. Any blood loss >500 ml for a vaginal delivery or >1,000 ml following cesarean section is considered abnormal. Definitions of major obstetrical hemorrhage vary, but it can be defined as a blood loss in excess of 1,500 ml, a hemoglobin drop of >4 g/dl, or an immediate transfusion of four units of red blood cells [1].

Bleeding during pregnancy is a leading cause of maternal death worldwide, including in developed countries [2, 3]. The latest Confidential Enquiry into Maternal and Child Health (CEMACH) report has it ranked in the top three major causes of maternal death in the UK, and it is a major cause of postpartum morbidity. CEMACH identified substandard care as a contributing factor to these deaths and highlighted the need for improved care for these women. It is also a persisting problem with an increasing mortality rate due to hemorrhage as evidenced in the last two reports [4]. This could be in part due to the increase in multiple births and the increasing cesarean section rate.

Few pregnant women require admission to intensive care units (<1% of intensive care admissions are parturients) [4]. However, a large proportion of these admissions to the ICU are because of obstetrical hemorrhage. Early recognition of the hemorrhage along with fast and effective resuscitation of the mother are the keys to good outcomes.

F. Plaat (✉)
Queen Charlotte's and Chelsea Hospital, Department of Anaesthesia,
Hammersmith House, Hammersmith Hospital,
Du Cane Road, London, W12 0HS, UK
e-mail: felicity.plaat@imperial.nhs.uk

E. Sheiner (ed.), *Bleeding During Pregnancy: A Comprehensive Guide*,
DOI 10.1007/978-1-4419-9810-1_13, © Springer Science+Business Media, LLC 2011

Initial Resuscitation

The approach to resuscitation of any collapsed patient (be they pregnant or otherwise) should be structured, using the ABCDE approach (Table 13.1) to ensure that steps and signs are not missed and that all members of the team are following the same protocol. This approach incorporates the simultaneous assessment and treatment of potentially life-threatening problems as they are identified [5].

From approximately 20 weeks' gestation, the pregnant woman is at risk of aortocaval compression, which may render attempts at resuscitation ineffective. This can be alleviated by manually displacing the uterus to the left, putting the patient in the left lateral position, and inserting a wedge under the patient's right flank (or if in the operating theater tilting the operating table 45° to the left).

A *call for help* is essential as obstetrical hemorrhage cannot be managed single-handedly. All obstetrical units should have a major hemorrhage protocol that can be activated to ensure that all the members of the management team are called. Obstetrical hemorrhage can be rapid and torrential. Early involvement of senior anesthesia and obstetrical staff is crucial. Frequent effective communication between all specialties is vital. Hematological advice should be sought early to aid the mobilization of blood products as they are required.

The *head-down tilt* should be instituted when possible to increase venous return, increase cardiac output, and ultimately improve systemic blood pressure.

Airway

A patient's airway must be open to allow inhalation of oxygen and expiration of carbon dioxide. Patients with impaired consciousness may have airway compromise, which should be rectified by opening of the airway. This can initially be managed by simple maneuvers such as a chin lift and jaw thrust. If the patient is unconscious, the airway needs to be secured by endotracheal intubation with a cuffed tube. This is especially important in pregnant women who have an increased risk of aspirating gastric contents. Intubation should be performed by experienced staff (i.e., an anesthetist) as pregnancy is also associated with an increased risk of difficult and failed intubation compared with that of the normal population [6].

Table 13.1 Approach to resuscitation of the pregnant patient

A – Airway
B – Breathing and ventilation
C – Circulation
D – Disability
E – Exposure and environmental control

Breathing and Ventilation

High-flow oxygen should be administered at a rate of 10–15 ml/min via a facemask with a nonrebreathing bag to increase the concentration of oxygen inspired (approximately 60% with this device). Initial assessment of the adequacy of breathing and ventilation involves measuring the respiratory rate, looking for other signs of respiratory distress (i.e., abnormal chest movements), auscultation, and measuring oxygen saturation. Oxygen therapy should be titrated to maintain an oxygen saturation >95%.

The respiratory rate should be monitored in all bleeding women. A rising respiratory rate is one of the earliest signs of shock – it begins to increase after approximately 15% of the blood volume is lost [7].

Circulation

Assessment of the circulation includes measuring the heart rate, blood pressure, peripheral perfusion (warmth of peripheries and capillary refill time), conscious level, and urinary output.

During pregnancy, the circulating blood volume is increased, reaching approximately 100 ml/kg at term (vs. 70 ml/kg in a nonpregnant individual). Cardiac output also increases throughout pregnancy, reaching 50% at term. This gives the pregnant patient a degree of physiological reserve; and as a result signs and symptoms of hypovolemia develop later. Signs may not be evident until 1,500 ml blood has been lost (30–35% of the circulating blood volume). Hypotension is a very late sign, occurring only once blood loss is in excess of 2 L. Finding a "normal" blood pressure should not be reassuring. An early physiological change is a fall in pulse pressure (i.e., decreased difference between diastolic and systolic pressures) due to peripheral vasoconstriction. Note that this change may be missed if no baseline recordings exist.

The resting heart rate also increases during pregnancy, by approximately 15–20 beats per minute (bpm), so a resting heart rate of around 90–100 bpm may be normal. Heart rates of ≥100 bpm should be investigated. Tachycardia may be absent despite hypovolemia in certain circumstances. Patients taking β-blockers, those with pacemakers, those who have congenital heart block, and those with naturally low resting heart rates (athletes) do not develop tachycardia. Signs of shock can also remain undetected until later in pregnant women owing to the peripheral vasodilation and widened pulse pressure seen during pregnancy.

Shock

Shock is a state of inadequate end-organ perfusion resulting in reduced tissue oxygen delivery, anaerobic metabolism, and buildup of metabolic waste products.

Resuscitation is required to maintain or restore tissue oxygen delivery and prevent irreversible end-organ damage. There are four stages of hypovolemic shock, as described in Table 13.2. Although Table 13.2 applies to the nonpregnant state, it can be applied to the pregnant patient, keeping in mind that blood loss is greater in each class during pregnancy. Recognizing shock in the pregnant patient can be difficult owing to the physiological changes. However, it is vital that staff members are trained to identify early indicators.

Vascular Access

Wide-bore intravenous cannulas are recommended for immediate intravenous access. For the treatment of hemorrhage regardless of cause, the insertion of two short wide-bore cannulas, preferably 14 gauge, is recommended. Tests have shown the use of a 14G opposed to 16G cannula increases maximum flow rate by approximately 50% [8]. Access can be difficult to obtain in a hypovolemic, peripherally shut-down patient; and other techniques of vascular access may be required.

Venous cutdown into a peripheral vein, such as the antecubital vein or proximal or peripheral long saphenous vein, has been described as a technique for difficult intravenous access in obstetrics [5]. Although peripheral cutdown can be performed quickly and have few complications, a randomized study of 78 trauma patients comparing saphenous vein cutdown and femoral cannulation found that the former took significantly longer [9].

Intraosseous access has conventionally been used in children, but its use is being encouraged for adult resuscitation when intravenous access is difficult. semi-Automatic "gun" systems have been developed to allow access into the tibia or humerus and appear to make the procedure easier and more effective [10]. The use of the intraosseous route has yet to be described in the obstetrical literature.

Central venous access via the internal jugular or subclavian vein has the advantage of not only securing intravenous access, it allows monitoring of central venous pressures and administration of vasoactive drugs. However, in the hypovolemic patient it can be technically challenging and associated with a not negligible risk, especially in a coagulopathic patient. Complications include pneumothorax, hemothorax, subcutaneous emphysema, and air embolism as well as damage to nearby structures such as the common carotid artery, brachial plexus, phrenic nerve, thoracic duct, and sympathetic chain.

Ultrasonographic (US) guidance is now recommended to aid the insertion of central venous catheters [11]. Catheter-related infection and sepsis are serious hazards mandating a strictly aseptic technique for insertion and subsequent accessing of the line. Electrocardiographic (ECG) monitoring must be used during insertion to detect arrhythmias if the catheter tip is inserted too far. Although potentially easier to insert, femoral central venous lines require a palpable femoral arterial pulse (although this

Table 13.2 Classification of hypovolemic shock in nonpregnant patients

Parameter	Class I	Class II	Class III	Class IV
Circulating volume lost (%)	0–15	15–30	30–40	>40
Volume of blood loss for a 70-kg adult (ml)	<750	750–500	1,500–2,000	>2,000
Physiological changes	Blood diverted from splanchnic bed	Peripheral vasoconstriction	Failure of peripheral vasoconstriction to compensate for hypovolemia	Profound decompensation
Signs and symptoms	Mild tachycardia	Tachycardia Normal systolic blood pressure Narrowed pulse pressure Tachypnea	Fall in systolic blood pressure	Low urine output Altered mental status and eventual loss of consciousness

Reproduced from Grady C, Howell C, Cox C, editors. Managing obstetric emergencies and trauma. 2nd ed., 2007. With the permission of the Royal College of Obstetricians & Gynaecologists is less of an issue now with US availability). These lines carry a higher risk of infection, and in the obstetrical setting access to the line can be problematic.

Blood Sampling

Blood samples should be obtained as vascular access is secured and sent to the laboratory for a full blood count, a coagulation profile [prothrombin time (PT), activated partial thromboplastin time (aPTT), fibrinogen], a biochemistry profile (sodium, potassium, urea, creatinine, calcium, and glucose), and cross-match.

Fluid Resuscitation

There is still debate over the use of crystalloid vs. colloid for resuscitation (see below). The first priority is to restore the circulating volume. Rapid infusion of either should be commenced as soon as intravenous access is obtained and blood samples are obtained. If blood loss is ongoing or >2 L and/or there is hemodynamic instability, blood transfusion is likely required. If O-negative blood is instantly available, transfusion may be commenced while awaiting group-specific or cross-matched blood.

Pressure infusion devices can enhance rapid infusion of fluid. Such a device can be a simple pressure bag or for severe hemorrhage the Level 1 rapid infusion device (Level 1 Technologies, Rockland, MA, USA). The Level 1 incorporates a counter-current fluid warming system to warm the fluid. Risks associated with these devices include inadequate warming of fluid at high-flow rates, potential for fluid overload due to rapid administration, and a large venous air embolism [12].

Control of Bleeding

An important component of assessing circulation is to determine the site or cause of the bleeding and attempt to arrest it. Causes and specific treatments of peripartum hemorrhage have been outlined in earlier chapters. It is vital to have good communication between the obstetrical, anesthesia, and midwifery teams to aid resuscitation and expedite rapid treatment of the underlying cause of the bleeding.

Assessment of Blood Loss

Estimating blood loss is particularly difficult in obstetrics because of contamination with amniotic fluid and concealed losses (e.g., intrauterine clot or placental abruption).

Errors, particularly in the underestimation of blood loss, are common, especially when the blood loss is large and involves spills on the floor and absorption into surgical swabs. Such estimation can be improved with training [13, 14]. Swabs and drapes should be collected and weighed (remembering to subtract the dry weight). Suctioned fluid should be measured. Clinical parameters also play a role in ascertaining amount of blood lost.

Disability

Disability assessment refers to the patient's neurological status and is part of the initial resuscitation. There are several neurological scoring systems. One is the Glasgow Coma Score (GCS). Although widely used, the scoring system is not easily remembered if not used frequently. The AVPU (alert, responsive to voice, responsive to pain, unresponsive) scoring system is much simpler and can be used in its place (Table 13.3). The patient's pupils should also be assessed for size and reactivity as part of the disability assessment.

Table 13.3 AVPU and Glasgow Coma Score neurological assessment tools

AVPU Score
  A – Alert
  V – Responsive to voice
  P – Responsive to pain
  U – Unresponsive
Glasgow Coma Score
  Eye opening
    4 – Spontaneous
    3 – To voice
    2 – To pain
    1 – No opening
  Best verbal response
    5 – Orientated
    4 – Confused
    3 – Inappropriate words
    2 – Incomprehensible sounds
    1 – No response
  Best motor response
    6 – Obeys commands
    5 – Localizes to pain
    4 – Withdraws to pain
    3 – Flexion to pain
    2 – Extension to pain
    1 – No response
Total: 3–15/15

An AVPU Score of P or U or a GCS of ≤8 is evidence of coma and requires urgent intervention to secure the patient's airway. In cases of hemorrhage, a reduced conscious level indicates hypoperfusion of the brain.

"Exposure" and Environmental Control

Exposure in the setting of obstetrical hemorrhage refers to examining the patient to find the cause of the bleeding if it has not been attended to during the circulatory assessment. Throughout the whole resuscitation process, it is vital that the patient is kept warm by keeping her covered as much as possible, warming the room, the use of intravenous fluid warmers, and where available forced-air warming blankets. Hypothermia leads to increased oxygen consumption, reduced tissue oxygen delivery, and detrimental effects on coagulation. When active heating measures are being employed, the patient's core temperature should be monitored at least every 30 min [15].

Monitoring

Minimum monitoring for the resuscitation of peripartum hemorrhage includes pulse oximetry, ECG, noninvasive blood pressure measurement, fetal monitoring, and urinary catheterization. Pulse oximetry provides information of the women's oxygen saturation and pulse rate. Be aware that patients with poor peripheral perfusion may have inaccurate pulse oximetry readings. ECG provides assessment of the patient's heart rhythm and heart rate. It can also show evidence of myocardial ischemia, which may occur in situations of severe hypovolemia and anemia.

Noninvasive blood pressure monitoring can be of the automated or the manual variety. The automated system has the advantages of being hands-free and allows a timer to be set to allow regular monitoring. However, sometimes it is difficult to assess the pressure if there is patient movement or if the blood pressure is low. If this is the case the blood pressure should be determined manually by auscultation or palpation. If a reading is abnormal, believe it unless proved otherwise and repeat the reading.

Fetal heart rate monitoring such as with cardiotocography (CTG), provides information not only about the fetal condition but the hemodynamic status of the mother. Fetal compromise is a sensitive indicator of inadequate placental perfusion. Although resuscitation of the mother takes priority over that of the fetus, the fetus directly benefits from this resuscitation.

A urinary catheter should be inserted early in the assessment of obstetrical hemorrhage and hourly urine measurements recorded. In addition to these observations, the patient's respiratory rate should be determined and recorded. Her temperature should also be checked at regular intervals.

Fluid Therapy for Obstetrical Hemorrhage

Volume Replacement

Crystalloids

Crystalloid solutions exert no oncotic forces across the blood vessel membrane and therefore are able to cross freely from the intravascular space to the extravascular space. Approximately 70% is lost from the intravascular space, with a half-life of around 30 min; therefore, the volume expansion effect is not prolonged. Hence, administration of a 3:1 ratio of crystalloid to what is loss is recommended.

Crystalloids are inexpensive, readily available, and relatively free from allergic reactions and effects on coagulation. They can, however, cause peripheral and pulmonary edema when given in excess (a particular risk in obstetrics). Hartmann's solution (lactated Ringer's) and Plasma-Lyte have electrolyte compositions closer to physiological norms than other solutions. They are the preferred choices in this setting [16].

Saline 0.9% provides adequate volume replacement but in larger volumes causes hyperchloremia and metabolic acidosis, although the clinical significance of the acidosis is unclear. Dextrose 5% is unsuitable for volume replacement therapy. After infusion the dextrose is rapidly metabolized, leaving pure water in the intravascular space. The large proportion of it moves intracellularly, leaving a small proportion in the intravascular space to contribute to volume expansion.

Colloids

Colloid solutions do exert an osmotic force across the cell membrane due to the large-molecular-weight molecules they contain. As a result of these molecules, the solutions draw water intravascularly, thereby expanding the vascular volume by more than the initial volume infused. They are given in an infusion ratio of 1:1 of colloid to losses. In contrast to crystalloids, their volume expansion effect persists for many hours. Because smaller volumes are required than with crystalloids, the circulating volume can be more quickly restored, there is less risk of peripheral edema, and theoretically they have a more sustained effect on the circulating volume. Disadvantages include their allergenic potential and potential to interfere with coagulation.

Gelatins (Gelofusine, Haemaccel) are small-molecular-weight molecules derived from bovine collagen. They are less expensive than starch compounds and are generally used as the first-line colloid for fluid resuscitation. Disadvantages include a relatively short life (several hours) in the intravascular space, an association with anaphylaxis, and interference with coagulation.

Hydroxyethyl starches (HESs) are synthetic polysaccharides of variable molecular weight. They are more expensive than the gelatins but persist longer in the intravascular space (approximately 24 h). However, they also interfere with coagulation, although this effect appears to be less with HES/0.4 (Voluven) [17].

Dextrans are complex polysaccharide molecules not commonly used for volume resuscitation as they are associated with several serious side effects, including impaired coagulation, anaphylaxis, and acute renal failure.

Albumin solutions (5 and 25%) are sometimes used for fluid resuscitation of hypovolemic patients with low serum albumin levels. Otherwise, its use is uncommon for resuscitation.

Colloid vs. Crystalloid Debate

Colloids and cystalloids can each restore intravascular volume. The Australasian SAFE study (Saline vs. Albumin Fluid Evaluation), a large randomized controlled trial of almost 7,000 patients found that there were no differences in mortality, length of intensive care unit or hospital stay, mechanical ventilation, or renal replacement therapy for patients resuscitated with saline vs. albumin [18]. No advantage of colloids over crystalloids has been shown in terms of survival after resuscitation of critically ill patients [19].

Red Blood Cells

Transfusion of red blood cells (RBCs) is required to restore the oxygen-carrying capacity of blood. Commonly units of packed RBCs (packed cells, PCs) are provided by transfusion services rather than whole blood. These PCs are formed by removing plasma from whole blood, after which the RBCs are suspended in an additive solution to prolong storage time. Each unit has a volume of approximately 300 ml and a hematocrit of approximately 60%. Transfusion of one unit of PCs typically increases the hemoglobin level by 1 g/dl [20]. For major blood loss, RBC transfusion is typically required when blood loss is >30% of the circulating blood volume, although potentially earlier in an anemic patient.

Transfusion is generally not recommended if the hemoglobin level is >10 g/dl but is always recommended if it is <6 g/dl [21]. The patient's starting hemoglobin level, the rapidity and ongoing nature of the blood loss, preexisting co-morbidities, and access to blood products determine if transfusion is required.

The obstetrical population is generally young, fit, and healthy; but obstetrical hemorrhage can be rapid owing to the increased uterine blood flow during pregnancy. Hemorrhage can also be unexpected. Along with the increased oxygen demands associated with pregnancy, these factors may necessitate transfusion nearer the upper limit of the accepted triggers.

The optimal hemoglobin concentration is unknown. A lower hematocrit decreases blood viscosity and increases cardiac output, thus improving tissue oxygen delivery [22]. Healthy, normovolemic patients are able to tolerate hemoglobin concentrations around 7 g/dl quite well. However, RBCs also influence coagulation. They have prothrombotic effects on platelets, enhancing platelet activation and marginalization [23]. Therefore, maintenance of reasonable hemoglobin levels may be required in the bleeding patient.

Packed RBCs require rigorous cross-matching to ensure the highest levels of compatibility with the receiving patient's blood group, a process that may take up to 1 h or longer if atypical antibodies are detected. In an emergency there may not be time to wait for this process to take place, and unmatched units may have to be given. As highlighted earlier, blood should be administered via a warming device.

O-negative blood should be used when bleeding is immediately life-threatening with no time to wait for any form of matching. Ideally, two units of O-negative blood should be stored on or in close proximity to the delivery suite for this purpose. Group-specific blood should be issued in an emergency as soon as the blood group is known. This blood is not cross-matched either but is a closer match to the patient's blood. This process takes 10–30 min after a sample is received. Fully cross-matched blood can take up to an hour to be issued. In patients with known RBC antibodies, the risk of a hemolytic transfusion reaction must be balanced against the risks of withholding transfusion.

Blood Substitutes

There has been much research into the development of blood substitutes that would require no cross-matching, have no risk of disease transmission, are less allergenic, have long shelf lives, and are potentially usable in the prehospital setting. As yet, none is in clinical or is likely to be available in the near future.

One study has thrown more questions on the clinical safety of these solutions. A meta-analysis of 16 clinical trials of hemoglobin-based substitutes used in a variety of clinical settings (including trauma) found a marked increase in the risk of death and myocardial infarction [24]. This finding appeared to be independent of blood substitute used and the clinical indication for use. In addition, both types substitute have been shown to interfere with the accuracy of laboratory testing of blood samples, which also limits their usability [25].

Hemostatic Resuscitation

Fresh Frozen Plasma

As the name suggests, fresh frozen plasma (FFP) is the plasma portion of whole blood that is removed and then frozen for storage. One unit comprises approximately 250–300 ml. FFP is given in a dose of 10–15 ml/kg, which is at least four units for an average adult. Guidelines recommend transfusing to aim for a PT and an aPTT <1.5 times the control levels [21]. It should be remembered that it needs 30 min to thaw, so transfusion services should be alerted early. It has been suggested that in the presence of major hemorrhage FFP should be given in a ratio close to 1:1 with PCs to minimize the dilutional coagulopathy [26]. Disadvantages of large volumes of FFP include the risk of transfusion-related acute lung injury (TRALI) and pathogen transmission.

Platelets

Pooled platelets are obtained from the blood of four to six donors, with each pooled unit having a volume of approximately 300 ml [20]. Transfusion should be instituted to maintain a platelet count $>50 \times 10^9$/L. The need for platelets should be anticipated after two blood volume replacements [21]. Platelets are difficult to store compared with other products, requiring continuous agitation at room temperature. Not all blood banks have stores and therefore need to be alerted early. A count of $75-100 \times 109$/L should trigger a request for platelets to avoid delay. There is currently insufficient evidence to recommend proactive administration of platelets for obstetrical hemorrhage situations, although a study of proactive administration for nonobstetrical bleeding showed a lesser drop in the platelets count and reduced mortality with that regimen [27].

Cryoprecipitate

Cryoprecipitate is obtained from thawed FFP. It is a concentrated source of fibrinogen as well as fibrinectin, factor VIII, von Willebrand factor (VWF), and factor XIII. It is provided in units of approximately 100 ml. Consensus guidelines recommend transfusion to keep fibrinogen levels at >1.0 g/dl [21]. Interestingly, fibrinogen levels <2.0 g/dl have been shown to be predictive of severe postpartum hemorrhage [28]. Like FFP, cryoprecipitate needs to be thawed, a process that taked approximately 30 min.

Fibrinogen Concentrates

Fibrinogen concentrates are derived from human donor plasma that undergoes a pasteurization process. Use of cryoprecipitate is declining due to concerns about a lack of viral inactivation of the units. Cryoprecipitate is currently not available in Europe, leading to increased use of concentrates. Other advantages of the concentrates include a smaller volume and no need for thawing – hence more rapid access and administration. Retrospective studies have shown that when given to patients with major hemorrhage fibrinogen concentrates improve coagulation parameters and reduce transfusion requirements [29]. Successful use has also been described in those with obstetrical hemorrhage [30]. The commercially available concentrate is Haemocomplettan P. Typically, a 2-g dose increases the fibrinogen concentration by 1 g/L. Prothrombin complex concentrates are also available.

Hypotensive Resuscitation

Regarding resuscitation from trauma, there is mounting evidence that administration of excess fluid during resuscitation can actually worsen bleeding and may lead to poorer patient outcomes. The mechanisms postulated are that fluid administration increases ventricular preload and arterial blood pressure, which is thought to reverse the compensatory vasoconstriction, thus worsening the patient's hemodynamic status. Expansion and dilution of the intravascular space with clear fluids is also detrimental in that it reduces the oxygen-carrying capacity of the blood, leading to dilutional coagulopathy and worsening of hypothermia. This situation, in turn worsens the coagulopathy. Actual expansion of the blood vessels by fluid can also lead to mechanical disruption of clots.

Studies carried out in patients with penetrating trauma have shown that the use of low-volume, hypotensive resuscitation strategies are associated with increased survival rates as well as reduced complications and shorter hospital stays [31]. This survival benefit is not seen after blunt trauma [32].

Hypotensive resuscitation is not recommended in a pregnant woman with a dependent placental circulation. It may, however, have a place in situations where the baby has already been delivered. In this setting fluid administration should be more cautious until bleeding is controlled surgically.

Whole Blood

The use of whole blood is still advocated by some as the ideal component for resuscitation from hemorrhage. Its advantages are that transfusion is simple and a large volume can be given readily to restore intravascular volume. Whole blood contains all of the coagulation factors and platelets so dilutional coagulopathy is less of a risk. It also reduces the number of donor exposures, thereby reducing the risk of transfusion reactions and complications. The use of whole blood for obstetrical hemorrhage was revisited in a large observational study of 1,540 parturients who suffered hemorrhage that required transfusion. Women were transfused with whole blood, RBCs, or RBCs with other blood products. Women treated with RBCs alone had a higher rate of acute tubular necrosis, and those treated with whole blood had higher rates of pulmonary edema [33].

Recombinant Factor VIIa

Recombinant factor VIIa (NovoSeven) is derived from hamster kidneys. It was originally developed and used to treat hemophilia. Today, it is widely used "off-label" in a variety of surgical specialties where it has been shown to reduce transfusion requirements during major hemorrhage. There is a growing body of experience of its use and success in the treatment of obstetrical hemorrhage that is resistant to traditional therapeutic measures.

The optimum dose during hemorrhage has not been determined. The most commonly described dose is 90–100 µg/kg given intravenously over 5–0 min. Liaison with hematologists is recommended. Coagulation factors, platelets, and fibrinogen levels need to be optimized prior to its administration. Platelet counts $>50 \times 10^9/L$ and fibrinogen levels $\times 1.0$ g/L prior to its administration optimize the effect [34]. Hypothermia and acidosis undermine the efficacy. More recent experience with the drug has indicated that it should be used early in the treatment pathway as it may reduce the need for total blood products and for interventional procedures [35]. It has also been proposed for use as a "bridge" treatment while transferring a bleeding patient to a definitive treatment site (i.e., to interventional radiology). There is currently a large multicenter randomized controlled trial underway to evaluate its use for postpartum hemorrhage [36]. Initial worries about a potential increased risk of thrombosis has not been proven [37].

Tranexamic Acid

Tranexamic acid is an antifibrinolytic agent that acts by inhibiting the breakdown of plasminogen to plasmin, hence inhibiting clot breakdown. Its use in the treatment of obstetrical hemorrhage has yet to be fully determined. A meta-analysis of three randomized controlled trials of 461 patients undergoing cesarean section or vaginal delivery showed that tranexamic acid given before delivery had reduced overall postpartum blood loss and there was a lower incidence of postpartum hemorrhage [38]. There are currently no randomized controlled trial data for its use in the treatment of postpartum hemorrhage, although a large multicenter trial is underway, the WOMAN (World Maternal Antifibrinolytic) trial [39]. Despite a lack of concrete evidence for its use, the World Health Organization (WHO) guidelines state that a dose of tranexamic acid is reasonable if other measures have failed [40]. The dose in clinical use is 1 g given by slow intravenous injection, which can be repeated after 30–60 min if there is ongoing bleeding.

Complications of Blood Transfusion

The complications of blood transfusion are listed in Table 13.4.

Table 13.4 Complications of blood transfusion

Hemolytic transfusion reaction
Nonhemolytic febrile reaction
Transfusion-related acute lung injury (TRALI)
Infection
  Bacterial contamination of units
  Disease transmission (bacterial, viral, prion)
Graft-vs.-host disease
Coagulopathy
  Dilutional
  Disseminated intravascular coagulation
Biochemical abnormalities
  Hyperkalemia
  Hypocalcemia
  Acidosis/alkalosis
Hypothermia
Fluid overload/pulmonary edema
Air embolism

Hypothermia

Hypothermia as the result of quick infusion of cold blood products has many effects. It worsens coagulopathy by decreasing coagulation factor synthesis, increasing fibrinolysis and impairing platelet function [7]. These effects are reversible with the correction of the hypothermia. It shifts the oxyhemoglobin dissociation curve to the left, impairing oxygen delivery to the tissues. It also causes shivering resulting in increased oxygen consumption. The result is metabolic (lactic) acidosis. Cardiac arrhythmias are induced at lower temperatures.

Biochemical Abnormalities

Hyperkalemia is due to cell lysis in stored RBCs. Potassium leaks from the cells and the potassium levels rise, contributing to the potential for hyperkalemia during a massive transfusion. Progressive ECG changes are the most frequent manifestation. Treatment should be started if the potassium level is >6.5 mmol/L. Calcium gluconate 10% (5 ml) is used to stabilize the myocardial membrane. Administration of an insulin-dextrose infusion or salbutamol nebulizers also rapidly lower the potassium concentration.

Hypocalcemia may be due to the citrate contained in stored blood products (RBCs less than the others). The citrate binds calcium in plasma thereby reducing ionized calcium levels. Signs of hypocalcemia include hypotension associated with ECG changes such as ST flattening and QT prolongation. Treatment is with 5 ml of 10% calcium gluconate given by slow intravenous injection.

Acid–base abnormalities also occur. Metabolic acidosis may result from the citric and lactic acid in transfused blood, but it may also be due to hypovolemia and reduced peripheral perfusion. Metabolic alkalosis can also occur due to the metabolism of the citrate to bicarbonate in the liver.

These biochemical changes highlight the importance of frequent blood gas and electrolyte analyses during and immediately after resuscitation.

Transfusion-Related Acute Lung Injury

Estimating the exact incidence of TRALI is difficult as it varies depending on the type of blood product transfused. Plasma is the triggering factor and hence FFP is associated with a higher rate of reactions, followed by platelets and then RBCs. It presents as acute respiratory distress with an onset during the blood transfusion or within the 6 h immediately following it, and it can be severe, even fatal [41]. The UK Serious Hazards of Transfusion Committee (SHOT) has identified TRALI as the leading cause of morbidity and mortality related to transfusion in the UK [42].

It is caused by an immune response to either leukocyte antibodies in the plasma of donor units, or in cases where no antibodies are detected it is thought to be triggered by reactive lipids released from the donor blood cell membranes. It is also more common in multiparous women due to prior exposure to antibodies via the placenta in previous pregnancies [41].

Cell Salvage

For cell salvage, hemorrhaged blood is collected from the surgical field, filtered, and then separated and washed in a centrifuge to provide autologous blood suitable for reinfusion back into the patient. More blood for reinfusion can be obtained from the washing of blood-stained swabs in saline and suction collection of the resulting fluid. Reinfusion of autologous blood reduces the need for allogenic blood and thus reduces risks associated with transfusion. During the washing and centrifugation, plasma, platelets, coagulation factors and complement are removed so allogenic coagulation factors may be needed.

In general usage, cell salvage has been shown to reduce transfusion requirements by 40% without causing adverse effects [43]. The use of cell salvage in obstetrics has been held up by concerns of potential amniotic fluid embolism, contamination of maternal blood by fetal squames, and rhesus sensitisation. However, to date, there have been no reported cases of amniotic fluid contamination or rhesus alloimunization. Use in obstetrics in the USA has been endorsed by the American Society of Anesthesiologists [44]. In the UK, the National Institute of Clinical Excellence (NICE) [45], the Obstetrics Anaesthetists Association (OAA), and the Association of Anaesthetists of Great Britain and Ireland (AAGBI) have endorse the use of cell salvage in obstetrics [46].

A few modifications of the traditional setup are recommended in obstetrics, including a separate suction unit for use from amniotomy until the placenta is delivered to reduce the volume of amniotic fluid collected. Leukodepletion filters reduce the amount of fetal squames present to nearly zero [47]. Maternal blood may be contaminated with small volumes of fetal blood. Therefore, for Rh-negative women, Kleihauer-Betke testing should be undertaken and an appropriate dose of anti-D immunoglobulin administered as soon as possible after delivery [48].

The limitations of this technique for treating obstetrical hemorrhage include the initial cost outlay for equipment, ongoing costs of consumables, ongoing training and skill retention of staff, and the difficulty of predicting when major bleeding may occur.

The use of autologous blood not only avoids the risks of allogenic transfusion but has higher levels of 2,3-diphosphoglycerate (2,3-DPG), thereby improving oxygen transport and lowering potassium levels. Use of cell salvage can reduce the amount (and cost) of donated blood and is acceptable to many Jehovah's Witness patients. It is useful in patients with rare antibodies for whom obtaining matched blood is difficult.

Point-of-Care Testing

Because of the inevitable delay in receiving laboratory results, point-of-care testing is recommended in emergency situations such as major hemorrhage. The clinical picture initially determines management but can be refined within minutes as results from bedside tests are obtained.

HemoCue

HemoCue is a handheld device that estimates hemoglobin concentration at the bedside. All it requires is a small sample of peripheral blood taken from the patient's arm or foot or eveb from another sample that is being taken. The HemoCue has been validated for use in obstetrical patients [49]. Its use has been described for estimating the hemoglobin of suction fluid during elective cesarean section, thereby allowing a more accurate prediction of blood loss [50].

Blood Gas Analysis

Blood gas analyzers are widely available They require small amounts of venous or arterial blood that can be analyzed within minutes for the acid–base status, hemoglobin, electrolytes, and glucose; and frequently lactate estimations are available. Blood gas analysis provides a good guide to the degree of tissue perfusion and adequacy of resuscitation through monitoring the base excess and lactate [51].

Thromboelastography

Thromboelastography (TEG) provides a global picture of the coagulation status. With it, the viscoelastic properties of a clot are measured over time. TEG has been used extensively for cardiac and liver surgery. For cardiac surgery, its use has been shown to decrease transfusion requirements and accurately predict rebleeding [52]. It has not yet been validated for use for an obstetrical hemorrhage. However, given its ability to give coagulation information in less than an hour (less time than conventional coagulation testing), it has potential to be useful in guiding transfusion of coagulation products in a delivery suite.

PT and aPTT Monitoring

A number of handheld instruments are available to measure PT INR and aPTT quickly. They are generally used to monitor heparin and warfarin therapy. Their efficacy in obstetrical care has not been investigated.

Despite the obvious advantages of point-of-care testing, commonly the machines are not cared for by laboratory personnel and may be not properly or routinely calibrated or indeed properly maintained. In addition, staff using these devices may not all be properly trained in their use, which may affect the results produced.

Anesthesia

The choice of anesthetic employed in cases of obstetrical hemorrhage depends on the experience and skill level of the anesthetist, the degree of maternal cardiovascular instability, prior fluid resuscitation of the mother, the urgency of the procedure, and of course evidence of fetal compromise. In all cases, intravenous access should be secured and fluid resuscitation underway preoperatively.

Regional Anesthesia

Regional anesthesia is the preferred option for most obstetrical procedures owing to its avoidance of potential for aspiration and airway difficulties. However, in a bleeding, hypovolemic patient, sympathetic blockade and resulting vasodilation may cause precipitous hypotension. Thus, regional anesthesia may be used when bleeding is controlled and there is no hemodynamic instability. However, the potential for coagulopathy must be considered, especially in cases of presumed placental abruption.

If the patient already has a functioning epidural, a slow, cautious, controlled top-up may be instituted. In addition, evidence suggests that there is reduced blood loss if regional anesthesia is used at cesarean section vs. general anesthesia [53].

In all cases in which there is a particular risk of hemorrhage, it is essential that the patient be warned about the possibility of conversion to a general anesthetic during the procedure. Conversion may be required because of maternal anxiety, impaired conscious level due to hypovolemia, or inadequate anesthesia.

General Anesthesia

General anesthesia is advocated in cases of hypovolemia-associated hemodynamic instability, severe hemorrhage with ongoing blood loss, coagulopathy, an uncertain diagnosis, complicated surgical intervention, and when regional anesthesia is contraindicated. It is also indicated when the airway is at risk because of a patient's reduced conscious level.

Consideration should be given to awake fiberoptic intubation followed by general anesthesia in patients at very high risk of a difficult/impossible intubation.

When inducing general anesthesia, propofol and thiopentone can cause profound peripheral vasodilation and hypotension in a hypovolemic patient. Ketamine (1–2 mg/kg) and etomidate (0.1–0.3 mg/kg) are more hemodynamically stable and may be preferable for induction. Vasopressors such as phenylephrine or metaraminol and ephedrine should be at hand for induction in case of cardiovascular collapse. Volatile anesthetic agents have a relaxant effect on uterine tone and worsen atony, so care must be taken to limit their concentration to <1.0 MAC. Nitrous oxide is still frequently used for obstetrical general anesthesia and helps supplement the anesthetic.

If uterine relaxation is needed to aid delivery, this can be achieved by either increasing the concentration of the anaesthetic volatile agent or by giving inhaled salbutamol or glyceryl trinitrate sublingually or intravenously (with cardiovascular monitoring).

In all cases of major obstetrical hemorrhage, especially those severe or urgent enough to warrant emergency general anesthesia, early calls for a senior anesthetist and indeed other speciality assistance are recommended.

Invasive Monitoring

Invasive monitoring of major obstetrical hemorrhage is frequently required. However, insertion of an invasive monitor is not an immediate treatment priority and should not delay resuscitation. Ideally, it can be undertaken once help arrives.

Central Venous Pressure Monitoring

The central venous pressure (CVP) is measured via a catheter whose tip lies in the superior vena cava just above the right atrium. The CVP gives an approximation of right heart filling pressures and thus an idea of the patient's volume status. It also allows administration of vasoactive drugs. Common sites of insertion are the internal jugular vein or subclavian vein. Although a femoral approach may be used, it is not as useful a measurement tool.

A stand-alone reading provides little clinical information, with trends over time and response to treatment being more informative. Readings can be affected by postural changes and transducer position. Coexisiting disease, such as pulmonary hypertension, right ventricular abnormalities, and left ventricular failure, can also make readings unreliable.

Arterial Monitoring

Peripheral arterial cannulation allows continuous beat-by-beat monitoring of the arterial blood pressure and allows frequent blood sampling without repeated skin punctures. Arterial lines are commonly 20-gauge or occasionally 22-gauge catheters and are inserted most commonly into the radial artery, although the brachial, femoral, and dorsalis pedis arteries can be used. Complications include bleeding, hematoma formation, arterial damage, distal limb ischemia, and infection.

Advanced Hemodynamic Monitoring

In hemodynamically unstable patients, more advanced methods of assessing hemodynamic variables – volume status, response to fluid therapy, cardiac function – may be required.

Pulmonary Artery Flotation Catheter

In recent times, use of pulmonary artery flotation catheters as means of monitoring cardiac output and fluid status has declined. Studies in adult intensive care patients have shown that these monitors are associated with reduced survival benefit and associated with several serious complications [54]. Aside from complications related to central venous puncture and long-term catheter placement, patients are at risk of arrhythmias, damage to cardiac structures and the pulmonary artery, pulmonary infarction and hemorrhage, and catheter entanglement [55].

Doppler Ultrasonography

Doppler US can provide continuous real-time cardiac output monitoring by measuring the velocity of blood flow in the descending thoracic aorta. In comparison with other methods of cardiac output monitoring, such as thermodilution, it has been validated and its accuracy has been proven [56]. The esophageal Doppler is one type of imaging. The device is a flexible probe with a small US transducer at its tip. The transducer sends and receives US waves directed at the descending aorta. The probe is inserted into the esophagus of the anesthetized patient and allows continuous imaging of aortic blood flow and cardiac output. Suprasternal Doppler imaging has also been developed to measure aortic blood flow via a handheld probe above the suprasternal notch [57].

Pulse Contour Analysis

Another, less-invasive form of cardiac output monitoring is pulse contour analysis. With this technique, venous (central or peripheral) and arterial lines are inserted. It involves two methods of cardiac output evaluation. The first is intermittent transpulmonary indicator dilution, whereby the indicator is injected into a vein and then measured at the arterial line. The injectate can be thermal (cold) or lithium. Continuous cardiac output monitoring can also be obtained through mathematical analysis of the arterial waveform. This provides beat-by-beat measurement of the stroke volume, which when combined with the heart rate allows determination of the cardiac output. The intermittent transpulmonary technique allows calibration of the continuous analysis. Again, these devices have reasonable agreement when compared to the gold standard measuring techniques [58, 59].

Transthoracic Echocardiography

The use of transthoracic echocardiography (TTE) is becoming more widespread in the fields of anesthesia and intensive care owing to advances in portable technology and increasing availability of equipment. TTE can assess volume status, filling pressures, left and right ventricular function, valvular function, and cardiac output. It is a noninvasive technique and quick to perform, although assessment techniques require technical training and practice. However, basic skills in assessing the simple hemodynamic parameters can be learned quickly. There is also no continuous monitoring of cardiac status with TTE.

The use of TTE has been described for use during obstetrical anesthesia, and the Rapid Obstetric Screening Echocardiogram (ROSE scan) has been developed to allow the obstetrical team members to have a simple systematic scan to assess cardiovascular status in parturients [60]. TTE provides information different from that other hemodynamic monitors and is a good complementary device for monitoring.

Ongoing Monitoring

Resuscitation of major hemorrhage requires ongoing reevaluation of the patient at regular intervals and after intervention to assess response to treatment and to detect deterioration. Early warning scoring systems have been shown to improve detection of worsening physiological parameters in nonobstetrical patients and have been adapted for use in obstetrics [61]. Their use is recommended by CEMACH. The Modified Early Obstetric Warning System (MEOWS) has physiological variables adjusted for pregnancy. The charts themselves vary but usually involve monitoring around six physiological variables. Each set of observations generate a score. If the score is high enough, it is evidence of patient deterioration and prompts a review by the medical staff. However, the system is effective only if the high score triggers a response. Although useful for ongoing monitoring of the bleeding patient, it is designed for use on every pregnant patient admitted to the hospital to detect signs of serious illness.

Transfer of the Unwell Mother

It is not uncommon for a woman having suffered an obstetrical hemorrhage to require transfer to another site, be it to an intensive care unit, an interventional radiology suite, or indeed another hospital to allow definitive treatment or a higher level of care. It is essential that the transfer is well planned from the outset, with good communication between teams. Accompanying staff should be trained and experienced in transfer of the critically ill and be able to deal with any complications that may occur en route. Minimum monitoring should include ECG, noninvasive blood pressure, pulse oximetry and urine output (Table 13.5). End-tidal carbon dioxide monitoring is mandatory in patients who are intubated and ventilated. he potential for deterioration en route should be considered. The patient may benefit from being intubated electively before transfer, and insertion of invasive monitoring such as central venous and arterial lines should also be considered. Noninvasive blood pressure monitoring may be inaccurate en route due to vibration. Units usually have a transfer bag that is equipped with the essentials required for transfer. This equipment should be checked and restocked regularly as well as after each transfer.

The estimated arrival time should be communicated to the receiving team to allow preparations to take place. Patient notes, copies of all investigations, and a transfer letter from the referring team should accompany the patient. On arrival a verbal handover should occur between the accompanying team and the nursing and medical staff of the receiving team. Communication with the patient's family should not be forgotten and is an important and essential part of the transfer process [62, 63].

Table 13.5 Transfer checklist

Functioning monitor with enough battery power
Ventilator (check settings and battery power)
One full and one spare oxygen cylinder (with appropriate attachments)
Alternative means of ventilation (i.e., self-inflating bag)
Airway equipment and drugs required for intubation or reintubation (thiopentone, suxamethonium, nondepolarizing muscle relaxant)
Portable suction unit
Infusion pumps with adequate battery power
Extra syringes of infusion drugs should they run out en route
Resuscitation drugs (including vasopressors, atropine, epinephrine)
Additional bags of crystalloid/colloid or any issued blood products
Methods of keeping the patient warm en route
Patient notes, copies of investigations, a transfer letter (?)

Placement After Definitive Care

Intensive Care Unit

In the last CEMACH report. 0.9% of all admissions to intensive care units (ICUs) were obstetrical [4]. Fewer than half of these ICU admissions required ventilatory support and only a small number of those admitted required prolonged ventilation or inotropes. Admissions are frequently for less than 48 h [64]. Postpartum hemorrhage is one of the most common causes for admission to the ICU peripartum, along with preeclampsia [64].

Indications for admission to the ICU include the need for invasive or in some cases noninvasive ventilation, multiple organ failure, renal support, or underlying severe cardiorespiratory co-morbidities. In practice, not all patients admitted to the ICU need that level of care per se, but it is frequently the location in any hospital where close monitoring can be provided. For the pregnant patient, there can be many disadvantages of admission to an ICU, including inexperience in monitoring the fetus antenatally, unfamiliarity with peripartum care, and separation of mother and baby. These problems can be overcome with close liaison between the intensive care personnel and the obstetrical and midwifery teams.

If a patient is likely to need intensive monitoring following hemorrhage, early liaison with the intensivists and the ICU is recommended. The level of care required can be provided in a normal operating theater environment until a bed becomes available. Standard monitoring can be continued and an ICU chart commenced Ventilation may be continued if required. If invasive lines are not inserted but will be required, they can be done at this time. Attention should be paid to maintaining the patient's temperature as well as thromboprophylaxis once bleeding is controlled and coagulation normalized.

High-Dependency Care

Following a major obstetrical hemorrhage, many women require a period of monitoring and closer observation than a standard ward can provide but not at a level as intensive as in the ICU. Many obstetrical units now have or are developing high-dependency units jointly run by obstetricians and anesthetists with a 1:2 nurse/midwifery to patient ratio of 1:2. Hemodynamic and respiratory variables and other clinical observations should be monitored hourly.

Communication

With obstetric care being a highly multidisciplinary area, good communication and teamwork are essential for promoting good care and outcomes after obstetrical hemorrhage. Delivery suites should have protocols for the management of major obstetrical hemorrhage, and the protocols should be closely followed. Good working relationships and communication systems should be developed with transfusion services. CEMACH reports have also highlighted the value and importance of regular team-based training drills, scenarios, and simulation for the management of major obstetrical hemorrhage.

Summary

The material in this chapter is summarized in the following outline.

1. Call for immediate help.
2. Uterine displacement: Place the patient in the left lateral position or insert a wedge (if still antenatal). Consider head-down tilt.
3. Follow the ABCDE protocol.

   Airway

   – Check if airway is patent and intervene if not.

   Breathing

   – Give high-flow oxygen via a facemask.

   Circulation

   – Insert two wide-bore intravenous cannulas (14 gauge).
   – Send blood for cross-match, coagulation screen, and full blood count.
   – Start rapid intravenous fluid administration (warmed) (Hartmann's 2 L then continue with colloid 1–2 L until blood is available).

- Consider using a rapid transfusion device.
- Attach monitoring equipment (ECG, noninvasive blood pressure monitor, pulse oximetry).

Disability

- Check for neurological problems.

  AVPU Score
  Glasgow Coma Score

Exposure and environmental control

- Activate major hemorrhage protocol (if available).
- Obtain blood as soon as possible for cross-matching (give O-negative blood in a dire emergency).
- Liase closely with the hematology department.
- Administer other blood products (FFP and platelets) as dictated by situation.
- Treat the cause of bleeding.
- Consider invasive monitoring in severe cases (it should not delay resuscitation).
- Regularly and frequently reassess parameters.

  Observations
  Blood gases (hemoglobin, electrolytes, acid–base status)
  Ongoing blood loss and replacement

- Placement after definitive care to other departments or facilities.

  High-dependency unit
  Intensive care unit
  Interventional radiology suite

- Liase with the intensive care team early.

Caution Box

Call for senior help early.
Do not forget the possibility of uterine displacement.
Hypotension is a very late sign, so normal blood pressure should not be reassuring.
Blood loss is frequently underestimated.
Treatment of the mother takes priority over that of the fetus.
Keep the patient warm.
Consider early use of FFP and other blood products.

References

1. Shevell T, Malone FD. Management of obstetric haemorrhage. Semin Perinatol. 2003;27: 86–104.
2. Ronsmans C, Graham W. Maternal mortality: who, when, where and why. Lancet. 2006;368:1189–200.
3. Khan K, Wojdyla D, Say L, et al. WHO analysis of causes of maternal death: a systematic review. Lancet. 2006;367:1066–74.
4. Confidential Enquiry into Maternal and Child Health (CEMACH). Saving Mothers' Lives: reviewing maternal deaths to make motherhood safer – 2003–2005. In: Lewis G, editor. The seventh report on confidential enquiries into maternal deaths in the United Kingdom. London: CEMACH; 2007.
5. Grady K. Structured approach to emergencies in the obstetric patient. In: Grady K, Howell C, Cox C, editors. Managing obstetric emergencies and trauma: The MOET course manual. 2nd ed. London: RCOG Press; 2007. p. 13–6.
6. Samsoon GL, Young JRB. Difficult tracheal intubation: a retrospective study. Anaesthesia. 1987;42:487–90.
7. Plaat F. Anaesthetic issues related to postpartum haemorrhage (excluding antishock garment). Best Pract Res Clin Obstet Gynaecol. 2008;22:1043–56.
8. Stoneham MD. An evaluation of methods of increasing the flow rate of i.v. fluid administration. BJA. 1995;75:361–5.
9. Westfall MD, Price RK, Lambert M, et al. Intravenous access in the critically ill trauma patient: a multicentred, prospective, randomised trial of saphenous cutdown and percutaneous, femoral access. Ann Emerg Med. 1994;23:541–5.
10. Brenner T, Bernhard M, Helm M, et al. Comparison of two intraosseous infusion systems for adult emergency medical use. Resuscitation. 2008;78:314–99.
11. National Institute for Clinical Excellence. TA49. Central venous catheters – ultrasound locating devices: guidance 2002. http://www.nice.org.uk/nicemedia/pdf/Ultrasound_49_GUIDANCE.pdf. Accessed 21 June 2010.
12. Adhikary GS, Massey SR. Massive air embolism: a case report. J Clin Anaesth. 1998;10: 70–2.
13. Toledo P, McCarthy RJ, Hewlett BJ, et al. The accuracy of blood loss estimation after simulated vaginal delivery. Anesth Analg. 2007;105:1736–40.
14. Bose P, Regan F, Paterson-Brown S. Improving the accuracy of estimated blood loss at obstetric haemorrhage using clinical reconstructions. BJOG. 2006;113:919–24.
15. National Institute for Clinical Excellence. CG65. Management of inadvertent perioperative hypothermia in adults: guidance 2008. http://www.nice.org.uk/nicemedia/pdf/CG65NICEGuidance.pdf. Accessed 5 Aug 2010.
16. Boldt J. The balanced concept of fluid resuscitation. Br J Anaesth. 2007;99:312–5.
17. Langeron O, Doelberg M, Ang ET, et al. Voluven®, a lower substituted novel hydroxyethyl starch (HES 130/0.4), causes fewer effects on coagulation in major orthopedic surgery than HES 200/0.5. Anesth Analg. 2001;92:855–62.
18. Finfer S, Bellomo R, Boyce N, et al. A comparison of albumin and saline for fluid resuscitation in the intensive care unit. N Engl J Med. 2004;350:2247–56.
19. Perel P, Roberts I, Pearson M. Colloids versus crystalloids for fluid resuscitation in critically ill patients. Cochrane Database Syst Rev. 2007;4:CD000567.
20. UK Blood Transfusion and Tissue Transplantation Services. Professional Guidelines, best practice and clinical information. http://www.transfusionguidelines.org.uk. Accessed 10 Aug 2010.
21. Stainsby D, Maclennan S, Thomas D, et al. Guidelines in the management of major blood loss. British Committee for Standards in Haematology, 2006.
22. Van der Linden P, Gilbart E, Paques P, et al. Influence of hematocrit on tissue O_2 extraction capabilities during acute hemorrhage. Am J Physiol. 1993;264:1942–7.

23. Hardy J-F, de Moerloose P, Samama CM. Massive transfusion and coagulopathy: pathophysiology and implications for clinical management. Can J Anaesth. 2006;53:S40–58.
24. Cohn CS, Cushing MM. Oxygen therapeutics: perfluorocarbons and blood substitute safety. Crit Care Clin. 2009;25:399–414.
25. Natanson C, Kern SJ, Lurie P, et al. Cell-free hemoglobin-based blood substitutes and risk of myocardial infarction and death. JAMA. 2008;299:2304–12.
26. Ho AMH, Karmakar MJ, Dion PW. Are we giving enough coagulation factors during major trauma resuscitation? Am J Surg. 2005;190:279–84.
27. Johansson PI, Stensballe J. Hemostatic resuscitation for massive bleeding: the paradigm of plasma and platelets – a review of the current literature. Transfusion. 2007;47:593–8.
28. Charbit B, Mandelbrot L, Samain E, et al. The decrease of fibrinogen is an early predictor of the severity of postpartum hemorrhage. J Thromb Haemost. 2007;5:266–73.
29. Fenger-Eriksen C, Lindberg-Larsen M, Christensen Q, et al. Fibrinogen concentrate substitution therapy in patients with massive haemorrhage and low plasma fibrinogen concentrations. Br J Anaesth. 2008;101:769–73.
30. Bell SF, Rayment R, Collins PW, et al. The use of fibrinogen concentrate to correct hypofibrinogenaemia rapidly during obstetric haemorrhage. Int J Obstet Anesth. 2010;19:218–34.
31. Bickell WH, Wall Jr MJ, Pepe PE, et al. Immediate versus delayed fluid resuscitation for hypotensive patients with penetrating torso injuries. N Engl J Med. 1994;331:1105–9.
32. Dutton RP, Mackenzie CF, Scalea TM. Hypotensive resuscitation during active hemorrhage: impact on in-hospital mortality. J Trauma. 2002;52:11416.
33. Alexander J, Sarode R, McIntire D, et al. Whole blood in the management of hypovolemia due to obstetric hemorrhage. Obstet Gynecol. 2009;113:1320–6.
34. McMorrow RCN, Ryan SM, Blunnie WP, et al. Use of recombinant factor VIIa in massive post-partum haemorrhage. Eur J Anesthesiol. 2008;25:293–8.
35. Ahonen J, Jokela R. Recombinant factor vIIa for life-threatening post-partum haemorrhage. Br J Anaesth. 2005;94:592–5.
36. Recombinant human activated factor VII as salvage therapy in women with severe post partum haemorrhage. http://clinicaltrials.gov/ct2/show/NCT00370877. Accessed 7 Aug 2010.
37. Franchini M, Franchi M, Bergamini V, et al. A critical review on the use of recombinant factor VIIa in life-threatening obstetric postpartum hemorrhage. Semin Thromb Hemost. 2008;34:104–12.
38. Ferrer P, Roberts I, Sydenham E, et al. Antifibrinolytic agents in post-partum haemorrhage; a systematic review. BMC Pregnancy Childbirth. 2009;9:29.
39. Shakur H, Elbourne D, Gulmezoglu M, et al. The WOMAN Trial (World Maternal Antifibrinolytic Trial): tranexamic acid for the treatment of postpartum haemorrhage: an international randomised, double blind placebo controlled trial. Trials. 2010;11:40.
40. WHO recommendations for the prevention of postpartum haemorrhage. Geneva: World Health Organization, 2009.
41. Barrett NA, Kam PCA. Transfusion-related acute lung injury: a literature review. Anaesthesia. 2006;6:777–85.
42. Serious Hazards of Transfusion (SHOT): 2009 Report. http://www.shotuk.org/wp-content/uploads/2010/07/SHOT2009.pdf. Accessed 1 Oct 2010.
43. Carless PA, Henry DA, Moxey AJ, et al. Cell salvage for minimising perioperative allogeneic blood transfusion. Cochrane Database Syst Rev. 2010;4:CD001888.
44. American Society of Anesthesiologists. Practice guidelines for obstetric anesthesia. Anesthesiology 2007;106:843–63.
45. National Institute for Clinical Excellence. IPG144. Intraoperative blood cell salvage in obstetrics: guidance 2005. http://guidance.nice.org.uk/nicemedia/live/11038/30690/30690.pdf. Accessed 15 Aug 2010.
46. OAA/AAGBI Guidelines for Obstetric Anaesthetic Services. Revised Edition. London: OAA/AAGBI; 2005:25.
47. Sullivan I, Faulds J, Ralph C. Contamination of salvaged maternal blood by amniotic fluid and fetal red cells during elective Caesarean section. Br J Anaesth. 2008;101:225–9.

48. Catling SJ, Williams S, Fielding AM. Cell salvage in obstetrics: an evaluation of the ability of cell salvage combined with the leucocyte depletion filtration to remove amniotic fluid from operative blood loss at caesarean section. Int J Obstet Anesth. 1999;8:79–84.

49. Yau R, Kathigamanathan T, Plaat F, et al. Evaluation of the Haemocue for measuring haemoglobin concentrations in the obstetric population. Int J Obstet Anesth. 2002;11(Suppl):8.

50. Gupta A, Wrench IJ, Feast MJ, et al. Use of the Hemocue® near patient testing device to measure concentration of haemoglobin in suction fluid at elective Caesarean section. Anaesthesia. 2008;63:531–4.

51. Rossaint R, Bouillon B, Cerny V, et al. Management of bleeding following major trauma: an updated European guideline. Crit Care. 2010;14:R52.

52. Shore-Lesserson L, Manspeizer HE, De Perio M, et al. Thromboelastography-guided transfusion algorithm reduces transfusions in complex cardiac surgery. Anesth Analg. 1999;88: 312–9.

53. Afolabi BB, Lesi FE, Merah NA. Regional versus general anaesthesia for caesarean section. Cochrane Database Syst Rev. 2006;18:CD004350.

54. Harvey S, Young D, Brampton W, et al. Pulmonary artery catheters for adult patients in intensive care. Cochrane Database Syst Rev. 2006;3:CD003408.

55. Evans DC, Doraiswamy VA, Prosciak MP, et al. Complications associated with pulmonary artery catheters: a comprehensive clinical review. Scand J Surg. 2009;98:199–208.

56. Dark PM, Singer M. The validity of trans-esophageal Doppler ultrasonography as a measure of cardiac output in critically ill adults. Int Care Med. 2004;30:2060–6.

57. Gan T. The esophageal doppler as an alternative to the pulmonary artery catheter. Curr Opin Crit Care. 2000;6:214–21.

58. Rocca GD, Costa MG, Pompei L, et al. Continuous and intermittent cardiac output measurement: pulmonary artery catheter versus aortic transpulmonary technique. Br J Anaesth. 2002;88:350–6.

59. Rauch H, Muller MJ, Fleischer F, et al. Pulse contour analysis versus thermodilution in cardiac surgery patients. Acta Anaesthesiol Scand. 2002;46:424–9.

60. Dennis, A. Transthoracic echocardiography and obstetric critical illness. Australian and New Zealand College of Anaesthetists Annual Scientific Meeting 2009. http://www.anzca.edu.au/events/asm/asm2009/abstracts/transthoracic-echocardiography-in-obstetric.html. Accessed 12 Aug 2010.

61. Chatterjee MT, Moon JC, Murphy R, et al. The "OBS" chart: an evidence based approach to re-design of the patient observation chart in a district general hospital setting. Postgrad Med J. 2005;81:663–6.

62. Australian and New Zealand College of Anaesthetists. Minimum standards for intrahospital transport of critically ill patients. Professional document: PS39. February 2003.

63. The Neuroanaesthesia Society of Great Britain and Ireland and The Association of Anaesthetists of Great Britain and Ireland. Recommendations for the transfer of patients with acute head injuries to neurosurgical units. December 1996.

64. Zeeman GG. Obstetric critical care: a blueprint for improved outcomes. Crit Care Med. 2006;34:S208–14.

Index

E. Sheiner (ed.), *Bleeding During Pregnancy: A Comprehensive Guide,*
DOI 10.1007/978-1-4419-9810-1, © Springer Science+Business Media, LLC 2011